The Conceptual Evolution of DSM-5

The Conceptual Evolution of DSM-5

Edited by
Darrel A. Regier, M.D., M.P.H.
William E. Narrow, M.D., M.P.H.
Emily A. Kuhl, Ph.D.
David J. Kupfer, M.D.

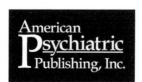

American Psychiatric Publishing, Inc.

Washington, DC
London, England

If you would like to buy between 25 and 99 copies of this or any other APPI title, you are eligible for a 20% discount; please contact APPI Customer Service at appi@psych.org or 800-368-5777. If you wish to buy 100 or more copies of the same title, please e-mail us at bulksales@psych.org for a price quote.

Copyright © 2011 American Psychiatric Publishing, Inc.
ALL RIGHTS RESERVED

Manufactured in the United States of America on acid-free paper
14   13   12   11   10   5   4   3   2   1
First Edition

Typeset in Caecilia and Cantoria.

American Psychiatric Publishing, Inc.
1000 Wilson Boulevard
Arlington, VA 22209-3901
www.appi.org

Library of Congress Cataloging-in-Publication Data
The conceptual evolution of DSM-5 / edited by Darrel A. Regier ... [et al.]. — 1st ed.
      p. ; cm.
   Includes bibliographical references and index.
   ISBN 978-1-58562-388-4 (pbk. : alk. paper)
   1. Diagnostic and statistical manual of mental disorders. 2. Mental illness—Diagnosis. 3. Mental illness—Classification. I. Regier, Darrel A.
   [DNLM: 1. Diagnostic and statistical manual of mental disorders. 2. Mental Disorders—diagnosis. 3. Mental Disorders—classification. WM 141]
   RC469.C654 2011
   616.89′075—dc22

                                                                                    2010026845

British Library Cataloguing in Publication Data
A CIP record is available from the British Library.

Contents

PART I

Diagnostic Spectra:
Assessing the Validity of Disorder Groupings

PART II

Integrating Dimensional Concepts Into a Categorical System

PART III

Assessing Functional Impairment for Clinical Significance and Disability

PART IV

Identifying Important Culture- and Gender-Related Expressions of Disorders

PART V

Incorporating Developmental Variations of Disorder Expression Across the Lifespan

Contributors

Jamie M. Abelson, M.S.W.
Institute for Social Research, University of Michigan, Ann Arbor, Michigan

Sergio Aguilar-Gaxiola, M.D., Ph.D.
Professor of Internal Medicine and Director, Center for Reducing Health Disparities, University of California, Davis School of Medicine, Sacamento, California

Jordi Alonso, M.D., Ph.D.
Senior Investigator and Head, Health Services Research Group, IMIM-Institut de Recerca, Hospital del Mar, Parc de Salut Mar

Gavin Andrews, M.D.
Professor of Psychiatry, Clinical Research Unit for Anxiety and Depression, University of New South Wales at St. Vincent's Hospital, Sydney, NSW, Australia

Katja Beesdo, Ph.D.
Assistant Professor, Institute of Clinical Psychology and Psychotherapy, Technische Universitaet Dresden, Dresden, Germany

Patricia A. Berglund, M.B.A.
Institute for Social Research, University of Michigan, Ann Arbor, Michigan

Guilherme Borges, M.Sc., Dr.Sc.
Professor, Department of Epidemiological Research, Division of Epidemiological and Psychosocial Research, National Institute of Psychiatry (Mexico) & Metropolitan Autonomous University

Mark Oakley Browne, Ph.D.
Professor, Discipline of Psychiatry, School of Medicine, University of Tasmania

Ronny Bruffaerts, Ph.D.
Associate Professor, Department of Neurosciences , Katholieke Universiteit Leuven

Giovanni B. Cassano, M.D.
Professor and Chair, Department of Psychiatry, Neurobiology, Pharmacology, and Biotechnology, University of Pisa, Pisa, Italy

Lee Anna Clark, Ph.D.
Professor, Department of Psychology, University of Notre Dame, Notre Dame, Indiana

Diana E. Clarke, Ph.D.
Research Statistician, American Psychiatric Association; Adjunct Assistant Professor, Johns Hopkins School of Public Health, Baltimore, Maryland

E. Jane Costello, Ph.D.
Professor, Department of Psychiatry and Behavioral Sciences, Center for Developmental Epidemiology, Duke University Medical School, Durham, North Carolina

Michelle G. Craske, Ph.D.
Professor, UCLA Anxiety Disorders Research Center, Department of Psychology, UCLA, Los Angeles, California

Ron Dahl, M.D.
Professor of Psychiatry and Pediatrics, University of Pittsburgh School of Medicine, Western Psychiatric Institute & Clinic, Pittsburgh, Pennsylvania

Giovanni de Girolamo, M.D.
Scientific Director, IRCCS —St. John of God, Clinical Research Centre

Madeleine Delves
Clinical Research Unit for Anxiety and Depression, University of New South Wales at St. Vincent's Hospital, Sydney, NSW, Australia

Michael Dewey, Ph.D.
Professor, Health Service and Population Research Department, Institute of Psychiatry, London, United Kingdom

Nicholas R. Eaton, M.A.
Graduate Student, Department of Psychology, University of Minnesota, Minneapolis, Minnesota

Warachal Eileen Faison, M.D.
Medical Director, Primary Care Neuroscience, Pfizer Inc., New York, New York

Ellen Frank, Ph.D.
Professor, Departments of Psychiatry and Psychology, University of Pittsburgh School of Medicine, Western Psychiatric Institute and Clinic, Pittsburgh, Pennsylvania

Richard Gater, M.D.
Mental Health and Neurodegeneration Research Group, University of Manchester, Manchester, England

Andrew T. Gloster, Ph.D.
Assistant Professor, Institute of Clinical Psychology and Psychotherapy, Technische Universitaet Dresden, Dresden, Germany

Nick Glozier, Ph.D.
Associate Professor, Disciplines of Psychiatry and Sleep Medicine, Sydney Medical School, The University of Sydney, Brain and Mind Research Institute, Camperdown, NSW, Australia

David Goldberg, D.M., F.R.C.P.
Professor Emeritus, Institute of Psychiatry, London, England

Oye Gureje, M.D., Ph.D., D.Sc.
Professor and Head of Department , Department of Psychiatry, University of Ibadan, University College Hospital

Josep Maria Haro, M.D., M.P.H., Ph.D.
Director of Research, Parc Sanitari Sant Joan de Déu

John E. Helzer, M.D.
Professor Emeritus, Department of Psychiatry, University of Vermont College of Medicine, Burlington, Vermont

Michael Höfler, Ph.D.
Researcher, Institute of Clinical Psychology and Psychotherapy, Technische Universitaet Dresden, Dresden, Germany

Steven E. Hyman, M.D.
Provost, Harvard University, Cambridge, Massachusetts

James S. Jackson, Ph.D.
Director and Research Professor, Institute for Social Research, and Daniel Katz Distinguished University Professor of Psychology, University of Michigan, Ann Arbor, Michigan

Regina James, M.D.
Director, Division of Special Populations, National Institute of child Health & Human Development, Bethesda, Maryland

Ronald C. Kessler, Ph.D.
Professor, Department of Health Care Policy, Harvard Medical School, Boston, Massachusetts

Rachel G. Klein, Ph.D.
Fascitelli Family Professor of Child and Adolescent Psychiatry, New York University Child Study Center, New York, New York

Stanislav Kostyuchenko, M.D.
Assistant, Department of Psychiatry, National Medical Academy of Postgraduate Education

Robert F. Krueger, Ph.D.
Hathaway Distinguished Professor, Department of Psychology, University of Minnesota, Minneapolis, Minnesota

Emily A. Kuhl, Ph.D.
Science Writer, Division of Research, American Psychiatric Association, Arlington, Virginia

David J. Kupfer, M.D.
Thomas Detre Professor, Department of Psychiatry, University of Pittsburgh and Western Psychiatric Institute & Clinic, Pittsburgh, Pennsylvania; Chair, DSM-5 Task Force

James F. Leckman, M.D.
Neison Harris Professor of Child Psychiatry and Pediatrics, Yale University School of Medicine, Yale Child Study Center, New Haven, Connecticut

Sing Lee, M.B., B.S., F.R.C.Psych.
Professor, Department of Psychiatry, The Chinese University of Hong Kong

Ellen Leibenluft, M.D.
Chief, Section on Bipolar Spectrum Disorders, Emotion and Development Branch, Mood and Anxiety Program, National Institute of Mental Health, Bethesda, Maryland

Daphna Levinson, Ph.D.
Director, Research and Planning, Ministry of Health, Mental Health Services

Viviane Kovess Masféty, M.Sc., M.D., Ph.D.
Professor and Directrice, Département of Epidémiologie; Directrice, Fondation MGEN; Head, L'Université Paris Descartes Research Unit, Ecole des Hautes Études en Santé Publique, Paris, France

Herbert Matschinger, Ph.D.
Senior Researcher, Department of Psychiatry and Psychotherapy, University of Leipzig

Briana Mezuk, Ph.D.
Department of Epidemiology and Community Health, Virginia Commonwealth University School of Medicine, Richmond, Virginia

Zeina Mneimneh, M.P.H., M.Sc.
Survey Director, University of Michigan/Survey Research Center, Institute for Social Research, Ann Arbor, Michigan

William E. Narrow, M.D., M.P.H.
Associate Director, Division of Research, American Psychiatric Association, Arlington, Virginia; Research Director of the DSM-5 Task Force

Johan Ormel, Ph.D.
Professor of Psychiatric Epidemiology, University Medical Center Groningen

Daniel S. Pine, M.D.
Chief of Developmental Studies, Mood and Anxiety Disorders Program, National Institute of Mental Health, Bethesda, Maryland

José Posada-Villa, M.D.
Professor, Instituto Colombiano del Sistema Nervioso, Clinica Montserrat

Martin Prince, M.D.
Professor, Centre for Public Mental Health, Health Service and Population Research Department, Institute of Psychiatry, London, United Kingdom

Judith L. Rapoport, M.D.
Chief, Child Psychiatry Branch, National Institute of Mental Health, Bethesda, Maryland

Darrel A. Regier, M.D., M.P.H.
Executive Director, American Psychiatric Institute for Research and Education and Director, Division of Research, American Psychiatric Association, Arlington, Virginia; Vice-Chair, DSM-5 Task Force

Paola Rucci, Dr.Stat.
Visiting Research Assistant Professor, Department of Psychiatry, University of Pittsburgh School of Medicine, Western Psychiatric Institute and Clinic, Pittsburgh, Pennsylvania; Fellow, Department of Medicine and Public Health, University of Bologna, Bologna, Italy

Norman Sartorius, M.D., Ph.D., F.R.C.Psych.
President, Association for the Improvement of Mental Health Programmes, Geneva, Switzerland

Michael Schoenbaum, Ph.D.
Senior Advisor, Office of the Director, Division of Services & Intervention Research, National Institute of Mental Health, Bethesda, Maryland

Susan K. Schultz, M.D.
Professor of Psychiatry, University of Iowa Carver College of Medicine, Iowa City, Iowa

Soraya Seedat, M.B.Ch.B., F.C.Psych., Ph.D.
Co-Director, Medical Research Council Unit on Anxiety and Stress Disorders, Cape Town, South Africa

David Shaffer, M.D.
Irving Philips Professor of Child Psychiatry and Professor of Pediatrics, Child & Adolescent Psychiatry, New York State Psychiatric Institute, New York, New York

Leonard J. Simms, Ph.D.
Associate Professor, Department of Psychology, University at Buffalo, The State University of New York, Buffalo, New York

Renata Sousa, Ph.D.
Psychologist and Researcher, Health Service and Population Research Department, Institute of Psychiatry, London, United Kingdom

Susan C. South, Ph.D.
Assistant Professor, Department of Psychological Sciences, Purdue University, West Lafayette, Indiana

Hisateru Tachimori, Ph.D.
Section Chief, National Institute of Mental Health, National Center of Neurology and Psychiatry

Eric Taylor, M.A., M.B.
Emeritus Professor, King's College London, Institute of Psychiatry, London, United Kingdom

Myriam Torres, M.S.
Institute for Social Research, University of Michigan, Ann Arbor, Michigan

Adley Tsang, B.So.Sci.
Senior Research Assistant, Hong Kong Mood Disorders Center, Prince of Wales Hospital

T. Bedirhan Üstün, M.D.
Coordinator Classifications Terminologies & Standards, World Health Organization, Geneva, Switzerland

Michael Von Korff, Sc.D.
Senior Investigator, Group Health Research Institute, Seattle, Washington

Philip S. Wang, M.D., Dr.P.H.
Deputy Director, National Institute of Mental Health, Bethesda, Maryland

Hans-Ulrich Wittchen, Ph.D.
Chairman and Director, Institute of Clinical Psychology and Psychotherapy, and Professor, Technische Universitaet Dresden, Dresden, Germany

Kimberly A. Yonkers, M.D.
Professor, Department of Psychiatry, Yale School of Medicine, New Haven, Connecticut

Charles H. Zeanah, M.D.
Professor, Department of Psychiatry, Tulane University, New Orleans, Louisiana

Rong Zhang, Ph.D.
Blue Cross Blue Shield of Michigan

Disclosure of Competing Interests

The following contributors to this book have indicated a financial interest in or other affiliation with a commercial supporter, a manufacturer of a commercial product, a provider of a commercial service, a nongovernmental organization, and/or a government agency, as listed below:

Darrel A. Regier, M.D., M.P.H.—The author, as Executive Director of the American Psychiatric Institute for Research and Education, oversees all federal and industry-sponsored research and research training grants in APIRE but receives no external salary funding or honoraria from any government or industry.

Lee Anna Clark, Ph.D.—The author receives research support and royalties from the University of Minnesota Press for the Schedule for Adaptive and Non-adaptive Personality (SNAP) measure.

Warachal Eileen Faison, M.D.—The author is a full-time employee at Pfizer Inc. and owns stock in Pfizer Inc.

Ellen Frank, Ph.D.—The author receives royalties from Guilford Press. The author is on the Advisory Board for Servier International.

Nick Glozier, Ph.D.—The author has received research support from the Australian Research Council, the National Health and Medical Research Council, Servier Laboratories, BOHRF, Beyond Blue, and the Heart Foundation. The author conducts medico-legal disability assessments for NSW Fire Brigades, NSW Police, RailCorp, the Worker's Compensation Commission, and several law firms, both appellant and respondent. The author is a member of the NSW Worker's Compensation Commission medical appeal panel for disability compensation.

Steven E. Hyman, M.D.—The author is a member of the Novartis Science Board but does not receive direct payment of honorarium.

Ronald C. Kessler, Ph.D.—The author has been a consultant for GlaxoSmithKline, Kaiser Permanente, Pfizer Inc., Sanofi-Aventis, Shire Pharmaceuticals, and Wyeth-Ayerst. The author has served on the advisory boards for Eli Lilly & Company and Wyeth-Ayerst. The author has received research support from Bristol-Myers Squibb, Eli Lilly & Company, GlaxoSmithKline, Johnson & Johnson, Ortho-McNeil Pharmaceuticals Inc., Pfizer Inc., and Sanofi-Aventis.

James F. Leckman, M.D.—The author receives research support from the National Institutes of Health, Tourette Syndrome Association, and Klingenstein Third Generation Foundation. The author receives royalties from John Wiley and Sons, McGraw Hill, and Oxford University Press.

Paola Rucci, Dr.Stat.—The author has received research support from Forest Research Institute and Fondazione IDEA.

Susan K. Schultz, M.D.—The author has received research support from the National Cancer Institute and the National Institute of Aging, with partnership from Baxter Healthcare. The author receives support from the American Psychiatric Association for editorial duties with the *American Journal of Psychiatry*.

Soraya Seedat, M.B.Ch.B., F.C.Psych., Ph.D.—The author has received research support from GlaxoSmithKline, Lundbeck, AstraZeneca, and Servier.

Michael Von Korff, Sc.D.—The author receives research support from Johnson and Johnson.

Kimberly A. Yonkers, M.D.—The author has received research support from Eli Lilly. The author has received publishing royalties from Up to Date Inc.

Charles H. Zeanah, M.D.—The author has received royalties from Guilford Press.

The following contributors to this book have indicated no competing interests to dsiclose during the year preceding manuscript submission:

Jamie M. Abelson, M.S.W.
Sergio Aguilar-Gaxiola, M.D., Ph.D.
Jordi Alonso, M.D., Ph.D.
Gavin Andrews, M.D.
Katja Beesdo, Ph.D.
Patricia A. Berglund, M.B.A.
Guilherme Borges, M.Sc., Dr.Sc.
Mark Oakley Browne, Ph.D.
Ronny Bruffaerts, Ph.D.
Diana E. Clarke, Ph.D.
E. Jane Costello, Ph.D.
Michelle G. Craske, Ph.D.
Ron Dahl, M.D.
Giovanni de Girolamo, M.D.
Madeleine Delves
Michael Dewey, Ph.D.
Nicholas R. Eaton, M.A.
Richard Gater, M.D.
Andrew T. Gloster, Ph.D.
David Goldberg, D.M., F.R.C.P.
Oye Gureje, M.D., Ph.D., D.Sc.
Josep Maria Haro, M.D., M.P.H., Ph.D.
John E. Helzer, M.D.
Michael Höfler, Ph.D.
James S. Jackson, Ph.D.
Regina James, M.D.

Rachel G. Klein, Ph.D.
Stanislav Kostyuchenko, M.D.
Robert F. Krueger, Ph.D.
Emily A. Kuhl, Ph.D.
David J. Kupfer, M.D.
Sing Lee, M.B., B.S., F.R.C.Psych.
Ellen Leibenluft, M.D.
Daphna Levinson, Ph.D.
Viviane Kovess Masféty, M.Sc., M.D., Ph.D.
Herbert Matschinger, Ph.D.
Briana Mezuk, Ph.D.
Zeina Mneimneh, M.P.H., M.Sc.
William E. Narrow, M.D., M.P.H.
Johan Ormel, Ph.D.
Daniel S. Pine, M.D.
José Posada-Villa, M.D.
Martin Prince, M.D.
Judith L. Rapoport, M.D.
Norman Sartorius, M.D., Ph.D., F.R.C.Psych.
Michael Schoenbaum, Ph.D.
David Shaffer, M.D.
Leonard J. Simms, Ph.D.
Renata Sousa, Ph.D.
Susan C. South, Ph.D.
Hisateru Tachimori, Ph.D.
Eric Taylor, M.A., M.B.
Myriam Torres, M.S.
Adley Tsang, B.So.Sci.
T. Bedirhan Üstün, M.D.
Philip S. Wang, M.D., Dr.P.H.
Hans-Ulrich Wittchen, Ph.D.
Rong Zhang, Ph.D.

Introduction

Darrel A. Regier, M.D., M.P.H.
William E. Narrow, M.D., M.P.H.
Emily A. Kuhl, Ph.D.
David J. Kupfer, M.D.

Over the past 30 years, there has been a continuous testing of multiple hypotheses that are inherent in the *Diagnostic and Statistical Manual of Mental Disorders,* from the third edition (DSM-III; American Psychiatric Association 1980) to the fourth (DSM-IV; American Psychiatric Association 1994). Although DSM-III was the first official classification from the American Psychiatric Association (APA) to embrace these hypotheses, their intellectual origin is more properly attributed to Eli Robins and Samuel Guze's landmark 1970 article on the establishment of diagnostic validity in psychiatric illness (Robins and Guze 1970) and the subsequent 1972 release of the St. Louis "Feighner diagnostic criteria" (Feighner et al. 1972). These formed the basis for the 1978 Research Diagnostic Criteria (Spitzer et al. 1978), which were used in the longitudinal collaborative study on the psychobiology of depression supported by the National Institute of Mental Health (Rice et al. 2005) and ultimately were the prototypical diagnoses adopted in DSM-III in 1980.

The expectation of Robins and Guze (1970) was that each clinical syndrome described in the Feighner criteria, Research Diagnostic Criteria, and DSM-III would ultimately be validated by its separation from other disorders, common clinical course, genetic aggregation in families, and further differentiation by future laboratory tests—which would now include anatomical and functional imaging, molecular genetics, pathophysiological variations, and neuropsychological testing.

Reprinted from Regier DA, Narrow WE, Kuhl E, Kupfer DJ: "The Conceptual Development of DSM-V." *American Journal of Psychiatry* 166:645–650, 2009. Copyright 2009, American Psychiatric Association. Used with permission.

To the original validators Kendler (1990) added differential response to treatment, which could include both pharmacological and psychotherapeutic interventions.

After almost 40 years of testing these hypotheses, we are impressed by the remarkable advances in research and clinical practice that were facilitated by having explicit diagnostic criteria that produced greater reliability in diagnosis across clinicians and research investigators in many countries. The benefit of using explicit criteria to increase reliability in the absence of etiological understanding was an outcome predicted by the British psychiatrist Ervin Stengel (1959). However, as these criteria have been tested in multiple epidemiological, clinical, and genetic studies through slightly revised DSM-III-R (American Psychiatric Association 1987), DSM-IV, and DSM-IV-TR (American Psychiatric Association 2000) editions, the lack of clear separation of these syndromes became apparent from the high levels of comorbidity that were reported (Boyd et al. 1984; Regier et al. 1990). A particularly clear discussion of the inability to identify "zones of rarity" between mental disorders was presented by Kendell and Jablensky (2003). In addition, treatment response became less specific as selective serotonin reuptake inhibitors were found to be effective for a wide range of anxiety, mood, and eating disorders and atypical antipsychotics received indications for schizophrenia, bipolar disorder, and treatment-resistant major depression.

More recently, it was found that a majority of patients with entry diagnoses of major depression in the Sequenced Treatment Alternatives to Relieve Depression (STAR*D) study had significant anxiety symptoms, and this subgroup had a more severe clinical course and was less responsive to available treatments (Howland et al. 2009). The lack of clear separation between current disorders defined by DSM-IV-TR was clearly illustrated in a survey of primary care patients (Lowe et al. 2008), which found that among individuals with the most severe ratings of depression, anxiety, or somatization, more than one-half in each syndrome group also had at least one, if not both, of the other two disorders. Furthermore, the combined influence of the three syndromes on functional impairment was far more significant than any of their individual effects. Likewise, we have come to understand that we are unlikely to find single gene underpinnings for most mental disorders, which are more likely to have polygenetic vulnerabilities interacting with epigenetic factors (that switch genes on and off) and environmental exposures to produce disorders.

In retrospect, it is interesting that there was such a strict separation of mood, anxiety, psychotic, somatic, substance use, and personality disorder symptoms for the original Feighner diagnoses (Regier et al. 2005). It is clear that an hierarchy was present that tended to suppress the significance of lower-order symptoms in the syndrome definitions in order to achieve such pure types. This hierarchical arrangement of disorders was implicit in the Kraepelinean classification tradition of ranking organic mental disorders, nuclear schizophrenia, manic-depressive illness, and neurotic illnesses from higher- to lower-order conditions (Surtees and Kendell 1979). It was followed by an explicit statement of Jaspers (1963): "The principle of medical diagnosis is that all the disease-phenomena should be characterized within a single diagnosis…in any one person" (p. 611). Although the idea of a strict hierarchy, in which the presence of any disorder could cause manifestations of disorders lower in the hierarchy, was explicitly abandoned for DSM-III-R after publication and review (Regier 1987) of the article by Boyd et al. (1984), the strict separation of symptoms and disorder types has persisted through DSM-IV-TR. Some remnants of the hierarchy persist in a few areas, such as the diagnosis of autistic disorder (299.00), in which there is still an explicit exclusion of a diagnosis of attention-deficit/hyperactivity disorder (ADHD) if autistic disorder is present. The practical effect of this exclusion is that insurance reimbursement is often denied for co-occurring symptoms of ADHD in the presence of a diagnosis of autism. To support this strict separation, we now have a plethora of comorbidity—because patients do not usually have only mood, somatic, or anxiety symptoms but tend to come with a mix from multiple symptom groups. Hence, we have heterogeneous conditions within single diagnostic groups, a remarkably high rate in specialty mental health settings of "not otherwise specified" diagnoses that do not quite fit the existing criteria, as well as high rates of "subsyndromal" mixed anxiety-mood-somatic disorders in primary care settings.

How then are we to update our classification to recognize the most prominent syndromes that are actually present in nature, rather than in the heuristic and anachronistic pure types of previous scientific eras? A serious consideration from the aforementioned study by Lowe et al. (2008) is that some patients with clinically significant distress and impairment might have only a few symptoms from mood, anxiety, and somatic diagnostic criteria sets that do not qualify for a formal diagnosis in any one disorder, although the aggregate burden requires a not-otherwise-specified diagnosis and treatment. A more important clinical consideration is that the clinical course and treatment response for anxious depression, posttraumatic stress disorder with depression, and other mixed disorders cannot be predicted from clinical trials of medications or psychosocial interventions that are based on outcomes with patient groups selected for pure categorical disorders or that contain an unknown heterogeneous mix of comorbid conditions. In addition, supraordinate dimensional measures may provide better phenotypic expressions for linkage to illness susceptibility substrates identified by neuroimaging and genetic studies. Common genetic determinants of schizophrenia and bipolar disorder have resulted in calls for a reappraisal of these disorders as distinct diagnostic entities (Lichtenstein et al. 2009; Owen and Craddock 2009).

As we began the DSM-5 developmental process in 1999, a major concern was to address a range of issues that had emerged over the previous 30 years. These included the basic definition of a mental disorder, the potential for adding dimensional criteria to disorders, the option of separating impairment and diagnostic assessments, the need to address the various expressions of an illness across developmental stages of an entire lifespan, and the need to address differences in mental disorder expression as conditioned by gender and cultural characteristics. The opportunity to evaluate the readiness of neuroscientific advances in pathophysiology, genetics, pharmacogenomics, structural and functional imaging, and neuropsychology was also a priority. All of these areas were summarized in a series of white papers published as *A Research Agenda for DSM-V* (Kupfer et al. 2002). A second volume of white papers was then commissioned by the APA to address developmental psychopathology issues across the lifespan (in very young children and in geriatric age groups) as well as gender-related differences in the occurrence and expression of mental disorders, titled *Age and Gender Considerations in Psychiatric Diagnosis: A Research Agenda for DSM-V* (Narrow et al. 2007).

In the next stage of DSM development, the American Psychiatric Institute for Research and Education was able to work jointly with the World Health Organization (WHO) and leaders of the World Psychiatric Association to develop a National Institute of Mental Health (NIMH) research conference grant application to review the research base for a wide range of mental disorder diagnoses. In addition to NIMH, the National Institute on Drug Abuse (NIDA) and the National Institute on Alcohol Abuse and Alcoholism (NIAAA) agreed to support this effort and to transform it into a cooperative agreement grant in which a steering committee was formed, consisting of representatives from the American Psychiatric Institute for Research and Education, each of the three National Institutes of Health institutes, and WHO. One of us (D.A.R.) was the principal investigator, and the coinvestigators included another author (W.E.N.) and Michael First, as well as Bridget Grant from NIAAA; Wilson Compton from NIDA; Wayne Fenton and then Bruce Cuthbert, followed by Michael Kozak, from NIMH; and Benedetto Saraceno, who designated Norman Sartorius to represent WHO. The 5-year grant from 2003 to 2008 supported 13 international conferences that have produced more than 100 scientific articles, many of which have now been compiled into monographs for use as reference volumes for the DSM-5 Task Force and the WHO ICD-11 Mental Disorders Advisory Group (Andrews et al. 2009; Helzer et al. 2008; Kupfer et al. 2002; Narrow et al. 2007; Philips et al. 2003; Saunders et al. 2007; Sunderland et al. 2007; Widiger et al. 2006). One consistent recommendation that emerged most strongly from the initial methods conference (Kraemer 2007; Kraemer et al. 2007), the conference on dimensional measures (Helzer et al. 2006), and the conference on public health was the call for better integration of categorical and dimensional assessment criteria for the next revision of DSM. Previous editions had questioned the clinical feasibility of establishing dimensional measures to assess thresholds and severity of disorders but had adopted "clinically significant distress or impairment" assessment requirements for all disorders in DSM-IV (pp. xxi–xxii). The only dimensional component of DSM-IV is Axis V, which mixes both symptoms and functional impairment for a Global Assessment of Functioning scale.

In April 2006, the DSM-5 Task Force chairperson (D.J.K.) and vice-chairperson (D.A.R.) were named by APA President Steven Sharfstein and Medical Director James Scully. This was followed by nominations of a substantial number of the task force members. However, before members of the task force could be fully approved, the Board of Trustees established principles for appointment that required limits on investments and income that could be received from pharmaceutical companies, the requirement that no more than two representatives from any one university participate in the task force or on the same work group, and a vetting and review process by a subcommittee of the board (www.dsm5.org). This process took almost 2 years to complete, with the task force members publicly announced in July 2007 and the work group members announced in May 2008. During the time needed to appoint and review the work group members, the task force was assigned the responsibility of addressing conceptual issues through study groups that would guide the overall development of revisions for specific diagnostic areas.

The focus of the study group on spectrum disorders included assessment of the spectra of mental disorder syndromes that cross existing diagnostic boundaries, recommendations for the overall structure of DSM categories, and identification of 11 potential criteria useful for testing the validity of mental disorder diagnoses—a marked expansion beyond the original criteria proposed by Robins and Guze (1970). A second study group, addressing developmental issues, focused on assuring attention to different expressions of mental disorders that might emerge at progressive ages and human developmental life stages. A third study group, on gender and culture, was established to assess the different expression or symptom equivalents of mental disorders that are mediated by gender and culture. A fourth study group, on the interface with general medicine, was formed to address approaches that would facilitate a better interface between general medical and mental disorder approaches to diagnosis.

A major initial concern identified by the fourth study group was the need to review disability assessment strategies and instruments that could apply across all of medicine and potentially replace the

Global Assessment of Functioning scale, which currently serves as Axis V of DSM-IV-TR. As a result of their recommendations, a fifth study group, for functional impairment and disability assessment, was formed that would specifically address the development of global impairment and disability assessment strategies. Finally, the need to address measurement and assessment issues in all of the diagnostic areas undergoing revisions resulted in the establishment of a sixth study group that will focus on diagnostic assessment instruments. Representatives from each of the work groups will work with a core group of diagnostic instrument experts who can evaluate methods for facilitating measurement-based care for clinicians, making clinical research assessments, and determining rates of mental disorder diagnoses in community populations for epidemiological studies. This final group had its first organizational meeting in January 2009 and will be working with each of the work groups to facilitate a bottoms-up approach for instrument development that will begin with the diagnostic criteria and determine how relevant dimensional metrics can facilitate measurement-based care (Trivedi et al. 2006).

Each of the 13 diagnostic area work groups has been responsible for conducting literature reviews that build on the relevant work from phases one and two of the DSM-5 development process. A research methods group has been established to review secondary data analyses proposed for funding by the APA to assess the evidence base for proposed revisions. The work group process has been supported by conference calls that occur at least monthly, with some work groups having subgroup meetings every 2 weeks. Face-to-face meetings have been supported at APA headquarters at least twice each year, and multiple work groups often meet simultaneously to facilitate cross-group collaborative discussions about issues of overlapping concern. Task force and work group members have participated actively in professional meeting presentations and town hall meetings, conducted surveys of published colleagues in their areas, provided summaries of major work group issues on the DSM-5 development Web site (www.dsm5.org), and received recommendations from the public and professional colleagues directed to the Web site.

As the DSM-5 process now moves into a field trial phase of secondary data analysis and primary data collection to test diagnostic options, there will be an intensification of the interactions between the cross-cutting study groups and the diagnostic work groups. Of major concern will be an attempt to address the consequences of continuing to use the original Feighner criteria, Research Diagnostic Criteria, and DSM-III hierarchical structure of "pure" diagnostic categories. The high rate of co-occurrence, frequent use of the "not otherwise specified" designation, and heterogeneous mix of conditions within current diagnostic boundaries are all major problems that we would like to address with the revision in DSM-5. The original Robins and Guze validators have not confirmed the wisdom of the current structure. The expanded set of validators recommended by our study group on spectrum disorders provides a framework for considering how disorders might be grouped into larger, supraordinate categories in DSM-5.

Mental disorder syndromes will eventually be redefined to reflect more useful diagnostic categories ("to carve nature at its joints") as well as dimensional discontinuities between disorders and clear thresholds between pathology and normality. However, our immediate task is to set a framework for an evolution of our diagnostic system that can advance our clinical practice and facilitate ongoing testing of the diagnostic criteria that are intended to be scientific hypotheses, rather than inerrant Biblical scripture. The single most important precondition for moving forward to improve the clinical and scientific utility of DSM-5 will be the incorporation of simple dimensional measures for assessing syndromes within broad diagnostic categories and supraordinate dimensions that cross current diagnostic boundaries. Thus, we have decided that one of the major—if not *the* major—differences between DSM-IV and DSM-5 will be the more prominent use of dimensional measures in DSM-5.

The readiness of biological markers to serve as associated features, risk factors, or diagnostic criteria will be of major concern. Likewise, the clinical utility and validity of age-, gender-, and culture-related specifiers or subtypes of disorders will need to be assessed. Measurement-based approaches for field testing new criteria sets will need to be reviewed and selected as part of the field test procedures.

As chairpersons and coordinators of this revision process, we are keenly aware of the rapidly changing research base for the description and treatment of mental disorders that include neurodevelopmental, neurocognitive, and addictive disorders. We are reevaluating the structure of the manual itself to facilitate both clinical practice and better research criteria to guide clinical trials, genetics, imaging, and treatment guideline development. More specifically, we anticipate that we will have a structure that contains "receptors" for new biological, neurocognitive, and environmental risk factors as they emerge to guide future research and clinical practice (Hyman 2007). As a result, we expect that DSM-5 will be a living document with a permanent revision infrastructure to enable revisions of specific diagnostic areas in which new evidence is replicated and reviewed as ready for adoption.

Such regular revisions are already routine for practice guidelines, for the reviews of new diagnostic categories in *International Classification of Diseases,* 9th Revision, Clinical Modification (National Center for Health Statistics and Centers for Medicare and Medicaid Services 1997), and for the American Medical Association (2007) Current Procedural Terminology codes used by the Centers for Medicare and Medicaid Services and all of medicine.

We look forward to a vigorous interactive process over the coming years before the publication of DSM-5 in May 2013.

References

American Medical Association: Current Procedural Terminology, 4th Edition. New York, Oxford University Press, 2007

American Psychiatric Association: Diagnostic and Statistical Manual of Mental Disorders, 3rd Edition. Washington, DC, American Psychiatric Association, 1980

American Psychiatric Association: Diagnostic and Statistical Manual of Mental Disorders, 3rd Edition, Revised. Washington, DC, American Psychiatric Association, 1987

American Psychiatric Association: Diagnostic and Statistical Manual of Mental Disorders, 4th Edition. Washington, DC, American Psychiatric Association, 1994

American Psychiatric Association: Diagnostic and Statistical Manual of Mental Disorders, 4th Edition, Text Revision. Washington, DC, American Psychiatric Association, 2000

Andrews G, Charney DS, Sirovatka PJ, et al (eds): Stress-Induced and Fear Circuitry Disorders: Refining the Research Agenda for DSM-V. Arlington, VA, American Psychiatric Association, 2009

Boyd JH, Burke JD, Gruenberg E, et al: Exclusion criteria of DSM-III: a study of co-occurrence of hierarchy-free syndromes. Arch Gen Psychiatry 41:983–989, 1984

Feighner JP, Robins E, Guze SB, et al: Diagnostic criteria for use in psychiatric research. Arch Gen Psychiatry 26:57–63, 1972

Helzer JE, Kraemer HC, Krueger RF: The feasibility and need for dimensional psychiatric diagnoses. Psychol Med 36:1671–1680, 2006

Helzer JE, Kraemer HC, Krueger RF, et al (eds): Dimensional Approaches in Diagnostic Classification: Refining the Research Agenda for DSM-V. Arlington, VA, American Psychiatric Association, 2008

Howland RH, Rush AJ, Wisniewski SR, et al: Concurrent anxiety and substance use disorders among outpatients with major depression: clinical features and effect on treatment outcome. Drug Alcohol Depend 99:248–260, 2009

Hyman SE: Can neuroscience be integrated into the DSM-V? Nat Rev Neurosci 8:725–732, 2007

Jaspers K: General Psychopathology, 7th Edition. Translated by Hoenig J, Hamilton MW. Manchester, UK, Manchester University Press, 1963

Kendell R, Jablensky A: Distinguishing between the validity and utility of psychiatric diagnoses. Am J Psychiatry 160:4–12, 2003

Kendler KS: Towards a scientific psychiatric nosology: strengths and limitations. Arch Gen Psychiatry 47:969–973, 1990

Kraemer HC: DSM categories and dimensions in clinical and research contexts. Int J Methods Psychiatr Res 16(suppl):S8–S15, 2007

Kraemer HC, Shrout PE, Rubio-Stipec M: Developing the diagnostic and statistical manual V: what will "statistical" mean in DSM-V? Soc Psychiatry Psychiatr Epidemiol 42:259–267, 2007

Kupfer DJ, First MB, Regier DA (eds): A Research Agenda for DSM-V. Washington, DC, American Psychiatric Association, 2002

Lichtenstein P, Yip BH, Björk C, et al: Common genetic determinants of schizophrenia and bipolar disorder in Swedish families: a population-based study. Lancet 373:234–239, 2009

Lowe B, Spitzer RL, Williams JBW, et al: Depression, anxiety and somatization in primary care: syndrome overlap and functional impairment. Gen Hosp Psychiatry 30:191–199, 2008

Narrow WE, First MB, Sirovatka PJ, et al (eds): Age and Gender Considerations in Psychiatric Diagnosis: A Research Agenda for DSM-V. Arlington, VA, American Psychiatric Association, 2007

National Center for Health Statistics and Centers for Medicare and Medicaid Services: The International Classification of Diseases, 9th Revision, Clinical Modification (ICD-9-CM). Salt Lake City, UT, Medicode Publications, 1997

Owen MJ, Craddock N: Diagnosis of functional psychoses: time to face the future. Lancet 373:190–191, 2009

Philips KA, First MB, Pincus HA (eds): Advancing DSM: Dilemmas in Psychiatric Diagnosis. Arlington, VA, American Psychiatric Association, 2003

Regier DA: Introduction, part VII: nosologic principles and diagnostic criteria, in Diagnosis and Classification in Psychiatry: A Critical Appraisal of DSM-III. Edited by Tischler GL. New York, Cambridge University Press, 1987, pp 399–401

Regier DA, Farmer ME, Rae DS, et al: Comorbidity of mental disorders with alcohol and other drug abuse: results from the Epidemiologic Catchment Area (ECA) study. JAMA 264:2511–2518, 1990

Regier DA, Narrow WE, Rae DS, et al: Advancing from reliability to validity: the challenge for DSMV/ICD-11 revisions, in Psychopathology in the Genome and Neuroscience Era. Edited by Zorumski CF, Rubin EH. Washington, DC, American Psychiatric Publishing, 2005, pp 85–96

Rice J, Andreasen NC, Coryell W, et al: NIMH Collaborative Program on the Psychobiology of Depression: clinical. Genet Epidemiol 6:179–182, 2005

Robins E, Guze SB: Establishment of diagnostic validity in psychiatric illness: its application to schizophrenia. Am J Psychiatry 126:983–987, 1970

Saunders JB, Schuckit MA, Sirovatka PJ, et al (eds): Diagnostic Issues in Substance Use Disorders: Refining the Research Agenda for DSM-V. Arlington, VA, American Psychiatric Association, 2007

Spitzer RL, Endicott J, Robins E: Research Diagnostic Criteria: rationale and reliability. Arch Gen Psychiatry 35:773–782, 1978

Stengel E: Classification of mental disorders. Bull World Health Organ 21:601–603, 1959

Sunderland T, Jeste DV, Baiyewu O, et al (eds): Diagnostic Issues in Dementia: Advancing the Research Agenda for DSM-V. Arlington, VA, American Psychiatric Association, 2007

Surtees PG, Kendell RE: The hierarchy model of psychiatric symptomatology: an investigation based on Present State Examination ratings. Br J Psychiatry 135:438–443, 1979

Trivedi MH, Rush AJ, Wisniewski SR, et al: Evaluation of outcomes with citalopram for depression using measurement-based care in STAR*D: implications for clinical practice. Am J Psychiatry 163:28–40, 2006

Widiger TA, Simonsen E, Sirovatka PJ, et al (eds): Dimensional Models of Personality Disorders: Refining the Research Agenda for DSM-V. Arlington, VA, American Psychiatric Association, 2006

PART I

Diagnostic Spectra: Assessing the Validity of Disorder Groupings

CHAPTER 1

Diagnosis of Mental Disorders in Light of Modern Genetics

Steven E. Hyman, M.D.

Historically, a pressing need for interrater reliability in psychiatric diagnosis has contributed to wide acceptance of operationalized diagnostic criteria, beginning with DSM-III (American Psychiatric Association 1980). As has long been noted, reliability became a priority at a time when validity could not be scientifically achieved. It was hoped, nonetheless, that further research on DSM-III disorders might ultimately yield a valid classification. It now appears that the accreting failures of the current diagnostic system cannot be addressed simply by revising individual criterion sets and certainly not by adding more disorders to DSM-5. The emerging field of genetics provides one useful window into the nature of mental disorders. Insights emerging from genetics and, increasingly, from neuroscience suggest that the exclusive use of categorical diagnoses and the predominant "splitting" approach of DSM-III and DSM-IV (American Psychiatric Association 1994) represent obstacles to the near-term development of a more scientifically and clinically satisfactory classification.

This chapter represents my personal viewpoint and does not represent an official position of the DSM-5 Task Force, of which I am a member, or of the International Advisory Group to the World Health Organization for the Revision of ICD-10, Chapter V (Mental and Behavioral Disorders), of which I am the chair.

3

Introduction and Background

Disease definitions that facilitate interrater reliability are the bedrock of replicable clinical investigation, including clinical trials. As a result, such definitions form the basis for rational treatment decisions and, indeed, all clinical communication. In general medicine, the wide availability of objective tests has meant that interrater reliability is often taken for granted. In contrast, the lack of objective tests for mental disorders has made reliability a significant challenge because diagnoses must be based on verbal reports and behavioral observations. DSM-III was the first systematic and relatively complete platform for psychiatric diagnosis that had a clear focus on interrater reliability. In the DSM-III approach to reliability, also adopted by the ICD-10 chapter on Mental and Behavioral Disorders (World Health Organization 1992), each diagnosis was based on a set of operationalized diagnostic criteria that had been field tested. This feature contributed to the rapid and widespread acceptance of DSM-III. DSM-III and its successor volumes—along with ICD-9 and ICD-10 (World Health Organization 1977, 1992)—have become global standards for the diagnosis of mental disorders. Although significant problems with reliability remained, the DSM-III approach contrasted markedly with the brief clinical descriptions provided by prior editions of the manual (see American Psychiatric Association 1952, 1968); these early descriptions gave little guidance as to how diagnoses should be applied.

The proximate intellectual foundation for DSM-III was the seminal work of Robins and Guze (1970), followed by two sets of diagnostic criteria for research, based on the Robins and Guze approach (Feighner et al. 1972; Spitzer et al. 1975). Using schizophrenia as their example, Robins and Guze (1970) argued that a *valid* diagnosis (presumably, a diagnosis that would represent a "natural kind," separable from other diagnostic entities), could be achieved by 1) identification of symptoms and signs that cluster together, 2) laboratory studies, 3) a clear separation of one disorder from another, 4) long-term follow-up studies to establish the stability of the diagnosis over time, and 5) family studies. A critical assumption underlying the work of Robins and Guze was that psychiatric disorders were best captured as discrete categories, discontinuous from each other and from health. These authors did not take an alternative approach—common in general medicine—that represents at least some disorders as quantitative deviations from health. Because quantitative (or dimensional) descriptions of disorder are continuous with a normal state, there must be thresholds—ideally set using outcomes data—that call for different levels of observation or treatment. Examples of disorders that are usefully represented as discontinuous categories are pneumococcal pneumonia or small cell carcinoma of the lung. Disorders better represented as quantitative dimensions are hypertension (the dimensions being systolic and diastolic blood pressure) or iron-deficiency anemia.

At the time of this writing, the diverse scientific approaches that will eventually explicate mental disorders remain in early, even embryonic, states. The etiological risk factors (genetic or nongenetic) for any common psychiatric disorder have not been established with an adequate level of certainty or completeness to be truly useful. Despite exciting recent developments in understanding the neural or genetic substrates of anxiety disorders (Delgado et al. 2008), addictive disorders (Hyman et al. 2006), autism (C.A. Walsh et al. 2008), depressive disorders (Mayberg et al. 2005), and schizophrenia (Cannon et al. 2002; T. Walsh et al. 2008), it would be premature to claim an understanding of the pathophysiology of these disorders. Indeed, as already noted, with few exceptions, there are still no objective medical tests for any disorder in DSM-IV. Objective tests do exist for some of the sleep disorders, but these are not listed among the DSM-IV or DSM-IV-TR (American Psychiatric Association 2000) criteria. Given the scientific hurdles that remain before us today, it is not surprising that the authors of DSM-III, working more than three decades ago, were not in a position to set "correct" boundaries for mental disorders. During the past three decades, profound changes occurred in the definitions of many general medical disorders, which could be addressed by a more mature science than that relevant to mental disorders. For example, in cancer, many diseases once thought to be singular, such as non-Hodgkin's lymphoma, have turned out to be multiple different diseases.

I argue, however, that our significant problems with DSM-IV are not addressable merely by achieving better definitions of existing disorders or by the addition of subtyping. Rather, there appear to be significant structural problems inherited from DSM-III, such as the exclusive use of categories and substantial degree of diagnostic splitting—for example, splitting fear-based anxiety disorders into agoraphobia, panic disorder, specific phobia, social phobia, posttraumatic stress disorder, acute stress disorder, and generalized anxiety disorder—that deserve reconsideration if DSM-5 is to pave the way for much-needed scientific progress.

In summary, lacking objective medical tests, the powerful need for interrater reliability drove the elaboration of rigid and highly specified criteria based on phenomenology. The need for shared diagnoses drove the wide global acceptance of the DSM and ICD systems and made them a clear benefit to research and clinical care. To our misfortune, the need for widespread diagnostic agreement collided with a very immature scientific base, leading to reification of what should have been a tentative and experimental system. If, for example, DSM-IV/DSM-IV-TR criteria must be used in order to satisfy granting agencies, journal reviewers, and regulatory agencies, it becomes very difficult to test hypotheses about other diagnostic approaches or to develop new treatments for conditions that do not match the criteria lists in the manual (Hyman and Fenton 2003). The strong forces that favor reification of DSM disorder definitions also call for a concerted effort to permit alternative approaches to be tested.

Challenges for the DSM-5 Task Force and Work Groups include:

1. Grappling with a scientific base still not up to the task of undergirding a valid classification;
2. Changing the classification in ways that will encourage, rather than inhibit, science that questions the boundaries and structuring of current DSM-IV diagnoses;
3. Making DSM-5 a living document so that well-replicated discoveries can be incorporated into the manual, without waiting many years for DSM-6; and
4. Doing all this without damaging clinical practice or administrative uses of DSM classification.

The difficulty of this prescription can be likened to performing substantial repairs on an airplane while it is still flying.

Emerging Concerns

It is easy to find flaws in DSM-IV and DSM-IV-TR; at the same time, for the major and well-studied disorders, there is a measure of reassuring evidence that their classifications pick out real, replicable features of psychopathology. The cross-cultural similarity of symptoms and course of many of the major disorders, such as autism (Wakabayashi et al. 2007), schizophrenia, bipolar disorder, obsessive-compulsive disorder (Matsunaga et al. 2008), and major depression, argues that the core features of these disorders are not the arbitrary creations of DSM-III work groups. In addition, for many of the major disorders, high levels of familial aggregation have been demonstrated (Kendler et al. 1997). Finally, twin studies suggest that autism, schizophrenia, and bipolar disorder have among the highest heritabilities of common, genetically complex disorders (for review, see Merikangas and Risch 2003; see also Hyman 2008). If the major disorders were mere chimaeras, such consistent family and genetic findings would not be expected (with the caveat that simple determinations of twin concordance do not distinguish between the inheritance of risk genes across generations vs. new mutations.)

In a short chapter such as this it is not possible to provide a thorough review of the data that raise concerns about DSM-IV classification. Concerns could be raised, however, not only in the formulation of individual diagnoses but also in basic structural elements—most notably, the categorical nature of all diagnoses (Cole et al. 2008; Fanous et al. 2001; Kendler and Gardner 1998). In the clinical realm, evidence for problems in classification includes the widespread need to rely on residual, "not otherwise specified" (NOS) diagnoses; the need to use categories that stubbornly resist even rudimentary validation; and the high degrees of comorbidity that accrue to many patients. The need to use NOS diagnoses varies according to disorder clusters and clinical communities but appears to represent a large fraction of diagnoses made in certain domains, including developmental and other childhood mental disorders, eating disorders, and personality disorders (de Bruin et al. 2007; Fairburn and Bohn 2005). In summary, a significant fraction of patients do not fit the highly specified criteria of named disorders. In this case, the rigidity of operationalized diagnostic criteria, based on phenomenology, trades interrater reliability for ability to capture the true heterogeneity of clinical populations.

A related problem of definition is the inability to establish even rough-and-ready validity for clinically employed categorical diagnoses such as schizoaffective disorder or schizophreniform disorder (Fanous et al. 2001; Laursen et al. 2005; Lichtenstein et al. 2009; Mahli et al. 2008).

Finally, the frequency of comorbidity among DSM-IV diagnoses is so great as to suggest underlying problems with the current classification. Certainly, an individual may have more than one illness or may have a condition that is a risk factor for another illness; for instance, the presence of mania may elevate the risk of substance use disorders (Regier et al. 1990). However, the high rates of comorbidity—for example, among disorders of childhood (Galanter and Leibenluft 2008; Goldstein and Schwebach 2004) or among mood, anxiety, and personality disorders (Kessler et al. 2005a, 2005b; McGlashan et al. 2000)—raise the question of whether too many disorders have been stipulated and whether the categorical approach is always the right one (Krueger and Markon 2006). The open question is whether different manifestations of a basic pathological process have been divided into multiple diagnostic silos, creating artifactual comorbidity in certain circumstances.

At a superficial level, the need for NOS diagnoses and the failure to validate certain other diagnoses, such as schizoaffective disorder, might simply indicate a need for additional disorder-specific research. However, the longstanding failure of such research to define useful boundaries among the pervasive developmental disorders (Happe et al. 2006) or, despite a substantial literature, to agree on how to classify patients with prominent symptoms of psychosis and mood disturbance points to deeper problems that are illuminated when family and genetic studies are taken into account (Craddock et al. 2005, 2006; Fanous et al. 2001; Laursen et al. 2005; Lichtenstein et al. 2009; Mahli et al. 2008). It may be that an effort to define a valid and clinically useful categorical disorder that corresponds to DSM-IV schizoaffective disorder cannot succeed. It may be that, only if we begin to think dimensionally, using clinical observation, clinical neuroscience, and genetics as our guide, will we begin to be able to classify such patients effectively (Hyman 2007). The anomalous findings that have emerged within the DSM "paradigm" will not be fixed by tinkering with sets of criteria or by adding or subtracting a few putative diagnoses at the margins. It is time to think deeply about the structure of the manual so that this structure does not impede movement toward a classification that will provide a better, even if imperfect, mirror of nature.

Problems Posed by Family and Genetic Studies

Far from providing the predicted validation of schizophrenia (or other disorders) as discrete categories (Robins and Guze 1970), findings of family and genetic studies have posed serious problems for a system that builds highly specified categories from phenomenological building blocks. In some (but not all) family studies of schizophrenia and bipolar disorder, salient symptoms have failed to co-segregate (Craddock et al. 2005, 2006). A single family may contain individuals with diverse psychiatric diagnoses, including schizophrenia, bipolar disorder, and intermediate conditions (Berrettini 2000; Cardno et al. 2002; Lichtenstein et al. 2009). In addition, shared genetic variants may contribute to risk of schizophrenia, bipolar disorder, and other conditions (Craddock et al. 2005; O'Donovan et al. 2008).

A DNA transposition initially associated with schizophrenia illustrates the complexity of psychiatric genetics. A large Scottish family was found to harbor a balanced translocation of a chromosomal segment that contained two genes on chromosome 1. Based on the phenotype of the proband, these genes were named Disrupted in Schizophrenia 1 and 2 (DISC1 and DISC2; Millar et al. 2000; St. Clair et al. 1990). DISC1 has emerged as a biologically interesting, well-studied positional candidate for risk of neuropsychiatric disorders (Mao et al. 2009). Even within the index Scottish family, however, the original translocation was found in individuals with different DSM-III diagnoses of schizophrenia, schizoaffective disorder, and recurrent major depression (St. Clair et al. 1990). In addition to the mutation found in the index family, DISC1 has been found to harbor multiple single-nucleotide polymorphisms in different families. DISC1 variants have been associated with schizophrenia, schizoaffective disorder, bipolar disorder, major depression, and both broad and narrow phenotypes of autism (Hennah et al. 2009).

These findings do not mean that cases of DSM-IV schizophrenia or bipolar disorder never breed true, or that Kraepelin's (1919/1971) distinction between dementia praecox (schizophrenia) and manic-depressive illness (bipolar disorder) is totally without merit (Fischer and Carpenter 2009). Instead, the findings may signify that schizophrenia and bipolar disorder, as we understand them clinically, might better be conceptualized as interactions among continuous dimensions—which might include psychosis, cognitive symptoms, mood disturbance, and perhaps negative or deficit symptoms—rather than as well-bounded categories.

Underlying the distinctly non-Mendelian patterns of familial segregation and the heterogeneity of even those psychiatric disorders most influenced by genes, such as autism, schizophrenia, and bipolar disorder, is the remarkable genetic complexity of common human illnesses. Robins and Guze (1970) developed their view of relatively simple categorical diagnoses at a time when this dizzying level of complexity was barely imagined.

At one extreme, genetic complexity can signify that the genetic components of risk for a disorder result from the interactions of genetic variants at multiple loci (which then interact with nongenetic factors). One version of this polygenic model, which posits that risks of common human illnesses arise from the infelicitous combinations of common genetic variants, is called the "common disease–common variant" hypothesis. The variants that contribute to common diseases are typically single nucleotide polymorphisms—that is, single-base changes in DNA sequence that are not individually harmful but produce risk through interaction with other variants. Individual common variants may not independently produce a phenotype (i.e., they have limited penetrance).

At the other extreme are diseases such as retinitis pigmentosa, in which each extended family member with the disorder has one rare mutation (of a large number of such mutations) that is transmitted in Mendelian fashion within that family (Pacione et al. 2003). Rare deleterious mutations produce harm by causing a loss of function, or a pathological gain of function, in a biologically significant RNA or protein. Such mutations are rare because they tend to cause reproductive disadvantage. These deleterious mutations, especially when they result from a deletion, duplication, or transposition affecting a large segment of DNA, are likely to be highly penetrant.

A large and accumulating body of data suggests that, like other common diseases such as type 2 diabetes mellitus (Zeggini et al. 2008), psychiatric disorders result from diverse combinations of genetic risk factors (Craddock et al. 2006; Freitag 2007; Happe et al. 2006) acting together with nongenetic factors, which may include environment, behavior, and chance (Hunter et al. 2008). No particular gene variant or locus may be necessary or sufficient to produce the common forms of these disorders. In the past few years evidence has emerged, most strongly for autism and schizophrenia, that significant genetic contributions to risk may depend both on common variants (Ferreira et al. 2008; O'Donovan et al. 2008) and on rare mutations (International Schizophrenia Consortium 2008; Morrow et al. 2008; T. Walsh et al. 2008; Weiss et al. 2008; Xu et al. 2008).

As our recognition of genetic complexity grows, with the data suggesting that heterogeneous combinations of large numbers of variants and mutations may be involved in at least some psychiatric disorders (Hyman 2008), the hope that genetic tests might play a significant role in diagnosis has begun to fade. An exception might be rarer forms of illness due to highly penetrant mutations. The importance of genetic discovery for common forms of illness, including psychiatric disorders, is more likely to lie in pointing toward pathophysiological mechanisms. Common genetic variants, discovered by methodologies such as genome-wide association, may each contribute relatively small increments of risk; nonetheless, "systems biology" approaches may be able to link apparently unrelated genetic findings to shared biological mechanisms. Certainly, the probability that risk genes will illuminate biology remains the main motivation for genetic studies. A significant result of these studies, for psychiatry, however, has been to undercut the hope of a "platonic ideal" for psychiatric disorders, represented by the Robins and Guze (1970) and DSM-III approaches (Kendler 2006). Put simply, the application of the five classic Robins and Guze validators will not converge on discrete, unitary categories.

What Is to Be Done?

The past decade has seen great progress in cognitive science, neuroscience, and genetics but only small, incremental steps in research that might positively influence the existing phenomenological criteria of DSM-IV and DSM-IV-TR. An important exception to the generally modest progress in this domain is the emerging consensus that schizophrenia is characterized by impairing cognitive deficits that map to the prefrontal cortex (Tan et al. 2006) and that deserve to be a focus of treatment development (Freedman et al. 2008). The lack of inclusion of this important symptom complex in DSM-III and DSM-IV was an error that slowed the development of therapeutics (Hyman and Fenton 2003). This example notwithstanding, the DSM revision process should be extremely conservative with respect to existing categorical disorders, because even small changes in wording could produce significant disruptions to epidemiology, clinical trials inclusion criteria, and laboratory research; such disruptions would militate against tinkering without very strong justification. A more important goal for DSM-5 is to make structural alterations that will facilitate discoveries that hasten the development of usefully valid diagnoses, new treatment approaches, and a sounder basis for clinical and translational research.

As I have previously written (Hyman 2007), a possible way forward would be to retain the categorical diagnoses for now but regroup them to facilitate diagnostic experiments, including the use of dimensions that might, in many cases, span multiple current disorders, or the reconceptualization of disorders hypothesized to be etiologically or pathophysiologically related into spectra that could be reanalyzed dimensionally or categorically based on emerging scientific data. The Spectra Study Group of the DSM-5 Task Force has elaborated a set of 11 "external validators" for the regrouping of disorders in DSM-5 (Table 1–1). These validators are meant to be used very differently from the five suggested by Robins and Guze (1970), even though there is overlap. The proposed validators are not meant to converge on categorical diagnoses but rather to be used as a checklist for deciding how to cluster now-separate disorders. The study group could not find strong enough justification for assigning specific weights to these validators and recognizes that some currently are "empty boxes" for many disorders. My view, however, is that some of the validators are potentially very strong justifications for clustering—for example, hypothesized pathophysiology (or shared neural circuitry), causal environmental factors, or shared genetic risk factors. Other validators, such as shared treatment response, are worth noting but have weak justifications for clustering. The study group also suggested that several possible clusters be examined for regrouping into spectra in DSM-5 (Table 1–2). The results of these analyses are not yet complete.

The construction of a larger grouping or spectrum, and its possible utility, can be illustrated with schizophrenia, related disorders, and subthreshold symptoms complexes in the family members of affected individuals. As should be clear from this discussion, based on the emerging genetics of schizophrenia, the category called schizophrenia in DSM-IV would be, at best, heuristic, even if it included appropriate recognition of cognitive symptoms. Even relatively classic presentations of schizophrenia differ among families in important respects, as would be expected from the genetic information available to date. This complexity will only grow as knowledge of genetics progresses and as environmental factors are better integrated into etiological models. Schizophrenia—like many general medical disorders such as type 2 diabetes, inflammatory bowel diseases, or hypertension—would seem not to represent a unitary disorder but a family of closely related symptom complexes with a

TABLE 1–1. External validators for clustering of disorders into putative spectra, proposed by the Spectra Study Group of the DSM-5 Task Force

Shared neural substrates (e.g., fear or reward circuitry)
Shared biomarkers
Shared temperamental antecedents
Shared cognitive and emotional process in abnormalities
Shared genetic risk factors
Familiality (e.g., disorders related to familial interactions)
Causal environmental risk factors
Symptom similarity (not as sole criterion)
High rates of comorbidity among disorders, as currently defined
Course of illness
Treatment response

shared pathophysiological mechanism. Based on family and genetic studies, schizophrenia is related to a variety of other disorders, some of which are confusingly classified separately from schizophrenia in DSM-IV and DSM-IV-TR.

As far back as the adoption studies of Kety et al. (1971), it was recognized that individuals with schizophrenia had blood relatives who did not have psychosis but did exhibit schizophrenia-like symptoms, including social isolation, suspiciousness, eccentric beliefs, and magical thinking. When such symptoms are chronic and impairing, a diagnosis of schizotypal personality disorder is warranted. Although a genetic relationship to schizophrenia has been confirmed (Fanous et al. 2001), this constellation of symptoms is classified as a personality disorder in DSM-IV. Such misplacement invites searches for superficial or spurious connections to other personality disorders rather than to a schizophrenia spectrum that might be characterized, inter alia, by the gray-matter thinning and cognitive deficits that have been demonstrated in relatives of individuals with schizophrenia (Brans et al. 2008; Cannon et al. 2002). Overall, the more DNA sequences a person shares with a person with schizophrenia, the greater the probability of structural prefrontal cortical deficits and cognitive impairments. Given the polygenic mode of inheritance of schizophrenia, it would seem likely that these quantitative differences in brain structure and function might reflect quantitative differences in genetic risk. Such analyses invite a dimensional approach to the diagnosis of schizophrenia and related disorders (Fanous et al. 2001; Tsuang et al. 2003) rather than a categorical approach. If, in addition to dimensions that measure psychosis, cognitive symptoms (or gray-matter deficits) and, possibly, deficit symptoms—a mood dimension—were to be added, it

TABLE 1–2. Possible candidate spectra proposed by the Spectra Study Group of the DSM-5 Task Force

SPECTRUM	COMPOSITION
Obsessive-compulsive disorder (OCD)	OCD plus tics and Tourette's disorder (putative disorders of striatal-thalamic-cortical circuitry)
Mood disorders	Mood disorders, including diverse presentations of depression and (perhaps) generalized anxiety disorder
Fear-based anxiety disorders	Disorders characterized by increased reactivity and slowed adaptation of amygdala circuitry
Schizophrenia	Schizophrenia plus cognitive and prefrontal structural abnormalities in otherwise unaffected family members; schizotypal personality disorder; nonaffective psychoses in schizophrenia families or those with characteristic gray matter loss, schizotypal disorder
Autism	Autism, including pervasive developmental disorder
Addictive disorders	Addiction and other disorders of reward circuitry and prefrontal inhibitory control, such as pathological gambling

might be possible to solve the problem of how to define schizoaffective disorder.

In a short essay such as this it is not possible to extend this analysis or to provide other examples (see, e.g., Table 1–2). It is important, however, to include important caveats. Elaboration of dimensions will be a challenging project that will involve constructing and testing quantitative scales, setting thresholds, and ideally, being able to apply some dimensions across clusters. For example, the same mood dimension would have to be applicable to both the schizophrenia spectrum and a bipolar spectrum, or else the problem of psychosis with prominent mood symptoms will not be solved. Clinical utility will be a fundamental issue that will undoubtedly present difficult challenges. In the end, a disease classification cannot sacrifice scientific validity, but if it is not useful to clinicians, it will not serve its major purpose in society.

In summary, the DSM-5 Task Force might usefully focus its attention on large groupings of disorders and engage in some diagnostic experiments of the sort I have sketched here. If DSM-5 becomes a living document, as it should be, perhaps with an editorial board structure to oversee its evolution, these diagnostic findings could be added, altered, or declared failures over time. While these experiments are undergoing thorough investigation, the corresponding categories could remain so that the world of clinical medicine continues to operate. None of this will be easy, but to remain prisoners of a highly specified, phenomenologically based categorical system would seem increasingly scientifically untenable. Genetics and neuroscience have not been kind to these categories, nor have these reified categories been kind to science. DSM-III was a brilliant advance; it is now time to move on.

References

American Psychiatric Association: Diagnostic and Statistical Manual: Mental Disorders. Washington, DC, American Psychiatric Association, 1952

American Psychiatric Association: Diagnostic and Statistical Manual of Mental Disorders, 2nd Edition. Washington, DC, American Psychiatric Association, 1968

American Psychiatric Association: Diagnostic and Statistical Manual of Mental Disorders, 3rd Edition. Washington, DC, American Psychiatric Association, 1980

American Psychiatric Association: Diagnostic and Statistical Manual of Mental Disorders, 4th Edition. Washington, DC, American Psychiatric Association, 1994

American Psychiatric Association: Diagnostic and Statistical Manual of Mental Disorders, 4th Edition, Text Revision. Washington, DC, American Psychiatric Association, 2000

Berrettini WH: Are schizophrenic and bipolar disorders related? A review of family and molecular studies. Biol Psychiatry 48:531–538, 2000

Brans RGH, van Haren NEM, van Baal GCM, et al: Heritability of changes in brain volume over time in twin pairs discordant for schizophrenia. Arch Gen Psychiatry 65:1259–1268, 2008

Cannon TD, Thompson PM, van Erp, et al: Cortex mapping reveals regionally specific patterns of genetic and disease-specific gray-matter deficits in twins discordant for schizophrenia. Proc Natl Acad Sci USA 99:3228–3233, 2002

Cardno AG, Rijsdijk FV, Sham PC, et al: A twin study of genetic relationships between psychotic symptoms. Am J Psychiatry 159:539–545, 2002

Cole J, McGuffin P, Farmer AE: The classification of depression: are we still confused? Br J Psychiatry 192:83–85, 2008

Craddock N, O'Donovan MC, Owen MJ: The genetics of schizophrenia and bipolar disorder: dissecting psychosis. J Med Genet 42:193–204, 2005

Craddock N, O'Donovan MC, Owen MJ: Genes for schizophrenia and bipolar disorder? Implications for psychiatric nosology. Schizophr Bull 32:9–16, 2006 de Bruin EI, Ferdinand RF, Meester S, et al: High rates of psychiatric co-morbidity in PDD-NOS. J Autism Dev Disord 37:877–886, 2007

Delgado MR, Nearing KI, LeDoux JE, et al: Neural circuitry underlying the regulation of conditioned fear and its relation to extinction. Neuron 59:829–838, 2008

Fairburn CG, Bohn K: Eating disorder NOS (EDNOS): an example of the troublesome "not otherwise specified" (NOS) category in DSM-IV. Behav Res Ther 43:691–701, 2005

Fanous A, Gardner C, Walsh D, et al: Relationship between positive and negative symptoms of schizophrenia and schizotypal symptoms in nonpsychotic relatives. Arch Gen Psychiatry 58:669–673, 2001

Feighner JP, Robins E, Guze SB, et al: Diagnostic criteria for use in psychiatric research. Arch Gen Psychiatry 26:57–63, 1972

Ferreira MAR, O'Donovan MC, Ment YA, et al: Collaborative genome-wide association analysis supports a role for ANK3 and CACNA1C in bipolar disorder. Nat Genet 40:1056–1058, 2008

Fischer BA, Carpenter WT Jr: Will the Kraepelinian dichotomy survive DSM-V? Neuropsychopharmacology 34:2081–2087, 2009

Freedman R, Olincy A, Buchanan RW, et al: Initial phase 2 trial of a nicotinic agonist in schizophrenia. Am J Psychiatry 165:1040–1047, 2008

Freitag CM: The genetics of autistic disorders and its clinical relevance: a review of the literature. Mol Psychiatry 12:2–22, 2007

Galanter CA, Leibenluft E: Frontiers between attention deficit hyperactivity disorder and bipolar disorder. Child Adolesc Psychiatr Clin North Am 17:325–346, viii–ix, 2008

Goldstein S, Schwebach AJ: The comorbidity of pervasive developmental disorder and attention deficit hyperactivity disorder: results of a retrospective chart review. J Autism Dev Disord 34:329–339, 2004

Happe F, Ronald A, Plomin R: Time to give up on a single explanation for autism. Nat Neurosci 10:1218–1220, 2006

Hennah W, Thompson P, McQuillin A, et al: DISC1 association, heterogeneity and interplay in schizophrenia and bipolar disorder. Mol Psychiatry 14:865–873, 2009

Hunter DJ, Altshuler D, Rader DJ: From Darwin's finches to canaries in the coal mine: mining the genome for new biology. N Engl J Med 358:2760–2763, 2008

Hyman SE: Can neuroscience be integrated into the DSM-V? Nat Rev Neurosci 8:725–732, 2007

Hyman SE: A glimmer of light for neuropsychiatric disorders. Nature 458:890–893, 2008

Hyman SE, Fenton WS: What are the right targets for psychopharmacology? Science 299:350–351, 2003

Hyman SE, Malenka RC, Nestler EJ: Neural mechanisms of addiction: the role of reward-related learning and memory. Annu Rev Neurosci 29:565–598, 2006

International Schizophrenia Consortium: Rare chromosomal deletions and duplications increase risk of schizophrenia. Nature 455:237–241, 2008

Kendler KS: Reflections on the relationship between psychiatric genetics and psychiatric nosology. Am J Psychiatry 163:1138–1146, 2006

Kendler KS, Gardner CO Jr: Boundaries of major depression: an evaluation of DSM-IV criteria. Am J Psychiatry 155:172–177, 1998

Kendler KS, Davis CG, Kessler RC: The familial aggregation of common psychiatric and substance use disorders in the National Comorbidity Survey: a family history study. Br J Psychiatry 170:541–548, 1997

Kessler RC, Berglund P, Demler O, et al: Lifetime prevalence and age-of-onset distributions of DSM-IV disorders in the National Comorbidity Survey Replication. Arch Gen Psychiatry 62:593–602, 2005a

Kessler RC, Chiu WT, Demler O, et al: Prevalence, severity, and comorbidity of 12-month DSM-IV disorders in the National Comorbidity Survey Replication. Arch Gen Psychiatry 62:617–627, 2005b

Kety SS, Rosenthal D, Wender PH, et al: Mental illness in the biological and adoptive families of adopted schizophrenics. Am J Psychiatry 128:302–306, 1971

Kraepelin E: Dementia Praecox and Paraphrenia (1919). New York, RE Krieger, 1971

Krueger RF, Markon KE: Reinterpreting comorbidity: a model-based approach to understanding and classifying psychopathology. Annu Rev Clin Psychol 2:111–113, 2006

Laursen TM, Labouriau R, Licht RW, et al: Family history of psychiatric illness as a risk factor for schizoaffective disorder: a Danish register-based cohort study. Arch Gen Psychiatry 62:841–848, 2005

Lichtenstein P, Yip BH, Bjork C, et al: Common genetic determinants of schizophrenia and bipolar disorder in Swedish nuclear families: a population-based study. Lancet 373:234–239, 2009

Malhi GS, Green M, Fagiolini A, et al: Schizoaffective disorder: diagnostic issues and future recommendations. Bipolar Disord 10:215–230, 2008

Mao Y, Ge X, Frank CL, et al: Disrupted in schizophrenia 1 regulates neuronal progenitor proliferation via modulation of GSK3beta/beta-catenin signaling. Cell 136:1017–1031, 2009

Matsunaga H, Maebayashi K, Hayashida K, et al: Symptoms structure in Japanese patients with obsessive-compulsive disorder. Am J Psychiatry 165:251–253, 2008

Mayberg HS, Lozano AM, Voon V, et al: Deep brain stimulation for treatment-resistant depression. Neuron 45:651–660, 2005

McGlashan TH, Grilo CM, Skodol AE, et al: The Collaborative Longitudinal Personality Disorders Study: baseline Axis I/II and II/II diagnostic co-occurrence. Acta Psychiatr Scand 102:256–264, 2000

Merikangas KR, Risch N: Genomic priorities and public health. Science 302:599–601, 2003

Millar JK, Wilson-Annan JC, Anderson S, et al: Disruption of two novel genes by a translocation co-segregating with schizophrenia. Hum Mol Genet 9:1415–1423, 2000

Morrow EM, Yoo S-Y, Flavell SW, et al: Identifying autism loci and genes by tracing recent shared ancestry. Science 321:218–223, 2008

O'Donovan MC, Craddock N, Norton N, et al: Identification of loci associated with schizophrenia by genome-wide association and follow-up. Nat Genet 40:1053–1055, 2008

Pacione LR, Szego MJ, Ikeda S, et al: Progress toward understanding the genetic and biochemical mechanisms of inherited photoreceptor degenerations. Annu Rev Neurosci 26:657–700, 2003

Regier DA, Farmer ME, Rae DS, et al: Comorbidity of mental disorders with alcohol and other drug abuse: results from the Epidemiologic Catchment Area (ECA) Study, JAMA 264:2511–2518, 1990

Robins E, Guze SB: Establishment of diagnostic validity in psychiatric illness: its application to schizophrenia. Am J Psychiatry 126:983–987, 1970

Spitzer RL, Endicott J, Robins E: Research diagnostic criteria. Psychopharmacol Bull 11:22–25, 1975

St. Clair D, Blackwood D, Muir W, et al: Association within a family of a balanced autosomal translocation with major mental illness. Lancet 336:13–16, 1990

Tan HY, Sust S, Buckholtz JW, et al: Dysfunctional prefrontal regional specialization and compensation in schizophrenia. Am J Psychiatry 163:1969–1977, 2006

Tsuang MT, Stone WS, Tarbox SI, et al: Insights from neuroscience for the concept of schizotaxia and the diagnosis of schizophrenia, in Advancing DSM: Dilemmas in Psychiatric Diagnosis. Edited by Phillips KA, First MB, Pincus HA. Arlington, VA, American Psychiatric Association, 2003, pp 105–128

Wakabayashi A, Baron-Cohen S, Uchiyama T, et al: Empathizing and systemizing in adults with and without autism spectrum conditions: cross-cultural stability. J Autism Dev Disord 37:1823–1832, 2007

Walsh CA, Morrow EM, Rubenstein JLR: Autism and brain development. Cell 135:396–400, 2008

Walsh T, McClellan JM, McCarthy SE, et al: Rare structural variants disrupt multiple genes in neurodevelopmental pathways in schizophrenia. Science 320:539–543, 2008

Weiss LA, Shen Y, Korn JM, et al: Association between microdeletion and microduplication at 16p11.2 and autism. N Engl J Med 358:667–675, 2008

World Health Organization: International Classification of Diseases, 9th Revision. Geneva, World Health Organization, 1977

World Health Organization: International Statistical Classification of Diseases and Related Health Problems, 10th Revision. Geneva, World Health Organization, 1992

Xu B, Roos JL, Levy S, et al: Strong association of de novo copy number mutations with sporadic schizophrenia. Nat Genet 40:880–885, 2008

Zeggini E, Scott LJ, Saxens T, et al: Meta-analysis of genome-wide association data and large-scale replication identifies additional susceptibility loci for type 2 diabetes. Nat Genet 40:638–645, 2008

CHAPTER 2

Integration of Dimensional Spectra for Depression and Anxiety Into Categorical Diagnoses for General Medical Practice

David Goldberg, D.M., F.R.C.P.
Leonard J. Simms, Ph.D.
Richard Gater, M.D.
Robert F. Krueger, Ph.D.

We have known for some time that in developed countries, the great majority of mental disorders are treated by general practitioners and hospital doctors rather than by specialist mental health services (Goldberg and Huxley 1980, 1992; Regier et al. 1978, 1993). In the developing world, this imbalance is even greater because there are markedly fewer mental health professionals available than in the developed world (World Health Organization 2005). However, despite the dominant role of general medical services in treating mental disorders throughout the world, the complex classificatory systems offered by both DSM-IV-TR (American Psychiatric Association 2000) and ICD-10 (World Health Organization 1992) are used only infrequently by these services; clinicians in hospitals and general practices appear to favor much less complex systems. The reason for this is that patients typically complain of untidy combinations of anxious, depressive, and somatic symptoms that are not always easy to assimilate into the complex conceptualizations of official classifications of mental disorders.

Problems With Categorical Diagnoses

A major problem with categorical diagnoses is the high rate of comorbidity observed among various common mental disorders, such as generalized anxiety disorder (GAD) and major depressive disorder (MDD). Internists and general practitioners appear to be reluctant to make multiple diagnoses when a patient with a given physical disorder is psychologically distressed. In terms of accepted classifications, comorbidity between these two diagnoses in community and primary care settings is substantial. Merikangas et al. (2003) reported that among Swiss community respondents in the Zurich cohort study, rates of comorbid anxiety and depression comfortably exceeded rates for either diagnosis alone and accounted for about two-thirds of such diagnoses each time the cohort was examined. In general medical settings, if one considers only current psychological symptoms, comorbidity between anxious and depressive symptoms is the rule, not the exception. Although both anxious and depressive symptoms can occur on their own, combinations of the two, often at subthreshold levels, are much more common.

In the National Comorbidity Survey, if the requirements for the duration of GAD were reduced from 6 months to 1 month, the prevalence of comorbidity between MDD and GAD rose by 42.8% (R.C. Kessler, personal communication, 2008). In the World Health Organization's study of mental illness in general health care, carried out in 11 countries (Üstün and Sartorious 1995), the effects of changing the duration required for GAD from 6 months to 1 month were dramatic, with the rate for comorbid GAD and MDD almost doubling (Table 2–1). The rate for "MDD only" fell because cases previously diagnosed as "MDD only" were transferred to the "comorbid" column. With the shorter duration, anxiety became the most common disorder, followed by comorbid anxiety and MDD, and the overall prevalence of these disorders increased by 4.3%. Hunt et al. (2002) found an even higher rate (44.9%) of comorbidity between GAD and "other affective disorders" in the Australian National Survey. Many authors have found substantial tetrachoric correlations between the diagnoses of MDD and GAD (Kendler et al. 2003; Krueger 1999; Slade and Watson 2006; Vollebergh et al. 2001).

Another problem with categorical diagnoses is that clinicians often use "not elsewhere classified" or "not otherwise specified" diagnoses—

TABLE 2–1.   Rates of anxiety and depressive disorders for 14 general-health care centers in 11 countries

REQUIRED DURATION OF GAD	DISORDER RATE (%)			
	GAD ONLY	MDD ONLY	COMORBID GAD–MDD	TOTAL
6 months	5.3	4.7	3.4	13.4
1 month	9.7	2.3	5.7	17.7

Note.   GAD=generalized anxiety disorder; MDD=major depressive disorder.
Source.   Üstün and Sartorius 1995.

instead of the definitions offered—perhaps because the clinician cannot remember the full list of symptoms required during a clinical interview, because the patient's idiosyncratic symptoms do not fit the exact rules specified by the nosology, or because the clinician has neglected to ask all the required questions. In any case, the system is not serving clinicians well. This is a consequence of the "shopping list" of symptoms offered by the DSM-IV (American Psychiatric Association 1994) system and would be eliminated if patients completed a simple dimensional scale that not only assessed all the symptoms but also estimated the severity of the disorder.

A third problem with categorical diagnoses is that they may lead to the clinician *ignoring sets of symptoms.* In MDD, the clinician is directed to pay attention to generalized anxiety symptoms only if they have lasted 6 months. In practice, a busy clinician in a general medical setting who is establishing a diagnosis of MDD may not even ask about anxiety symptoms. This may lead to a patient's anxieties about his or her current medical condition being ignored. In GAD, depressive symptoms are noted only if they exceed the number required for an MDD diagnosis, and in somatoform disorders, the symptoms of anxiety and depression may escape attention because they form no part of the diagnostic requirements.

Should Duration of Symptoms Be Measured?

The first problem in designing dimensional scales is deciding on the most appropriate symptom durations to be adopted. If the purpose of a scale is only to replicate current diagnostic practice, then anxious symptoms should have a much longer duration than depressive symptoms. Although it would be possible to build-in time durations for the various dimensions—for example, 2 weeks for MDD, 6 months for GAD, and so on—this would lose some of the advantages of a dimensional system, which should be responding to a patient's current symptoms, that is, symptoms within the past week or month. It would be up to the clinician using the dimensions to insert time durations afterwards. It is not in a patient's best interest if specified time durations lead—as they must in current diagnostic convention—to anxious symptoms of brief duration being ignored. It is the present contention that the diagnostic rules do not make sense in general medical settings. Anxiety of short duration is every bit as important as anxious symptoms of longer duration; indeed, it is often more so, because short-term anxiety is more likely to be related to a patient's presenting complaints.

Are There Advantages for a Patient in Discriminating Between Anxious and Depressive Symptoms?

The assessment of depressive symptoms is, of course, of prime importance in medical settings, because depressive symptoms will exacerbate pain, will cause greater disability, and above all may lead to suicide. This accounts for the numerous self-rated and clinician-rated depression scales that are widely used in general medical practice. Within a depressive dimension, different degrees of severity may attract different interventions. For example, a patient presenting with mild depression may warrant a combination of preventive advice and health information. However, with ascending degrees of severity, quite different interventions are appropriate, perhaps leading to inpatient hospitalization for the most severely depressed and suicidal patients (National Collaborating Centre for Mental Health 2004).

To some extent, anxious and depressive symptoms respond to the same interventions: the restoration of sleep, greater physical activity, various forms of psychological intervention, and of course medications, such as selective serotonin reuptake inhibitors, tricyclic antidepressants, and the newer antidepressants. However, if medication is to be given, the choice should be influenced by the intensity of anxious symptoms, because some medications are likely to exacerbate anxious symptoms in the short term.

Anxious symptoms on their own should attract different interventions than depressive symptoms. An inquiry about current sources of anxiety will quickly establish whether it is related to health anxiety, is related to a current life problem, or is longstanding and not getting any worse. Health anxiety often responds to accurate information and reassurance from the treating clinician, whereas anxiety related to other life problems may respond to problem solving from either the clinician or a counselor.

How Many Dimensions?

Factor analysis of diagnoses among community respondents in Holland revealed a three-dimensional symptom space consisting of a depressive or "distress" dimension, with diagnoses of MDD, dysthymic disorder, and GAD; a fear dimension, with diagnoses of phobias, posttraumatic stress disorder (PTSD), and panic disorder; and an externalizing dimension, with alcohol and drug dependence (Vollebergh et al. 2001). Slade and Watson (2006) reported broadly similar results for Australia, although in this study PTSD and neurasthenia loaded on the distress dimension, and obsessive-compulsive disorder loaded on the fear dimension. However, both these studies used a case-finding instrument (a version of the Composite International Diagnostic Interview [CIDI]) that did not include somatic symptoms, so somatization does not appear in the factor space.

Krueger et al. (2003) reported data from the Psychological Disorders in General Medical Care study, based on more than 5,000 CIDI-Primary Care interviews in 14 different countries, which did include somatic symptoms. Two three-dimensional models were fitted to the data. In the first of these models (three-factor A), symptom counts for depression, anxious worry, and anxious arousal loaded on the depression-anxiety factor, whereas somatization, hypochondriasis, and neurasthenia loaded on the somatization factor, and hazardous use of alcohol loaded on the alcohol-problems factor. The results for the second model (three-factor B) were the same, except that neurasthenia loaded on the depression-anxiety factor. These models were compared with a simple two-factor model that represented internalizing disorders on the one hand and alcohol problems on the other. In general, the two-factor model provided the best fit in 12 of the countries, although in the United States, the three-factor A produced the best fit, and in Germany the three-factor B provided the best fit. This solution merely reproduces the internalization-externalization higher-order distinction and reflects that fact that hazardous use of alcohol has an imperfect relation to emotional disorders. It will hardly suffice to reflect the different diagnoses that are common in this setting.

It can be seen that the addition of the somatic-symptoms parts of the CIDI (not used in previous studies) influenced the dimensional structure produced. Because somatic symptoms are one of the leading reasons that people across the world consult physicians, it is clearly important that such symptoms are taken into account.

At a finer-grained level, in general medical practice, analyses of factor patterns of psychological symptoms—if the research interview contains somatic symptoms (e.g., World Health Organization's Psychological Problems in General Health Care Survey)—are likely to find anxious and depressive symptoms on one dimension, fear symptoms on a second, and somatic symptoms on a third. However, there is no perfect factor invariance across countries, and there are arguments for distinguishing between anxious and depressive symptoms.

It would therefore appear, at first, as though a three-dimensional system (anxious depression, fear, and somatization disorders) would suit our purposes, with a fourth dimension of hazardous use of alcohol added in view of the medical importance of alcohol abuse. However, there is a problem in producing a single dimension for depressive and anxious symptoms, even though there are substantial correlations between the symptoms (Goldberg et al. 1987). Spitzer et al. (2006) confirmed that in primary care, comorbidity is substantial, but they argued that factor analysis confirmed the symptoms as distinct dimensions, with differing and independent effects on functional impairment and disability. However, it is notable that the "anxiety" dimension used in this work had GAD, social anxiety, PTSD, and panic disorder loading on it (Kroenke et al. 2007), so this dimension appears to be in some ways similar to the "fear" dimension reported earlier by Vollebergh et al. (2001) and Slade and Watson (2006). The Generalized Anxiety Disorder Scale–7 (Spitzer et al. 2006) is one of the better anxiety scales, but there are problems with supposing that a single scale can diagnose all the different anxiety disorders. Validity coefficients for the various anxiety disorders— GAD, social anxiety, PTSD, and panic disorder—were all high, with positive likelihood ratios for "any anxiety disorder" and GAD of 5.1– 5.5 and those for social anxiety disorder, PTSD, and panic disorder, 3.5–3.9. Three points are of interest:

1. No figures were given for phobias, so perhaps the dimension was not a fear dimension at all, but rather a dimension responding to the anxious component in the diagnoses mentioned.
2. The figures for the Generalized Anxiety Disorder Scale–2 were almost as good as those for the Generalized Anxiety Disorder Scale–7, so it is not clear that the longer version achieved very much (version 2 merely asks "Feeling nervous, anxious or on edge?" and "Not being able to stop or control worrying?").
3. The scale does not allow judgment to be made between the various anxiety disorders.

Zimmerman and Chelminski (2006) developed a set of 13 self-report scales that produces Axis I categories for psychiatric outpatient settings, but the various scales do not appear to be empirically derived and, in any case, are not designed for general medical clinics.

If the various somatoform disorders so common in general medical settings are to be taken into account, we are left with at least three symptom dimensions: depressive symptoms, fear and anxiety symptoms, and somatic symptoms. To these, it would appear sensible to add an alcohol dimension, not only because alcohol use is of great medical importance but also because this addition would permit easy conversion to a linear scale.

A First Way of Proceeding

One could produce dimensional scales simply by including the criteria in any revised diagnostic guidelines. This undoubtedly would allow ready translation from dimension to category (and is what some existing scales have done) and would achieve an excellent relationship with categorical diagnoses (e.g., consider the Patient Health Questionnaire-9 and Generalized Anxiety Disorder Scale–7). In a sense, this approach is bound to succeed, because it is essentially tautological. However, this approach would mean that the scale would consist largely of symptoms on the threshold of caseness rather than of a mix of mild, moderate, and severe symptoms. Thus, an increasing score on such a dimensional scale would indicate an increasing probability that the individual was indeed a "case," but it would not be a reliable indicator of the severity of disorder, nor would it indicate which anxiety disorder was present.

A Second Way of Proceeding

An alternative approach would be to derive dimensions from big data sets that have been collected from patients treated in general medical settings and fit these dimensions to modern latent-variable models. Such analyses would permit items to be selected that represent relatively homogeneous and distinctive symptom groups. Moreover, latent modeling approaches would facilitate selection of items that both discriminate well (i.e., have good slopes and factor loadings) and offer a range of severity thresholds. This approach would stand a better chance of identifying individuals with severe anxious and depressive symptoms (rather than just providing an increasing degree of likelihood that a given individual does indeed qualify for a categorical diagnosis).

Although the prominent measures of anxious and depressive symptoms (e.g., structured interviews and the Beck and Hamilton scales) largely have served the field well, these measures were developed without benefit of modern psychometric models, and this has resulted in a number of psychometric problems—most notably, heterogeneity of item content that fails to reflect the structural work over the past several decades (e.g., Brown et al. 1998; Clark and Watson 1991; Krueger and Finger 2001; Mineka et al. 1998; Simms et al. 2008). As described earlier, much factor analytic work has suggested more optimal ways of defining internalizing and externalizing symptomatology, and latent modeling approaches have proven to be well suited to exploiting the results of structural studies to facilitate development of modern measurement tools for clinical and research settings.

Item response theory (IRT; see, e.g., Embretson and Reise 2000; Hambleton and Swaminathan 1985; Lord 1980) refers to a broad range of latent-trait models that characterize psychological test items by one or more item parameters. IRT methods offer several advantages over classical test development methods, which have been used to develop most psychopathology measures to date. Relevant to our purposes here, the most notable advantage of IRT is its ability to describe the points along a symptom dimension, where measurement is most and least precise.

A complete account of IRT is well beyond the scope of this chapter; interested readers should see Embretson and Reise (2000), which is a reasonably accessible volume devoted to the theory and use of IRT. A variety of models have been proposed to represent both dichotomous (e.g., present vs. absent) and polytomous (e.g., ordinal scales of severity or frequency) response data. Of these, a two-parameter model, with parameters for *item threshold/severity* and *item discrimination,* has been applied most consistently to psychopathology measures. These item parameters can be combined to form an *item information curve* that specifies where along a given symptom dimension an item provides the greatest measurement precision. In general, the item threshold/severity determines the horizontal location of the curve's peak, whereas item discrimination influences the relative height of the peak compared with other items on the scale. Individual item information curves then can be summed to form a *test information curve* that provides an overall index of measurement precision for a given scale.

In Figure 2–1 we present four-item information curves as well as the test information curve, which represents the sum of the item curves. These curves depict the IRT characteristics of four hypothetical items, which vary in both threshold/severity and discrimination. Of these items, number 3 is the most discriminating item (as evidenced by the height of its peak), whereas number 4 reflects lower precision but has the highest threshold/severity of all items (because its peak is the furthest right along the severity dimension). Taken together, these items give rise to a test information curve that is moderately peaked and centered around zero on the severity dimension (which is on a z-score metric). Notably, the information value of these hypothetical items drops off quickly for individuals who are more than a standard deviation below or above the population mean for this dimension, which may not be ideal in clinical settings, where we wish to identify, with reasonable precision, those who are showing high levels of symptoms. Unfortunately, however, test information curves like the one in Figure 2–1 are the rule rather than the exception with most classically developed psychopathology measures.

So how is one to use IRT techniques to develop modern measures of the symptom dimensions as described? Development of measures, regardless of whether IRT methods are used, should proceed through a series of theory-informed steps, which have been described well elsewhere (Clark and Watson 1995; Loevinger 1957; Simms and Watson 2007). In some cases, items in existing measures and data sets could be used to form the basis for a structural model and measure of psychopathology. Indeed, this kind of study has formed the basis for much of the empirical evidence described here. However, ideal scales typically are built from scratch using the extant literature as a guide for development of a sufficiently large and broad item pool to tap all potentially relevant aspects of the diagnostic constructs to be measured.

Briefly, the empirical and theoretical underpinnings of dimensions to be measured, including operational definitions for each, must be fully explicated. Next, an overinclusive pool of items must be developed by teams of experts to tap all relevant aspects of the dimensions. Third, responses to the initial item pool must be collected in a sample that both broadly represents the type of sample in which the measure is designed to be useful later and is large enough to support structural analyses. Fourth, item responses must be subjected to classical and modern structural analyses, including common factor analyses and IRT methods, to confirm the dimensionality of the item pool. Traditional factor analyses can be used to ensure that items form homogeneous factors meaningfully differentiable from one another. IRT methods then would be useful to identify strongly discriminating items that vary along all severity levels among which one wishes to discriminate later. To that end, item and test information curves would be useful tools for making such decisions about the relative worth of candidate test items.

Interestingly, structural analyses might reveal problems in the item pool that require remediation (e.g., dimensions with too few strong markers or perhaps severity levels of the dimensions that re-

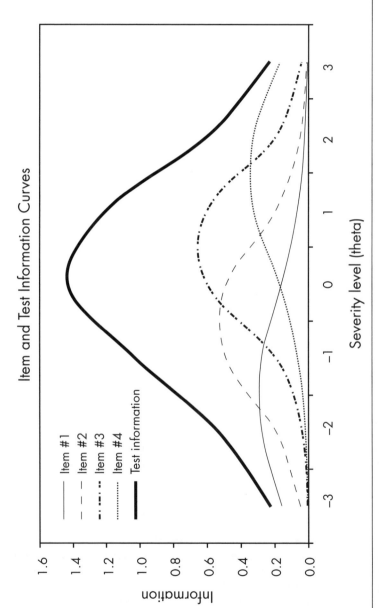

FIGURE 2–1.   Hypothetical item and test information curves.

quire additional items). Thus, the measure development process is likely to be iterative, with multiple rounds of item writing, data collection, and structural analyses as needed.

A possible factor pattern that might emerge from such a structural analysis of patients who consult physicians in general medical settings is shown in Figure 2–2. However, if these dimensions are to be useful in applied clinical settings, it may be necessary to combine them, to some extent, to form dimensions that more closely conform to existing nosological constructs. For example, structural depression research has suggested that anxious misery (i.e., negative affect) and anhedonia (i.e., low positive affect) combine to form the depressive phenotype (e.g., Clark and Watson 1991; Mineka et al. 1998). Thus, clinicians who wish to measure "depression," as a whole, rather than its constituent parts will need a method for doing so, regardless of what our fine-grained structural analyses suggest. Similarly, disorders such as panic disorder might be conceptualized as composites of anxious misery plus anxious arousal plus, in cases of agoraphobia, behavioral avoidance.

To handle such dimensional complexity, we are likely to have to adopt a more sophisticated IRT model for our analyses. Traditional IRT models assume that the dimensions under study are unidimensional, a condition that previous research indicates we are unlikely to find (Goldberg et al. 1987; Ormel et al. 1995). However, a number of multidimensional IRT models have been proposed and applied in recent years to handle complexity such as this. One model in particular, the *bifactor model* (Gibbons and Hedeker 1992; Gibbons et al. 2007), is attractive for application of IRT in psychopathology measurement research. In short, the bifactor model permits variables to load both on a general common factor and on one of several specific factors, thus allowing a direct fit of a hierarchical model in which a strong underlying dimension (e.g., depression) is marked by symptoms of varying levels of specificity (e.g., depressed affect, suicidality, anhedonia). A generic example of a bifactor structural model is presented in Figure 2–3.

Using such a model, we could readily apply all the benefits of IRT parameterization described earlier to the general factor while still accounting for the specific dimensions identified by our more-refined structural models. Simms and Watson (2007) presented an example of this method as applied to measurement of depression and anxiety in patient, community, and emerging-adult samples. In short, results of this study highlighted a strong general factor that corresponded to general distress or demoralization and was composed of a number of more specific factors (e.g., dysphoria, irritability, anxiety, low positive affect, suicidality) that varied considerably in the magnitudes of their relations to the underlying distress factor. In the present context, these results provide a foundation on which to build complex, ecologically valid models and measures of internalizing symptomatology.

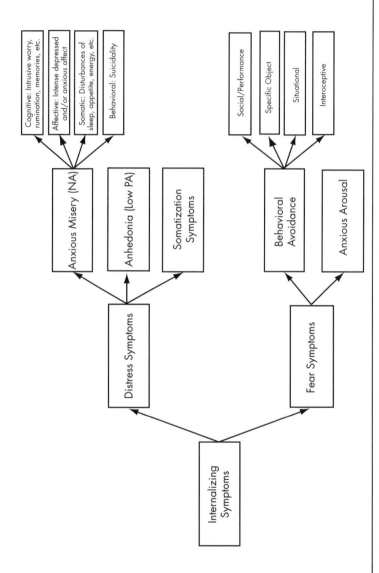

FIGURE 2–2.   Possible factor pattern of internalizing symptoms in general medical settings.

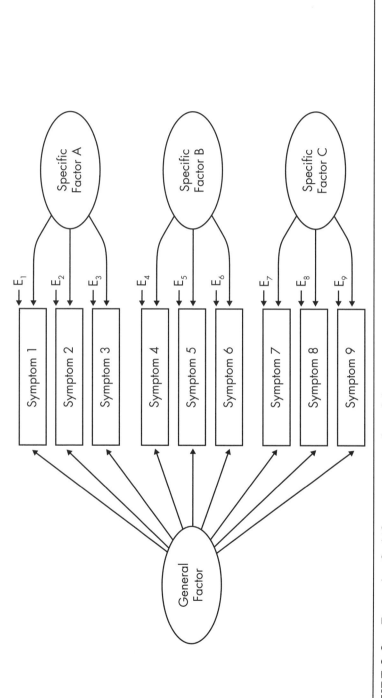

FIGURE 2–3. Example of a bifactor structural model.

Although this process can be time consuming and costly, such procedures will result in measures that cleanly tap a set of theoretically and empirically supported psychopathology dimensions. Moreover, IRT methods are useful for identifying biased items that function differently across certain subgroups of interest, such as groups that differ in gender, ethnicity, or diagnostic group (e.g., Santor and Coyne 2001; Santor et al. 1994). Finally, IRT has shown great promise as a basis for efficient computerized adaptive measures that result in equivalent clinical information while using only a fraction of the items of a traditional paper-and-pencil measure (e.g., Simms and Clark 2005).

Advantages and Limitations of Dimensions

Advantages

There would be several advantages of using dimensions in clinical practice. Dimensions would allow a severity measure of disturbance on a particular symptoms measure to be obtained and would permit thresholds on the dimension, where the benefits of an intervention exceed the soft (nonmonetary) costs, to be computed. Dimensions also could permit a range of different interventions to be placed on the dimension. Multiple dimensions could provide a more complete picture of a patient's symptoms.

Limitations and Drawbacks

It would be a mistake to suppose that a given set of dimensions ever would be adequate to encompass the full diversity of symptoms possible or even the dimensions that might be of relevance to a particular specialist clinic. Thus, one can postulate eating disorders as being dimensional, yet it would be absurd to impose their routine measurement on every medical clinic. Next, it may be difficult to extract categorical equivalents from some dimensions—for example, fear disorders—for which the various categorical disorders permit no easy transformation into a single, linear dimension. Fortunately, the general medical implications of phobic disorders are much less than those of anxious, depressive, or somatic symptoms. Obsessional disorders would be another example for which one would not expect the dimensions that have been considered thus far to provide diagnostic thresholds.

Uses of Dimensions

Categorical diagnoses tend to ignore symptoms that are not part of the definition of the diagnostic entity: thus major depressive disorder, generalized anxiety disorder, and somatoform disorders are all single-dimension disorders, yet the patient may have problems on other dimensions as well. With dimensional diagnoses, if each symptom has a fourfold frequency response scale, the clinician would have valuable information about severity and could use arbitrary cut points to decide on interventions. Furthermore, use of the somatic symptoms scale would cover a basic range of common symptoms otherwise dealt with in a systems review. For survey research in particular clinics or in specified physical disorders, dimensions would allow a much richer collection of data than would use of single, binomial, diagnostic categories.

References

American Psychiatric Association: Diagnostic and Statistical Manual of Mental Disorders, 4th Edition. Washington, DC, American Psychiatric Association, 1994

American Psychiatric Association: Diagnostic and Statistical Manual of Mental Disorders, 4th Edition, Text Revision. Washington, DC, American Psychiatric Association, 2000

Brown TA, Chorpita BF, Barlow DH: Structural relationships among dimensions of the DSM-IV anxiety and mood disorders and dimensions of negative affect, positive affect, and autonomic arousal. J Abnorm Psychol 107:179–192, 1998

Clark LA, Watson D: Tripartite model of anxiety and depression: psychometric evidence and taxonomic implications. J Abnorm Psychol 100:316–336, 1991

Clark LA, Watson D: Constructing validity: basic issues in scale development. Psychol Assess 7:309–319, 1995

Embretson SE, Reise SP: Item Response Theory for Psychologists. Mahwah, NJ, Erlbaum, 2000

Gibbons RD, Hedeker D: Full-information item bi-factor analysis. Psychometrika 57:423–436, 1992

Gibbons RD, Bock RD, Hedeker D, et al: Full-information item bifactor analysis of graded response data. Appl Psychol Meas 31:4–19, 2007

Goldberg D, Huxley P: Mental Illness in the Community: The Pathway to Psychiatric Care. London, Tavistock, 1980

Goldberg D, Huxley P: Common Mental Disorders: A Bio-Social Model. London, Tavistock, 1992

Goldberg DP, Bridges K, Duncan-Jones P, et al: Dimensions of neuroses seen in primary care settings. Psychol Med 17:461–470, 1987

Hambleton RK, Swaminathan H: Item Response Theory: Principles and Applications. Amsterdam, Kluwer Nijhoff, 1985

Hunt C, Issikadis C, Andrews G: DSM-4 generalised anxiety disorder in the Australian National Survey of Mental Health and Well-Being. Psychol Med 32:649–659, 2002

Kendler KS, Prescott CA, Myers J, et al: The structure of genetic and environmental risk factors for common psychiatric and substance use disorders in men and women. Arch Gen Psychiatry 60:929–937, 2003

Kroenke K, Spitzer RL, Williams JB, et al: Anxiety disorders in primary care: prevalence, impairment, comorbidity, and detection. Arch Intern Med 146:317–325, 2007

Krueger RF: The structure of common mental disorders. Arch Gen Psychiatry 56:921–926, 1999

Krueger RF, Finger MS: Using item response theory to understand comorbidity among anxiety and unipolar mood disorders. Psychol Assess 13:140–151, 2001

Krueger RF, Chentsova-Dutton YU, Markon KE, et al: A cross-cultural study of the structure of comorbidity among common psychopathological syndromes in the general health care setting. J Abnorm Psychol 112:437–447, 2003

Loevinger J: Objective tests as instruments of psychological theory. Psychol Rep 3:635–694, 1957

Lord FM: Applications of Item Response Theory to Practical Testing Problems. Hillsdale, NJ, Erlbaum, 1980

Merikangas KR, Zhang H, Avenevoli S, et al: Longitudinal trajectories of depression and anxiety in a prospective community study: the Zurich Cohort Study. Arch Gen Psychiatry 60:993–1000, 2003

Mineka S, Watson D, Clark LA: Comorbidity of anxiety and unipolar mood disorders. Annu Rev Psychol 49:377–412, 1998

National Collaborating Centre for Mental Health: Depression: Management of Depression in Primary and Secondary Care. London, England, RC Psych Publications, 2004. Available at: http://www.nice.org.uk/pdf/word/CG023. Accessed June 10, 2009.

Ormel J, Oldehinkel AJ, Goldberg DP, et al: How many dimensions of neurosis? Psychol Med 25:520–521, 1995

Regier DA, Goldberg ID, Taube CA, et al: The de facto US mental health services system: a public health perspective. Arch Gen Psychiatry 35:685–693, 1978

Regier DA, Narrow WE, Rae DS, et al: The de facto US mental and addictive disorders service system: epidemiologic catchment area prospective 1-year prevalence rates of disorders and services. Arch Gen Psychiatry 50:85–94, 1993

Santor DA, Coyne JC: Evaluating the continuity of symptomatology between depressed and nondepressed individuals. J Abnorm Psychol 110:216–225, 2001

Santor DA, Ramsay JO, Zurhoff DC: Nonparametric item analyses of the Beck Depression Inventory: evaluating gender item bias and response option weights. Psychol Assess 6:255–270, 1994

Simms LJ, Clark LA: Validation of a computerized adaptive version of the Schedule for Nonadaptive and Adaptive Personality (SNAP). Psychol Assess 17:28–43, 2005

Simms LJ, Watson D: The construct validation approach to personality scale construction, in Handbook of Research Methods in Personality Psychology. Edited by Robins RW, Fraley RC, Krueger RF. New York, Guilford, 2007, pp 240–258

Simms LJ, Grös DF, Watson D, et al: Parsing the general and specific components of depression and anxiety with bifactor modeling. Depress Anxiety 25:E34–E46, 2008

Slade T, Watson D: The structure of common DSM-IV and ICD-10 mental disorders in the Australian general population. Psychol Med 36:1593–1600, 2006

Spitzer RL, Kroenke K, Williams JB, et al: A brief measure for assessing generalized anxiety disorder: the GAD-7. Arch Intern Med 166:1092–1097, 2006

Üstün TB, Sartorius N: Mental Illness in General Health Care: An International Study. New York, Wiley, 1995

Vollebergh WA, Iedema J, Bijl RV, et al: The structure and stability of common mental disorders: the NEMESIS study. Arch Gen Psychiatry 58:597–603, 2001

World Health Organization: International Statistical Classification of Diseases and Related Health Problems, 10th Revision. Geneva, World Health Organization, 1992

World Health Organization: Mental Health Atlas 2005: Revised Edition. Geneva, Switzerland, World Health Organization, 2005. Available at: http://www.who.int/mental_health/evidence/atlas. Accessed June 9, 2009.

Zimmerman M, Chelminski I: A scale to screen for DSM-IV Axis 1 disorders in psychiatric out-patients: performance of the Psychiatric Diagnostic Screening Questionnaire. Psychol Med 36:1601–1612, 2006

CHAPTER 3

One Way Forward for Psychiatric Nomenclature

The Example of the Spectrum Project Approach

Ellen Frank, Ph.D.
Paola Rucci, Dr.Stat.
Giovanni B. Cassano, M.D.

The nosology embodied in DSM-IV (American Psychiatric Association 1994) and DSM-IV-TR (American Psychiatric Association 2000) represented a significant advance in diagnostic classification, especially when compared with DSM-II (American Psychiatric Association 1968); however, nosology in DSM-III (American Psychiatric

Portions of this chapter have been adapted from these reports: Fagiolini A, Frank E, Rucci P, et al.: "Mood and Anxiety Spectrum as a Means to Identify Clinically Relevant Subtypes of Bipolar I Disorder." *Bipolar Disorder* 9:462–467, 2007; Cassano GB, Mula M, Rucci P, et al.: "The Structure of Lifetime Manic-Hypomanic Spectrum." *Journal of Affective Disorders* 112:59–70, 2009; Cassano GB, Benvenuti A, Miniati M, et al.: "The Factor Structure of Lifetime Depressive Spectrum in Patients With Unipolar Depression." *Journal of Affective Disorders* 115:87–99, 2009.

Association 1980), as well as DSM-III-R (American Psychiatric Association 1987) and later editions, was based primarily on reliable clinical descriptions. Furthermore, because it had been determined that decisions needed to be either categorical or dimensional, the DSM approach did not allow any dimensional constructs within the classifications. One unintended consequence of this strictly categorical approach has been the high level of psychiatric comorbidity in patients presenting for treatment. Furthermore, our current diagnostic system frequently conflates symptom intensity, symptom duration, impairment, and distress under the general rubric of severity. Across diagnoses, we see marked inconsistencies in the numbers of concepts involved in the definition of a syndrome, with consequent differences in the determination of remission. Not surprisingly, there is often a failure of convergence of clinical and epidemiological data on prevalence and risk factors. Finally, and perhaps most important, our current diagnostic system is not well suited for the incorporation of new knowledge, especially with respect to validating criteria, such as genetic and other biological markers.

Since the 1990s, these problems have become more apparent, and some investigators have attempted to address them in various ways. Although there are no easy solutions that cross all diagnoses, the adoption of dimensional measures, to be used in concert with a categorical diagnostic system, may provide new strategies—within disorders and across groups of related disorders—and may help to address several of the problems outlined here. One major effort to resolve these problems has been the Spectrum Project, a collaboration between investigators in Italy and investigators in the United States. The concepts and methods developed by the Spectrum Project (www.spectrum-project.org), led by Giovanni B. Cassano of the University of Pisa, Italy, may provide a way forward for the next revision of DSM, DSM-5. In this chapter, we describe these concepts and methods, and then, using the mood spectrum as an example, we describe the specific advantages of the Spectrum Project approach.

Spectrum Project Approach

According to the conceptualization of the Spectrum Project, diagnostic criteria for DSM-IV-TR Axis I and ICD-10 (World Health Organization 1992) fail to describe fully the range of clinical features associated with the defined disorders. Clinical observations and myriad descriptive studies tell us that patients actually manifest a wide range of features that encompass variations in temperament and behavioral traits.

In order to develop a research agenda based on his initial observations (Cassano and Savino 1993), Dr. Cassano established the Spectrum Advisory Committee in 1995. The scientific collaborators he convened included the authors of this chapter and other researchers from the Universities of Pisa, Pittsburgh, and California at San Diego and Columbia University. This group sought to turn the clinical observations into measurable constructs replicable across populations. We began by developing measures that used the structured clinical interview format. When we were satisfied that the interviews performed well, we examined the feasibility of more efficient self-report methods.

The Spectrum Project conceptualizes psychopathology as occurring on a continuum with normality and provides a continuous or dimensional approach to measurement within the traditional DSM-IV categories of mood, anxiety, psychotic, eating, and substance use disorders. This approach considers both lifetime and recent experiences of symptoms, behavioral tendencies, and temperamental traits related to each of these categories, independent of the degree to which they cluster in time (Figure 3–1).

Not surprisingly, the spectrum model is characterized by a broader conceptualization of psychopathology and an integrated view of the currently accepted unipolar–bipolar dichotomy. Comorbidities may occur, either as full-blown disorders or as softer "spectrum" conditions. Attempting to address the fact that disorders rarely appear in the pure and seemingly isolated prototypes described in DSM-IV, the model incorporates both common symptoms, generally omitted from the psychiatric diagnostic criteria, and a more flexible method of clustering symptoms.

The Spectrum Project has developed assessments in formats that cover the respondent's lifetime or only the previous month. The lifetime measures also consider early precursors or prodromes, and both the lifetime and the last-month versions allow for the assessment of residual symptoms. Perhaps most important, the Spectrum Project conceptual framework allows for a more rational approach to the question of comorbidity through its capacity to determine the level of relatedness among disorders and/or subsyndromal representations thereof. This in turn allows for a more meaningful examination of connections to specific biological factors as well as developmental, gender, and cross-cultural differences.

Each spectrum measure is organized into relevant domains:

- *Mood spectrum domain:* includes mood-manic, mood-depressive, energy-manic, energy-depressive, cognition-manic, cognition-depressive, and rhythmicity.
- *Panic-agoraphobic spectrum domain:* includes typical panic, atypical panic, anxious expectation, typical agoraphobia, other phobias, reassurance sensitivity, substance sensitivity, stress sensitivity, and separation sensitivity.

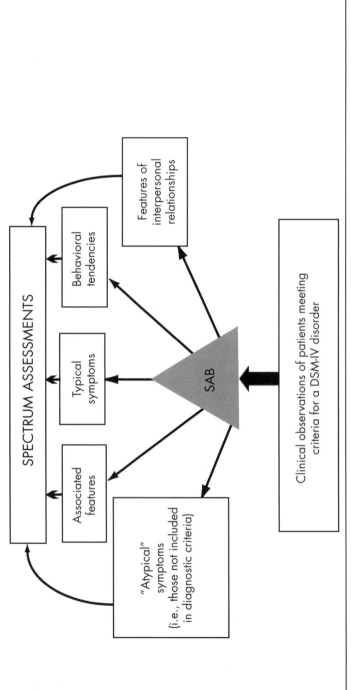

FIGURE 3–1.   Sources for spectrum assessments.

Note.   SAB=Spectrum Advisory Board.

- *Substance use spectrum domain:* includes substance use and improper use of drugs, sensitivity to drugs and substances, use of substances or drugs for self-medication, sensation seeking, attention deficit, and typical symptoms of substance abuse disorder.
- *Psychotic spectrum domain:* includes interpersonal sensitivity, paranoid, schizoid, misperceptions, and typical psychotic symptoms.
- *Anorexia-bulimia spectrum:* subdivided into attitudes and beliefs, weight history, self-esteem and satisfaction, phobias, avoidant and compulsive behaviors, weight maintenance, eating dyscontrol, associated features and consequences, and impairment and insight.
- *Obsessive-compulsive spectrum domain:* includes doubt, hypercontrol, attitude toward time, perfectionism, repetition and automation, and obsessive-compulsive themes.
- *Social anxiety spectrum domain:* includes social phobic traits during childhood and adolescence, interpersonal sensitivity, behavioral inhibition and somatic symptoms, and specific anxieties/phobic features.

Spectrum Measures: Reliability, Validity, and Clinical Utility

Summaries of reliability and validation studies of the spectrum assessment measures are shown in Table 3–1, and the full text of the studies cited is available at www.spectrum-project.org. These studies demonstrate the extent to which the individual spectra represent distinct psychopathological dimensions, the relationships between spectrum features and Axis II disorders, and the relationships of spectrum features to functional impairment. As shown in Table 3–1, reliability and validity varied moderately across the domains of each of the scales; however, all findings were generally in the acceptable-to-excellent range.

The spectrum measures have already demonstrated substantial clinical utility. For example, studies of the relation of lifetime panic spectrum to treatment outcome in trials of mood disorder, funded by the National Institute of Mental Health, show panic-spectrum features to be an otherwise hidden but important correlate of poor outcome of treatment (Frank et al. 2000a, 2000b). In a study involving a sequenced approach to treatment, among 61 patients with recurrent unipolar depression (Frank et al. 2000b), only 18% met criteria for lifetime panic disorder, while 38% exceeded a receiver operating characteristic (ROC) curve–defined threshold score of 35 on the lifetime Panic-Agoraphobic Spectrum Self-Report. Participants who scored above this threshold were significantly less likely to respond to interpersonal psychotherapy (IPT) monotherapy ($P < 0.05$). Furthermore, when the full acute treatment sequence (IPT followed by

TABLE 3–1. Reliability and validation studies for the spectrum approach

INSTRUMENT	SOURCE	POPULATION	RELIABILITY	VALIDITY
Structured Clinical Interview for Panic-Agoraphobia Spectrum (SCI-PAS)	Cassano et al. 1999; Shear et al. 2001	141 panic disorder patients 140 cardiovascular disease patients 141 healthy control subjects	Test-retest and interrater reliability ranges: 0.46–0.94 Internal consistency range: 0.75–0.89	*Convergent validity of domains:* Panic-like symptom domain and Beck Anxiety Inventory, $r=0.74$, $P<0.01$ Anxious expectation domain and Anxiety Sensitivity Index, $r=0.75$, $P<0.01$ Typical agoraphobia domain and Fear Questionnaire, $r=0.67$, $P<0.01$ Total SCI-PAS score and Panic Disorder Severity Scale, $r=0.70$, $P<0.01$ Separation sensitivity domain and Adult Separation Anxiety Disorder Scale, $r=0.75$, $P<0.01$ Separation sensitivity domain and Separation Anxiety Symptom Inventory, $r=0.74$, $P<0.01$

TABLE 3–1. Reliability and validation studies for the spectrum approach *(continued)*

INSTRUMENT	SOURCE	POPULATION	RELIABILITY	VALIDITY
Structured Clinical Interview for Substance Use Spectrum (SCI-SUBS)	Sbrana et al. 2003	67 patients with DSM-IV-TR disorders with or without substance use disorder comorbidity 33 control subjects	Internal consistency range: 0.64–0.93	*Discriminant validity:* Domain scores of substance use disorder patients were significantly higher than those of control subjects and patients without substance use disorder (P<0.05)
Structured Clinical Interview for Psychotic Spectrum (SCI-PSY)	Sbrana et al. 2005	351 patients with DSM-IV disorders with or without psychosis 102 control subjects	Internal consistency range: 0.77–0.94	*Discriminant validity:* All diagnostic groups had significantly greater (P<0.01) total SCI-PSY scores than those of control subjects
Structured Clinical Interview for Anorexic-Bulimic Spectrum (SCI-ABS)	Mauri et al. 2006	55 patients with eating disorders 118 students 114 gym attendees 58 obstetric/gynecology patients	Test-retest and interrater reliability ranges: 0.84–0.99 Internal consistency range: 0.41–0.93	*Convergent validity:* Range of correlations with Eating Attitude Test: 0.46–0.77 Range of correlations with Eating Disorder Inventory: –0.01–0.50 *Discriminant validity:* All domain scores significantly (P<0.01) discriminated eating disorder patients from all control groups

TABLE 3–1. Reliability and validation studies for the spectrum approach *(continued)*

INSTRUMENT	SOURCE	POPULATION	RELIABILITY	VALIDITY
Structured Clinical Interview for Obsessive-Compulsive Spectrum (SCI-OBS)	Dell'Osso et al. 2000	135 patients with psychiatric diagnoses, including obsessive-compulsive disorder (OCD) 119 control subjects	Test-retest and interrater reliability ranges: 0.94–0.98 Internal consistency range: 0.61–0.93	*Convergent validity:* Range of correlations with Checklist for Obsessions and Compulsions, current symptoms: 0.49–0.70 Range of correlations with Checklist for Obsessions and Compulsions, lifetime symptoms: 0.48–0.71 Range of correlations with the Yale-Brown Obsessive Compulsive Scale: 0.30–0.54
Structured Clinical Interview for Social Phobia (SCI-SHY)	Dell'Osso et al. 2000	50 patients with social phobia 50 patients with OCD 35 patients with major depressive disorder 119 control subjects	Test-retest range: 0.97–0.99 Internal consistency range: 0.87–0.94	*Convergent validity:* Range of correlations with Liebowitz Social Anxiety Scale: 0.48–0.83 *Discriminant validity:* All domain scores significantly (*P*<0.01) discriminated social phobia patients from other psychiatric patients and control subjects

TABLE 3–1. Reliability and validation studies for the spectrum approach *(continued)*

INSTRUMENT	SOURCE	POPULATION	RELIABILITY	VALIDITY
Structured Clinical Interview for Mood Spectrum (SCI-MOODS)	Fagiolini et al. 1999	112 patients with bipolar disorder 122 patients with recurrent unipolar depression 141 students 116 patients with gastrointestinal disorders	Test-retest range: 0.93–0.94 Internal consistency range: 0.79–0.92	*Discriminant validity:* All domain and subdomain scores of patients with mood disorders were significantly greater ($P<0.01$) than for control subjects Manic subdomain scores were significantly greater ($P<0.01$) in patients with bipolar disorder, compared with patients with recurrent unipolar depression

IPT plus selective serotonin reuptake inhibitor [SSRI] in IPT nonresponders) was considered, subjects with high Panic-Agoraphobic Spectrum Self-Report scores experienced a clinically and statistically significant delay in time to full response (18.1 weeks vs. 10.3 weeks; $P<0.05$). In an investigation of treatments for bipolar I disorder, among 66 patients, only 12% met criteria for DSM-IV-defined panic disorder, whereas 55% exceeded our ROC-defined threshold for clinically significant lifetime panic spectrum (Frank et al. 2002). In this group we observed a 27-week delay in time to sustained response of the index episode relative to those with lower levels of panic-spectrum features (44 weeks vs. 17 weeks; $P=0.002$). High panic-spectrum comorbidity in patients with bipolar disorder was also associated with greater number of lifetime depressive episodes and higher levels of current depressive symptoms.

Most recently, we carried out a two-site study at the Universities of Pittsburgh and Pisa in patients with unipolar depression. In this study, participants in an acute major depressive episode were randomly assigned to IPT-first or SSRI-first treatment sequences. Those who did not respond and whose symptoms subsequently remitted on one monotherapy had the other treatment added to their acute regimen. In this study, we found that participants with higher scores on the *need for medical reassurance* factor of the PAS-SR had more rapid remission with IPT than with SSRI monotherapy and that higher scores on the PAS-SR factors *panic symptoms, drug phobia, fear of losing control/depersonalization,* and *agoraphobia* predicted a longer time to remission with both treatments (Frank et al. 2010).

Identifying Subthreshold Conditions

Converging evidence from clinical and epidemiological studies, including the National Comorbidity Survey Replication (Kessler et al. 2003), confirms that subthreshold conditions are clinically relevant. Defining a cutoff for subthreshold conditions was therefore considered one of the priorities of the Spectrum Project. Usually this goal is approached analytically, using ROC analysis, which identifies a threshold that optimally balances sensitivity and specificity with respect to an external criterion (the "gold standard"). ROC analyses are commonly used on psychiatric research questionnaires to set a cutoff score that can be used for diagnostic screening in a two-phase survey. In this case, the cutoff was determined in a pilot study, with the diagnosis used as the gold standard. As mentioned, the spectrum instruments include the diagnostic criteria and other features that constitute the halo of a disorder. Moreover, the spectrum questions explore the lifetime experience of an individual. Therefore, using the lifetime diagnosis as a gold standard and assuming that the true cutoff score for a subthreshold condition would lie below that of the corresponding diagnosis, we obtained a first estimate of that score from the panic-agoraphobic spectrum by imposing the constraint that the sensitivity would be 70% or more (Frank et al. 2000b). Using large samples, including patients with the disorders of interest and control subjects, we similarly obtained a cutoff score for each spectrum condition using ROC analysis (Table 3–2). This procedure offers a starting point for distinguishing subjects with clinically meaningful lifetime spectrum subthreshold or full-blown psychopathology. Research is currently under way to demonstrate the clinical utility of identifying subthreshold conditions. Mood-spectrum psychopathology also has been associated with an increased likelihood of suicide attempts in patients with schizophrenia and mood disorders (Balestrieri et al. 2006), with poorer quality of life in individuals with rheumatoid arthritis (Piccinni et al. 2006), with a higher likelihood of developing a depressive episode during interferon treatment in patients with chronic hepatitis (Dell'Osso et al. 2007), and with a history of self-induced vomiting and suicidality in patients with anorexia nervosa (Wildes et al. 2007).

Setting Thresholds in Clinical Studies

One of the questions that might be addressed in clinical studies is whether a spectrum predicts time to respond to treatment (or remission). As noted earlier, we (Frank et al. 2000b, 2002) used panic-agoraphobic spectrum scores to predict time to response in mood disorders. The panic-agoraphobic spectrum was used for this purpose, both as a dimensional score (the count of positive items) in a Cox regression analysis and as a dichotomous variable (above or below the cutoff of 35 defined by ROC analysis), to generate Kaplan-Meier estimates of survival curves. In these studies, we found that the panic-agoraphobic spectrum significantly delays the response to treatment in major depression and bipolar disorder. The dimensional and categorical spectrum scoring provided consistent evidence that the information conveyed by the panic-agoraphobic spectrum is clinically useful above and beyond that provided by the presence/ absence of a comorbid diagnosis of panic disorder or agoraphobia.

Mood Spectrum as an Example of Opportunities for DSM-5

In the second half of this chapter, we explore various applications of the spectrum measures in mood disorders. Efforts by the Spectrum Project collaborators have been directed toward an empirical evaluation of the relationship of depressive and manic/hypomanic spectrum

TABLE 3–2. Thresholds for clinically significant spectrum psychopathology

SPECTRUM	THRESHOLD	SENSITIVITY, %	SPECIFICITY, %	AUC (95% CI)
Panic-agoraphobic	35	89	80	0.854 (0.808–0.900)
Mood				
Depression	22	93	70	0.907 (0.877–0.936)
Mania	22	87	70	0.861 (0.822–0.901)
Obsessive-compulsive	59	82	71	0.832 (0.744–0.890)
Social phobia	59	84	79	0.907 (0.870–0.943)
Anorexia/Bulimia	45	96	83	0.943 (0.920–0.967)
Psychotic	29	87	71	0.886 (0.845–0.926)
Substance use	25	91	71	0.905 (0.866–0.944)

Note. AUC=area under the curve.

phenomenology in patients with traditionally defined unipolar and bipolar disorders. These studies have enabled us to describe 1) the rate of lifetime manic/hypomanic symptoms reported by patients with recurrent unipolar disorder, 2) the relationship between the number and severity of lifetime manic/hypomanic symptoms and number and severity of depressive symptoms, and 3) the predictive value and clinical implications of various patterns of lifetime symptoms (as opposed to syndromes).

Function of Mood Spectrum Within a Group of Patients With Unipolar Disorders

Does a mood-spectrum assessment of unipolar disorders allow clinicians to understand aspects of the disorders that neither the DSM/Structured Clinical Interview for DSM Disorders approach nor conventional measures of severity (e.g., Hamilton Depression Scale, Inventory of Depressive Symptomatology) allow them to see in patients? Do patients with unipolar depression differ from patients with bipolar disorder in the lifetime experience of isolated manic/hypomanic symptoms? We argue that the field would benefit from a unitary and continuous approach to the assessment of both manic/hypomanic and depressive symptoms. On the basis of this unitary conceptualization of mood disorders, we hypothesized that patients with recurrent unipolar depression, without discrete lifetime hypomanic episodes, would nonetheless report lifetime hypomanic/manic symptoms and that the number of lifetime hypomanic/manic symptoms would be related to the number of lifetime depressive symptoms. We also hypothesized that manic/hypomanic symptoms would be associated with indicators of greater severity of depression.

We then examined the extent to which individuals with a lifetime diagnosis of recurrent unipolar disorder endorsed experiencing manic/hypomanic symptoms over their lifetimes and compared these reports with those of patients with bipolar disorder (Cassano et al. 2004). We tested these hypotheses in 223 patients with bipolar and recurrent unipolar mood disorders who were administered the Structured Clinical Interview for the Mood Spectrum (SCI-MOODS; Fagiolini et al. 1999). Patients with recurrent unipolar depression endorsed experiencing a substantial number of manic/hypomanic symptoms over their lifetimes. In both groups the number of manic/hypomanic items endorsed was related to the number of depressive items endorsed (see Figures 3–2 and 3–3). In the group with recurrent unipolar depression, the number of manic/hypomanic items was related to an increased likelihood of endorsing paranoid and delusional thoughts and suicidal ideation. In the bipolar group, the number of lifetime manic/hypomanic items was related to suicidal ideation and was just one indicator of psychosis. The presence of a significant number of manic/hypomanic items in patients with recurrent unipolar depression seems to challenge the traditional unipolar-bipolar dichotomy and to bridge the gap between these two categories of mood disorders.

Factor Structure of Mania/Hypomania Spectrum

The observation that bipolar disorders frequently go unrecognized prompted our group to consider use of a self-report version of the SCI-MOODS (MOODS-SR; Cassano et al. 2009b) to aid in the identification of bipolarity in clinical and nonclinical samples. The MOODS-SR was derived from the SCI-MOODS (Fagiolini et al. 1999) and is focused on the presence of manic and depressive symptoms, traits, and lifestyles that may characterize the "temperamental" affective dysregulation that makes up both fully syndromal and subthreshold mood disturbances. The subthreshold disturbances include symptoms, which are either isolated or clustered in time, and temperamental traits present throughout an individual's lifetime. The MOODS-SR consists of 161 items coded as present or absent for one or more periods of at least 3–5 days in the lifetime. Items are organized into three manic/hypomanic and three depressive domains—each exploring mood, energy, and cognition—plus a domain that explores disturbances in rhythmicity (i.e., changes in mood, energy, and physical well-being according to the weather, season, phase of menstrual cycle) and in vegetative functions, including sleep, appetite, and sexual function. The sum of the scores on the three manic/hypomanic domains constitutes the score for the manic/hypomanic component, whereas the sum of scores for the three depressive domains composes the depressive component.

We examined the 68 items of the MOODS-SR that explore cognitive, mood, and energy/activity features associated with mania/hypomania (Dell'Osso et al. 2002). Pooled data from 617 patients with bipolar disorders, recruited at the Universities of Pittsburgh and Pisa, Italy, were examined. Classical exploratory factor analysis, based on a tetrachoric matrix, was carried out, followed by an item response theory (IRT)–based factor-analytic approach. Nine factors were initially identified—psychomotor activation, creativity, mixed instability, sociability/extraversion, spirituality/mysticism/psychoticism, mixed irritability, inflated self-esteem, euphoria, and wastefulness/recklessness—that accounted overall for 56.4% of the variance of items. In a subsequent IRT-based bifactor analysis, only five of these factors (psychomotor activation, mixed instability, spirituality/mysticism/psychoticism, mixed irritability, euphoria) were retained. These anal-

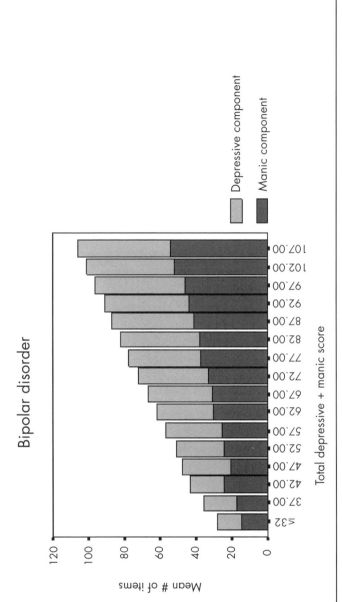

FIGURE 3–2. Association between the depressive and the manic/hypomanic spectrum components in patients with bipolar disorder.

Source. Cassano et al. 2004.

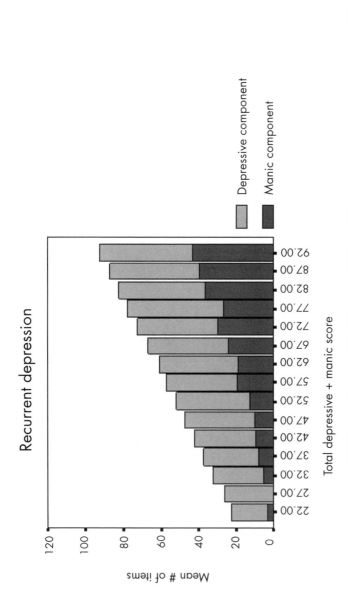

FIGURE 3–3. Association between the depressive and the manic/hypomanic spectrum components in patients with recurrent unipolar depression.

Source. Cassano et al. 2004.

yses confirm the central role of psychomotor activation in mania/hypomania and support the definitions of pure manic (psychomotor activation and euphoria) and mixed manic (mixed instability and mixed irritability) components, thus providing a potential opportunity to obtain better clinical and neurobiological definitions for patients with specific profiles.

Factor Structure of Depressive Spectrum

Using a similar strategy, we carried out a factor analysis of 74 items of the MOODS-SR that explored cognitive, mood, energy/activity, and neurovegetative features associated with depression (Cassano et al. 2009a). Data were collected from 598 patients with unipolar depression who were administered the instrument in Italian (*n*=415) or English (*n*=183). Six factors were identified—depressive mood, psychomotor retardation, suicidality, drug/illness-related depression, psychotic features, and neurovegetative symptoms—that accounted overall for 48.3% of the variance of items. A differential item functioning analysis revealed no quantitative gender differences in the factor scores but identified qualitative differences in the endorsement of items. These differences included "being indifferent about everything that happened" and "hearing voices," which were more frequent in males, and "crying very easily," "nothing you put on looked or felt right," "difficulty becoming sexually aroused," "being fatigued, weak, or tired for the smallest task," and "difficulty making even minor decisions," which were more frequent in females.

Clustering of Patients With Bipolar I Disorder According to Levels of Spectrum Psychopathology

In these analyses we sought to 1) use the lifetime mania and depressive spectrum assessments, along with assessments of anxiety spectrum conditions, to identify distinct subtypes of patients with bipolar disorder; 2) analyze the relationships of these subtypes with demographic and clinical variables collected at baseline; and 3) determine whether these subtypes are useful in predicting severity of illness, functioning, and quality of life during treatment (Fagiolini et al. 2007).

We performed a latent-class analysis of 261 adults with bipolar disorder, using four spectrum variables (i.e., depressive spectrum, mania/hypomania spectrum, panic spectrum, and obsessive-compulsive spectrum) dichotomized at the ROC-established thresholds for clinically significant spectrum psychopathology. Of this group, 127 patients were euthymic at study entry, and the remaining 134 were in a depressive ($n=94$), manic ($n=19$), mixed ($n=16$), hypomanic ($n=4$), or unspecified ($n=1$) state. Comorbidity, with syndromal obsessive-compulsive disorder and with panic disorder (with or without agoraphobia), according to DSM-IV, was found in 7 and 30 subjects, respectively. Latent-class analysis using four dichotomous variables supported a three-cluster solution that included, respectively, 126 (48%), 105 (40%), and 30 (12%) subjects. The profile plot of Figure 3–4 shows that participants assigned to Cluster 1 had high probabilities of having clinically significant depressive, manic, panic-agoraphobic, and obsessive-compulsive spectrum psychopathology. Participants assigned to Cluster 2 had probabilities close to 1.0 of having clinically significant depressive and manic spectrum, a 0.3 probability of having panic-agoraphobic spectrum, and virtually no probability of having clinically significant obsessive-compulsive spectrum psychopathology. Cluster 3 included subjects who, despite meeting criteria for bipolar disorder, had only a 0.4 probability of crossing the ROC-established threshold for clinically significant depressive spectrum and very low probability of having the other three spectrum conditions. Interestingly, we found clinical and demographic differences among the subtypes. Members of Class 1 were more likely to be female, to have an early onset of bipolar disorder, and to have greater severity of illness, both at study entry and during the study, as shown by Clinical Global Impression (CGI) scale scores. Compared with Class 1 members, those of Class 2 displayed a less-severe form of bipolar disorder and a higher quality of life and satisfaction. Members of Class 3 were more likely to be male, with a later age at onset of the disorder than the rest of the sample and better functioning, with a better quality of life and less-severe CGI scores than Class 1 members both at intake and during the study.

In contrast, a second latent-class analysis that used lifetime DSM-IV diagnoses of panic disorder, social phobia, generalized anxiety disorder, and obsessive-compulsive disorder, dichotomized as present or absent, supported a two-cluster model: one with 86.5% of subjects and a second with 13.5% of subjects. The presence of any comorbidity defined Cluster 2. Adding the patient's current clinical status (depressed vs. euthymic) as a covariate in the model improved the fit and resulted in a more parsimonious choice. Of the 436 patients with bipolar disorder, more than one-third ($n=149$, 34%) had comorbid anxiety, including 10.8% with panic disorder, 8.9% with social phobia, 3.6% with obsessive-compulsive disorder, and 19% with any of the three anxiety disorders. Euthymic patients were less likely to have comorbid anxiety.

We conclude that, in terms of defining phenotypes of bipolar depression, the spectrum-assessment approach provides more nuanced and probably more treatment-relevant information than simply inquiring about the presence of categorical diagnoses in the patient's history.

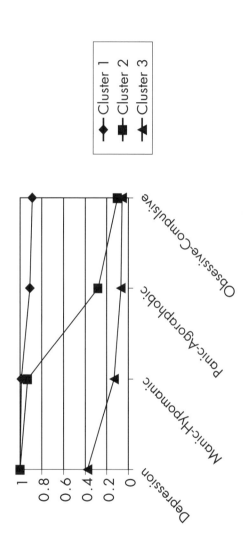

FIGURE 3–4. Profile plot showing the probability of exceeding the threshold for four lifetime spectra in three latent classes observed among patients with bipolar disorder.

Cluster 1: BIC=1063.8, L2=181.5378, *P*<0.0001, classification error=0; Cluster 2: BIC=943.2; L2=33.1540, *P*<0.001, classification error=0.0534; Cluster 3: BIC=938.8, L2=0.9499, *P*=0.51, classification error=0.1170.

Source.   Fagiolini et al. 2007.

Conclusion

We believe that the ultimate decision on how better to conceptualize a diagnosis should be strongly grounded on clinical utility and that the spectrum approach meets that test. We envisage the clinical utility of this approach in improving the diagnostic assessment, identifying groups for treatment response, identifying moderators of treatment response, characterizing subthreshold conditions for early identification and prevention, setting thresholds for functional and structural imaging changes, and establishing different levels of genetic vulnerability. Furthermore, in reviewing the evidence to date on the utility of the spectrum approach, it is apparent that spectra may have a place in DSM-5 alongside the current categorical diagnoses.

Dimensional measures can be applied to a variety of clinical and research questions, and we believe these can be adapted easily for screening, either as a lifetime measure or as a more current state. Such screening applications could provide important information for larger clusters of disorders and for determining overall level of severity. Specific categorical diagnostic determinations do not interfere with the spectrum approach but complement its usefulness. Spectrum measures can be adapted for epidemiological surveys yet enable the researcher to examine broader and more-specific phenotypic assessments, from clinical-outcome studies to a more precise characterization of patients with specific neurobiological findings.

We have anchored our theories in a promising set of measures that are potentially linked to biological variables and treatment outcome. These measures provide a better appreciation of patient variability (or phenotypes) and should enable the field both to improve its ability to produce durable recovery for patients with a range of disorders and to identify phenotypes related to specific genetic and brain structural or functional markers.

References

American Psychiatric Association: Diagnostic and Statistical Manual of Mental Disorders, 2nd Edition. Washington, DC, American Psychiatric Association, 1968

American Psychiatric Association: Diagnostic and Statistical Manual of Mental Disorders, 3rd Edition. Washington, DC, American Psychiatric Association, 1980

American Psychiatric Association: Diagnostic and Statistical Manual of Mental Disorders, 3rd Edition, Revised. Washington, DC, American Psychiatric Association, 1987

American Psychiatric Association: Diagnostic and Statistical Manual of Mental Disorders, 4th Edition. Washington, DC, American Psychiatric Association, 1994

American Psychiatric Association: Diagnostic and Statistical Manual of Mental Disorders, 4th Edition, Text Revision. Washington, DC, American Psychiatric Association, 2000

Balestrieri M, Rucci P, Sbrana A, et al: Lifetime rhythmicity and mania as correlates of suicidal ideation and attempts in mood disorders. Compr Psychiatry 47:334–341, 2006

Cassano GB, Savino M: Symptomatology of panic disorder: an attempt to define the panic-agoraphobic spectrum phenomenology, in Psychopharmacology of Panic. Edited by Montgomery SA. London, England, Oxford University Press, 1993, pp 38–57

Cassano GB, Banti S, Mauri M, et al: Internal consistency and discriminant validity of the Structured Clinical Interview for Panic-Agoraphobic Spectrum (SCI-PAS). Int J Methods Psychiatr Res 8:138–145, 1999

Cassano GB, Rucci P, Frank E, et al: The mood spectrum in unipolar and bipolar disorder: arguments for a unitary approach. Am J Psychiatry 161:1264–1269, 2004

Cassano GB, Benvenuti A, Miniati M, et al: The factor structure of lifetime depressive spectrum in patients with unipolar depression. J Affect Disord 115:87–99, 2009a

Cassano GB, Mula M, Rucci P, et al: The structure of lifetime manic-hypomanic spectrum. J Affect Disord 112:59–70, 2009b

Dell'Osso L, Cassano GB, Sarno N, et al: Validity and reliability of the Structured Clinical Interview for the Obsessive-Compulsive Spectrum (SCI-OBS) and for the Structured Clinical Interview for Social Phobia Spectrum (SCI-SHY). Int J Methods Psychiatr Res 9:11–24, 2000

Dell'Osso L, Armani A, Rucci P, et al: Measuring mood spectrum: comparison of interview (SCI-MOODS) and self-report (MOODS-SR) instruments. Compr Psychiatry 43:69–73, 2002a

Dell'Osso L, Rucci P, Cassano GB, et al: Measuring social anxiety and obsessive-compulsive spectra: comparison of interviews and self-report instruments. Compr Psychiatry 43:81–87, 2002

Dell'Osso L, Pini S, Maggi L, et al: Subthreshold mania as predictor of depression during interferon treatment in HCV+ patients without current or lifetime psychiatric disorders. J Psychosom Res 62:349–355, 2007

Fagiolini A, Dell'Osso L, Pini S, et al: Validity and reliability of a new instrument for assessing mood symptomatology: the Structured Clinical Interview for Mood Spectrum (SCI-MOODS). Int J Methods Psychiatr Res 8:71–81, 1999

Fagiolini A, Frank E, Rucci P, et al: Mood and anxiety spectrum as a means to identify clinically relevant subtypes of bipolar I disorder. Bipolar Disord 9:462–467, 2007

Frank E, Grochocinski VJ, Spanier CA, et al: Interpersonal psychotherapy and antidepressant medication: evaluation of a sequential treatment strategy in women with recurrent major depression. J Clin Psychiatry 61:51–57, 2000a

Frank E, Shear MK, Rucci P, et al: Influence of panic-agoraphobic spectrum symptoms on treatment response in patients with recurrent major depression. Am J Psychiatry 157:1101–1107, 2000b

Frank E, Cyranowski JM, Rucci P, et al: Clinical significance of lifetime panic spectrum symptoms in the treatment of patients with bipolar I disorder. Arch Gen Psychiatry 59:905–911, 2002

Frank E, Cassano GB, Rucci P, et al: Predictors and moderators of time to remission of major depression with interpersonal psychotherapy and SSRI pharmacotherapy. Psychol Med, April 12, 2010 (Epub ahead of print)

Kessler RC, Merikangas KR, Berglund P, et al: Mild disorders should not be eliminated from the DSM-V. Arch Gen Psychiatry 60:1117–1122, 2003

Mauri M, Borri C, Baldassari S, et al: Acceptability and psychometric properties of the Structured Clinical Interview for Anorexic-Bulimic Spectrum (SCI-ABS). Int J Methods Psychiatr Res 9:68–78, 2006

Piccinni A, Maser JD, Bazzichi L, et al: Clinical significance of lifetime mood and panic-agoraphobic spectrum symptoms on quality of life of patients with rheumatoid arthritis. Compr Psychiatry 47:201–208, 2006

Sbrana A, Dell'Osso L, Gonnelli C, et al: Acceptability, validity and reliability of the Structured Clinical Interview for the Spectrum of Substance Use (SCI-SUBS): a pilot study. Int J Methods Psychiatr Res 12:105–115, 2003

Sbrana A, Dell'Osso L, Benvenuti A, et al: The psychotic spectrum: validity and reliability of the Structured Clinical Interview for the Psychotic Spectrum. Schizophr Res 75:375–387, 2005

Shear MK, Frank E, Rucci P, et al: Panic-agoraphobic spectrum: reliability and validity of assessment instruments. J Psychiatr Res 35:59–66, 2001

Spectrum Project: The Spectrum Project: 1995–2006. Available at: http://www.spectrum-project.org. Accessed June 15, 2010.

Wildes JE, Gaskill JA, Ringham R, et al: Mood spectrum psychopathology in patients with anorexia nervosa. Compr Psychiatry 48:413–418, 2007

World Health Organization: International Statistical Classification of Diseases and Related Health Problems, 10th Revision. Geneva, World Health Organization, 1992

CHAPTER 4

Meta Effects of Classifying Mental Disorders

Norman Sartorius, M.D., Ph.D., F.R.C.Psych.

During a meeting convened by Joe Zubin in 1959, C.G. Hempel presented his paper on classification, and in the discussion that followed, A. Lewis suggested that it is necessary to distinguish two types of classifications of mental disorders (Fulford and Sartorius 2009). One type is *public* classifications: these should serve to improve communication between all concerned and might be the best to use in epidemiological and other research, where researchers want to make their findings comprehensible and comparable with findings of other scientists. The other type is *private* classifications, which serve the needs of particular groups that have reached agreement on the use of names for categories and their content. Public classifications should "eschew categories based on theoretical concepts" and be "operational and descriptive," because that would make it possible to communicate and compare results of epidemiological studies, for example.

A public classification of mental disorders has to satisfy scientific, public health, and practical requirements. Scientific requirements include a need to make the classification reflect scientific evidence; a need to satisfy taxonomic requirements (e.g., that the categories of the classification should be mutually exclusive and jointly exhaustive; i.e., they should allow the placement of each of the objects of the classification into a single category, and the total of categories should make it possible to place all objects that are being classified); and an effort to preserve continuity between the revisions of the classification so as to permit comparisons over time (Sartorius 1976, 1978). Practical and public health requirements include a need to make the classification easy to use in practice; a need to ensure that the public classification has links with "private" classifications (and that it can be translated into different languages and into classifications used by other professions, e.g., psychiatric nurses); and a need to reflect experience, particularly if evidence is not available. Until now, in the classification of mental disorders, the practical requirements have been easier to satisfy than the scientific: the knowledge about the pathogenesis of mental disorders is still insufficient to govern the structure of the classification, and satisfying some of the taxonomic requirements would have made the classification less easy to use and therefore unlikely to be generally used.

The purpose of the *International Classification of Diseases* (ICD), from its original version to its most recent revision, ICD-10 (World Health Organization 1992), has been to facilitate communication of, and comparisons among, findings. The ICD should be seen as a typical example of a public classification that classifies data in a manner that makes it possible for all those interested—governments, researchers, and practitioners—to understand and compare facts relevant to healthcare. In the beginning, the ICD was no more than a list of categories that grouped causes of death. Gradually the remit for the ICD was expanded to include diseases, reasons for contacting services, disability, health care interventions, and other facts of importance for planners and practitioners of health services (Sartorius 1995).

A classification of diseases, including the ICD, is produced to facilitate reporting about activities of health care services and epidemiological estimates of parameters of diseases (e.g., their frequencies) in populations. Classifications and their productions, however, also have other uses and effects. Classifications contribute to definitions of the medical disciplines, including psychiatry. They can be used as a basis for health insurance and related public health measures. They also can have significant effects on the images of medical disciplines and on the perceptions of people with diseases included in these classifications. Classifications, which are used as bases for training health personnel, usually become platforms for action and learning in later life. Finally, classifications also can define directions of research, sometimes restraining innovative scientific explorations of issues that cut across the categories of the classifications. In this chapter, I examine these remote effects of classifications of mental disorders. However, before doing so, I briefly discuss four problems that face the makers of classifications of mental disorders.

Problems Facing Makers of Classifications of Mental Disorders

What Should Be Grouped?

The English language has the luxury of choice of four terms for psychiatric maladies. These words are used loosely, but it is accepted generally that the word *illness* refers to the experience of a person who has the malady, the word *disease* to a medical substrate of the malady, and the word *sickness* to social recognition of the malady, for example, in determining sickness benefits (Sartorius 2002). The problem that plagues psychiatry—or at least is better recognized in psychiatry than in other medical disciplines—is that the areas covered by these three terms overlap only in part. Some people feel *ill*, although it is not possible to detect a medical substrate, a tissue damage, that would justify the use of the word *disease,* whereas some people with *diseases* who have major tissue damage or other medical findings do not feel *ill.* Some people are declared *sick* and given treatment even though they have no signs of *disease* and do not feel *ill,* a sad phenomenon that finds its acme in the abuse of psychiatry for political purposes. It is not always clear what should be grouped in a classification: ICD-10 has labeled the conditions seen in psychiatric practice *disorders,* a vague term that denotes the incomplete overlap of the three meanings of malady just described (World Health Organization 1992).

Caseness and Diagnoses

A second problem that psychiatry (and its classifications) has to face is that there is a difference between a psychiatric diagnosis and "caseness." Whether someone is a "case" depends on the purpose of this label. Thus, in epidemiological studies, a *case* might be defined differently from a "case" in assessment of psychiatric services or in estimation of the need for service or intervention. The difference between a "case" and a psychiatric diagnosis lies in the use of the three dimensions of "caseness": 1) the cluster of symptoms that psychiatry considers as the disease; 2) the distress that an individual who has the disease experiences[1]; and 3) the disability—the impairment of functioning—that the disease produces, in the context of an individual's life situation, personality traits, and, possibly, comorbid diseases. Here again, overlap between the syndrome, the distress, and functional impairment can be significant, partial, or nonexistent. Some people with a particular form of a disease are disabled by it, whereas others are not. Some people are severely distressed but do not show the symptoms necessary to satisfy the definition of a disease. A person who discovers a wart of black color might be severely distressed because he or she fears that the wart is an early stage of a melanoma that will spread rapidly, although he or she is neither disabled nor has a disease. Other persons might be disabled to a severe level but show few symptoms of a disease. The cluster of symptoms, the disability, and the distress can each be measured in terms of severity, and it is probable that extreme severity of any one of the three dimensions of caseness will make those persons (or their caregivers) seek help from health services or others who surround them even if they have no (symptomatic) diagnosis.

In some classifications of mental disorders—notably, the *Diagnostic and Statistical Manual of Mental Disorders* (DSM)—the definition of a mental disorder requires the presence of symptoms, disability, and distress. This is a problematic solution because of a growing amount of evidence that the impairment of functioning of people with mental disorders depends much more on social class, personal assets, cultural expectations, and other factors than on disease alone. The ICD recommends to users of the chapter on mental disorders that they should not use *disability* (*functional impairment* in the language of DSM) in making a diagnosis of mental disorders because disability depends, to a large extent, on the social environment of the person who has the disease. ICD, however, also uses impairment in the performance of basic functions (e.g., self-care) as a component criterion for some conditions (e.g., the dementias). Clinicians often attempt to help persons who seek help because they are severely distressed but are not disabled or showing sufficient symptoms to be diagnosed as having a mental disorder. The question that will have to be resolved soon, in order to inform the makers of ICD-11 and DSM-5, is whether the classifications should group diagnostic terms or "cases" seen in psychiatric and general medical practice.

Consequences of Ignorance About the Pathogenesis of Mental Disorders

Another major problem for makers of the classifications is that of the relationships between disorders that are to be grouped. Two, or more than two, morbid events can be considered as parts of the same disorder if their pathogenesis is the same. Thus, if the patho-

---

[1]In some instances, the distress is experienced by the family or others surrounding the person with the disease, not by the person; such is the case in the instance of manic episodes, during which patients often do not feel ill or distressed at all.

genesis of depression is the same as the pathogenesis of anxiety, the two conditions should be considered the same, not comorbid, despite the fact that their clinical pictures are different. For example, in ICD-10, retinopathy, peripheral neuropathy, polydypsia, and ketoacidosis are all grouped in categories assigned to diabetes because they share a common pathogenesis. The term *comorbidity* should be reserved for instances in which two morbid events of different pathogenesis exist in the same individual at the same time. The pathogenesis of most mental disorders is still a matter of speculation and remains largely unknown. Consequently, at present, the classification has different categories for conditions that might be the same in their pathogenesis and, vice versa, the classification wrongly groups disorders of different pathogenesis into the same category. The same situation applies to uncertainty about the way to deal with the reappearance of morbid events that have similar symptoms in the same person: if the pathogenesis of the morbid events results in the same clinical picture on each occasion, the classification should place them into the same category, counting them, for epidemiological and treatment purposes, as one disorder. If the pathogenesis is different on each occasion (although the clinical condition and symptoms may be the same), the events should not be counted as episodes of the same disorders but as independent diseases, somewhat like injuries that can occur for different reasons many times in the course of one's life.

For the time being, it has been decided to classify psychiatric disorders by their symptoms; this decision is not necessarily the best, but it seems to be the only one possible in the current state of our ignorance. This classification choice has the advantage that the grouping of disorders can be done reliably: among its disadvantages is that such a classification can be reified, taken to reflect the natural order of things, although it is no more than a hypothesis of the real nature of mental disorders created on the basis of evidence available at a point in time (Sartorius 1988). When this happens, the classification can, in fact, hamper the exploration of pathogenetic processes involved in the syndromes that modern operational criteria have placed together into categories.

Overlap Between Variants of Lifestyle, Impairment, and Mental Disorders

Variants of lifestyle and behavior that are seen in people with mental disorders may overlap. Persons, such as the famous "clochards" of Paris, who have chosen to live on the street without permanent abode and rely on charity often do not have demonstrable mental disorders; yet vagabondage has been included as a category in the classification of mental disorders in some countries. Also, in recent

years we have seen the exclusion of homosexuality from the classification of mental disorders in ICD-10 and in some national classifications, whereas in other classifications homosexuality still is seen
as a mental disorder that requires psychiatric treatment. Hermaph-
rodites have raised their voices, protesting that their condition is described as a disorder of sexual development (Karkazis and Feder
2008). People with intellectual disability are opposing the notion that
their conditions should be classified in the chapter on mental disorders in the ICD under the name of mental retardation. In some countries, hazardous driving has come to be seen as an expression of a
mental disorder that should be removed by psychotherapy. These
examples of conditions that have been placed into the classification
of mental disorders and/or removed from it illustrate a difficulty
that is specific for the makers of such classifications.

Areas of Mental Health Programs Affected by the Classification of Mental Disorders and Their Revisions

The Identity of Psychiatry

A medical discipline is defined by the disorders that it treats, by the
methods that it uses to treat such disorders, and by the length of
time necessary to learn how to use these treatment methods. Therefore, any discussion of a classification of mental disorders also is a
discussion of the identity of psychiatry. The classification indicates
whether a particular disorder "belongs" to psychiatry, and the total-
ity of the disorders placed in a classification of mental disorder de-
fines the limits of psychiatry. If all disorders that are currently classified in the classification of mental disorders were to be moved to
other chapters of a classification of diseases, psychiatry would cease
to exist.

This relationship between the classification of mental disorders
and the identity of psychiatry—and thus also of psychiatrists—makes
it certain that a discussion about classification will be of great interest to psychiatrists, raise emotions, and lead to intense discussions
and anxieties. Clinicians who represent other medical disciplines
are, of course, also interested in the matter, because the definition
of the territory of one discipline usually affects the territories of
others.

The controversy surrounding the concept of subthreshold disorders exemplifies the way in which classification of mental disorders

influences the definition of the discipline of psychiatry.[2] The existence of subthreshold disorders is a by-product of the use of operational criteria that define categories of mental disorders on the basis of a consensus rather than evidence. It places before psychiatrists a dilemma that will be difficult to resolve. As things stand, it is clear that psychiatrists who provide treatment to people who do not have a disease (but have a subthreshold disorder) could be seen as fraudulent charlatans because they treat people who do not have disorders. However, if these psychiatrists do not help people who come to them with subthreshold disorders—for example, people who do not show many symptoms but are very distressed—the psychiatrists are not fulfilling their roles of good physicians. Also, problems related to subthreshold disorders are close to problems related to states that show some similarity to mental disorders but are considered different from them and therefore should not receive psychiatric treatment, such as grief reactions as well as excessive religious zeal and related behavior (e.g., self-flagellation and even crucifixion).

Psychiatrists, as well as other physicians, often see patients who ask for help because of problems that might be causing distress or impaired functioning. Psychiatrists examine these patients, advise them, and provide treatment that is not necessarily different from treatment that would be provided to a patient who has an "above-the-threshold" disorder. These clinicians are helping people who are distressed or disabled but who do not have all the symptoms that have been selected to define a category. In other medical disciplines, the threshold of illness usually can be expressed in terms of laboratory findings or results of a variety of examinations that provide "hard data," such as those obtained by the use of X-ray or imaging apparatus. Psychiatry does not have that luxury, and helping people who do not meet criteria (set by psychiatrists!) of illness can easily lead to the accusation that psychiatry medicalizes the problems of daily living so that its practitioners can make money.[3]

Another example of the effect of changes of classification on the definition of the discipline of psychiatry is the removal of the "progressive paresis of the insane" from the classification of mental dis-

---

[2]The term *subthreshold disorders* came into existence when the classification of mental disorders was "operationalized"—that is, when the American Psychiatric Association published DSM-III (American Psychiatric Association 1980), in which each category of the classification was provided with a description of criteria that had to be satisfied, if a disorder was to be placed in that category.

[3]It is true that other medical disciplines deal with conditions for which diagnosis is based mainly on patients' complaints (e.g., migraine and some other forms of headache), but the numbers of such conditions in other chapters of the classification of diseases is much smaller than for psychiatry.

order (now placed with the communicable disease chapter, because it is a late form of syphilis). By removing the condition from the chapter "belonging" to psychiatry, the discipline has, in fact, unofficially been declared unable to deal with behavioral syndromes caused by a communicable disease.

The second descriptor of a discipline—a definition of methods that its practitioners will use—also depends on the definition of disorders and their grouping in the classification. If disorders that are grouped in a category (because presumably they have the same pathogenesis) do not react in the same way to the methods of treatment that define psychiatry, it is legitimate to doubt the effectiveness of such methods and, by implication, the justification for the existence of the discipline that uses them. Johannes Reil, who introduced the term *psychiaterie* some 200 years ago, argued that the discipline of psychiatry should be created in order to demonstrate that mental disorders are not moral failings or consequences of black magic but diseases like any others and that it is therefore necessary to create a medical discipline that will demonstrate that both diseases of the body and diseases of the mind are the legitimate subject of medicine (Marneros 2004). Methods used in the treatment of physical illnesses have similar effectiveness for all the disorders grouped in a category of the classification. If this does not hold for psychiatry, it becomes difficult to see psychiatry as a discipline similar to its sisters in the practice of medicine.

The vagueness of the limits of psychiatric disorders, and of the categories in which they are placed, as well as a reluctance to define precisely what methods of treatment psychiatrists should or should not use, has allowed the emergence of territorial disputes with practitioners of nonmedical disciplines and others—for example, practitioners of alternative medicine. These disputes are considerably more important in the field of psychiatry than in other parts of medicine. Such disputes are often settled politically, with decision-makers disregarding the option of assessing which professional group is best qualified to provide care and deciding, on the basis of that evidence, who should be doing what.

Financial Resources for Health Care of Persons With Mental Disorders

The recent decision to introduce parity in the reimbursement of health care expenses for mental and physical disorders in the United States was considered, justly, an important step to more equitable treatment of people with mental illness. People with conditions placed outside the DSM-IV (American Psychiatric Association 1994) chapter on psychiatry have not had any disadvantage in terms of reimbursement, even if their conditions were disorders that, in other classifications, would fall into the chapter that groups mental disorders (e.g., premenstrual dysphoric disorder and postviral fatigue syndromes). On the other hand, in some countries—for example, in Eastern Europe and Vietnam—*psychotic* mental disorders have been treated free of charge, whereas patients have had to pay for treatment of other mental, and most physical, disorders. Psychiatrists have often indicated that patients had psychosis so as to ensure that treatment was free even though the psychiatrists knew the patients had other conditions.

These examples indicate the influence of a classification on the funding of health care on an individual level. On the level of societies' decisions about health care, a classification also plays an important role. During the preparation of ICD-10, there was a long and intensive discussion about the placement of cerebrovascular disorders. Neurologists argued that the consequences of stroke made it highly probable that such patients would come under their care; cardiologists argued that the conditions were due to vascular damage, and therefore the disorders should be placed in the chapter on cardiovascular disorders. However, the background of the argument was not exclusively scientific. Many governments make decisions about the distribution of resources on the basis of mortality figures. Diseases that kill more people are given higher priorities in national health programs and thus receive more resources. Cerebrovascular disorders are a major cause of mortality; thus, their placement in the classification underlines the importance of the discipline that deals with people with the condition that causes death.[4]

In some instances, when it was too difficult to decide where to place a condition, a special arrangement was introduced into ICD-10: the same condition was placed in two chapters. One placement carried a sign of a dagger, indicating that death due to that disease should be coded in that chapter, whereas the other placement carried an asterisk, indicating that care provided to a person with the disease should be coded in that chapter. Thus, for example, dementia found its place as a cause of death in the chapter on neurological disorders and as a cause of treatment in the chapter on psychiatric disorders.

The definition of categories affects estimation of prevalence of disorders, another dimension that decision makers take into account when assessing the priority and financing of healthcare. A broad definition of a category will increase the total number of cases that can be considered as being in need of care; narrowing a category

---

[4]Finally stroke was placed into the chapter on cardiovascular diseases, and its consequences, such as hemiparesis, were placed into the chapter on neurology. As a result, in calculating mortality, stroke is reported as a cardiovascular illness.

(i.e., making criteria more stringent) will decrease prevalence and incidence estimations for conditions placed in that category and will have a negative influence on the priority given to the discipline responsible for the care of people with such diseases.

HIV/AIDS provides another example of the role that a classification might have on resource allocation. Although HIV is a neurotropic virus and persons with AIDS often experience depression and, later in the course of the illness, dementia, both HIV-related dementia and encephalopathy are included in the chapter on infectious diseases; depressive states observed in the course of the illness are not specifically identified. Resources given to the fight with HIV/AIDS have been vast, but it is not easy to direct a reasonable amount of these resources to research on psychiatric and neurological components of the syndrome or to the provision of care for people with psychiatric and neurological problems linked to their HIV/AIDS. Researchers in Africa will often include a reference to HIV/AIDS in proposals for mental health research and service support, because this will make the acquisition of funds considerably easier; they will get funds that they would not get if they wrote their proposals without mention of AIDS.

These examples illustrate the effect of a classification on reimbursement and on decisions about priority of health programs. In the eyes of the decision makers, psychiatry deals with disorders that are not very frequent, are long-lasting, and usually do not respond to treatment. Psychiatric disorders are not seen as contributing to mortality: suicide and violent acts linked to mental disorders are not placed in the chapter dealing with mental disorders but in a different chapter. Therefore, mortality due to these causes usually does not enter into the decision making as an argument for higher priority of mental health programs.

The Image of Psychiatry

For a long time, a majority of the population (including a sizeable part of health care workers and political decision-makers) considered most mental illnesses to be incurable. Persons who had a mental illness were seen as being of little value for society, and because they were not curable, it seemed logical that society should be reluctant to invest money in the provision of adequate care or to support a medical discipline that seemed incapable of diminishing the prevalences of mental diseases or improving their courses. The main reasons for providing any support, therefore, have been the obligation of a society to help its feeble members and the need to protect society from the evil deeds of the mentally ill. The ethical imperative—helping members of society who are feeble or in distress—often has lost in competition with other causes of social action. The second reason for action—protection of society—was satisfied by measures such as incarceration or involuntary hospitalization of mentally ill people, often under conditions that would speed up their demise. Psychiatrists were seen as ineffective in the treatment of mental illness and as serving primarily as guardians of patients in the institutions. With the advent of psychoanalysis, psychiatrists came to be seen as a luxury the rich could use to unburden their worries. Not infrequently, psychiatrists have been seen as having diseases similar to those seen in their patients: this opinion has been another part of the rather poor image of psychiatry.

The classification of mental disorders also plays a role in stigmatization of the discipline of psychiatry. This begins with a medical education and the puzzlement of medical students who do not understand why they have to learn about 670 disorders (currently the number of categories used for the classification of mental disorders, according to ICD-10) when there are so few types of medications (i.e., antidepressants, antipsychotics, tranquilizers, and stimulants) used for treatment of all these disorders. In the eyes of a medical student, psychiatrists who have produced such classification cannot be practice-oriented doctors, an impression that is further strengthened when students hear about matters such as the necessary duration of psychoanalytic psychotherapy and the abuse of psychiatry for political purposes. The vagueness of language used by some psychiatrists in describing the categories of their classification of mental disorders (and principles used to make the classification) is, for these students, further confirmation of the fact that psychiatrists are neither real doctors nor particularly useful consultants. Once students complete their medical training, graduates usually maintain their opinions about various disciplines of medicine, including psychiatry, and contribute to the dismal image that psychiatry has for the general public.

The removal of categories of mental disorders from the classification of mental disorders as soon as the cause of the mental disorder is found (e.g., the AIDS dementia and general paresis in the chapter on communicable diseases) further strengthens doubt that psychiatry is a medical discipline. If it were a real medical disclipline, the argument goes, then conditions that are presenting psychiatric symptoms, but are the result of a "real" (physical) illness, should be treated by psychiatrists, like other disorders for which there is no certainty about a physical cause as yet. Doubt about whether psychiatry is a part of medicine also is enhanced by the reluctance of psychiatrists to deal with physical illness. The existence of specialists of "consultation psychiatry" or "liaison psychiatry" is a sad confirmation of this attitude. There is no specialty of "consultation orthopedics" or "liaison ophthalmology": an orthopedic surgeon is supposed to know enough about orthopedic problems that might emerge in the practice of other doctors and the same is true for the ophthalmologist who is expected to be able to deal with issues concerning his or her discipline regardless of the ward on which the patient is located. Among psychiatrists, on the other hand, only a precious few—the liaison psychiatrists—seem to be able and willing to deal with mental illness in people who also have a somatic illness.

The media and the general public like classifications that are simple and tell them what kind of interventions are likely to be useful. Burns are divided by severity into four groups, defined by their risk to life and likelihood of reparation. Cancer, as well as cancer pain, has been classified in clear groups that are staged, and the stages have been linked to specific treatments. Communicable diseases are divided according to the bug that causes them. A number of bone and joint diseases have been precisely defined in a manner that facilitates treatment. Psychiatry, for a long time, did not produce clear and simple instructions about placement of diagnoses into categories of a classification of mental disorders. Several psychiatric disorders have been operationally defined in the past, but until the appearance of DSM-III there was no widely accepted classification that clearly stated criteria used to place a disorder into a category. DSM-III was a major step forward in improving the image of psychiatry. The next step, providing a clear specification of methods to be used for treatment of disorders that are clearly defined, has yet to be taken. It will not be easy to do this; although detailed guidelines for the treatment of mental disorders are numerous, these guidelines do not all say the same thing. Many of the guidelines express the views of their authors regardless of what other authors have said (or found); this is a situation similar to that which was described by Stengel in the 1960s, when he found that "any psychiatrist worth his salt produces a classification of mental disorders" (Stengel 1959). Half a century after Sir Aubrey Lewis's suggestion that a public classification should have operationally defined categories, there is almost universal agreement on the need to have a classification with operational definitions of mental disorders usable in everyday clinical practice, and there is a fair amount of agreement on criteria that should be used. It is to be hoped that agreement on treatment of these conditions will not take another 50 years.

Research Into the Pathogenesis of Mental Disorders

A classification of mental disorders should be a reflection of the current state of knowledge about relationships among events, conditions, or objects that are classified. As long as it is seen as a summary of past knowledge that guides all future exploration (rather than as a rigid framework), a classification is useful; once it gets reified and is seen as the governing frame, it will stifle investigation and reduce chances of discovery of relationships between conditions or their causal links and pathogenesis.

Unfortunately, this is already happening. Enthused by the precision of definition for categories of mental disorders produced in the latter part of the twentieth century, many people took the fact that diagnoses could be made more reliably as proof of their validity and of the validity of the classification that contained categories for the placement of such diagnoses. Editors of scientific journals no longer accepted papers that described research carried out on well-defined conditions unless the definitions used coincided with definitions in DSM-IV and DSM-IV-TR (American Psychiatric Association 2000). Authorities who approved the use of medications and other treatments requested proof that a new drug was useful in the treatment of a particular condition defined in DSM-IV. One could imagine a drug with a positive effect on a certain proportion of people (who perhaps share a genetic basis) with different clinical syndromes that are classified in different categories of DSM-IV: it would be difficult to carry out research on such "cross-category" effectiveness and even more difficult to get a license to market a drug that helps some patients in different categories of the classification. For pharmaceutical companies engaged in the search for new drugs, it has become foolish to carry out research on a dimension of illness present in several disorders that currently are placed in different categories of DSM or ICD, because it would be impossible to obtain a license for a drug not linked to the treatment of a condition with a particular diagnosis. In view of the fact that much of the research on psychopharmacology today is financed by pharmaceutical industry, the classification that is now officially recognized does impede innovative research.

The restrictive effect of the classification—clearly seen in the scarcity of publications that describe research on mental disorders across categories or of research on a particular dimension of mental functioning in physical and mental illness—will not necessarily be removed by a dimensional approach to the classification of mental disorders; but if that approach were to be accepted, it would, for a while, open new avenues of research (and possibly allow a different, less-stigmatizing organization of services for the mentally ill). Insofar as research is concerned, clearly it will be necessary to continue work on standardization of assessment of various aspects of mental disorders (e.g., symptoms, dimensions, or even more elementary descriptors of mental states), avoiding the obsessional adherence to diagnosis or criteria for categories of a classification. Such an approach will facilitate the discovery of pathogenetic mechanisms and thus more likely lead to classifications in which distinctions between mental illnesses are made on a scientific basis.

Stigmatization of People With Mental Illness

The classification of mental disorders plays an important role in attribution of stigma to a diagnosis and the individuals who have such a disorder. Mental disorders are stigmatized and generally seen as conditions that diminish the value of the affected individual for society. The image of a person with a mental illness is that of someone with symptoms, such as delusions and hallucinations, who is usually dangerous and unable to contribute to society; placement of a diagnosis in the chapter on mental disorders will make those with such a diagnosis share the negative image that frightens the public and results in many disadvantages.

Recent research on stigmatization of the mentally ill has brought evidence that stigmatization of mental illness is present in a vast majority of all societies and that the consequences of stigmatization are negative in all of these societies (Sartorius and Schulze 2005).[5] Therefore, it is not surprising that people with mental illness usually hide their diagnoses and that they try—whenever they become organized—to take their diagnoses from the chapter on mental disorders into some other chapter of the classification. Pressure groups (often composed of patients and their families) in some instances have succeeded in avoiding stigmatization by insisting on their diagnosis being placed in a category in a chapter "belonging" to another discipline. Thus, in ICD-10, the diagnosis "fatigue syndromes" is in the chapter on mental disorders, whereas the less-stigmatizing term "postviral fatigue syndrome" has been placed in the chapter on communicable diseases. Premenstrual dysphoric syndromes found their place in the chapter dealing with gynecological problems. The aforementioned HIV-related mental disorders are in the chapter dealing with infectious diseases. Attempted suicide is in a chapter separate from that dealing with mental disorders, although suicide and attempted suicide are usually associated with mental disorder. "Personality type A," regardless of its severity, is placed in the "reasons for contact" chapter, far away from the personality disorders group in the chapter on mental disorders. The diagnosis of homosexuality has vanished from the chapter on mental disorders, although it is still considered as an abnormality (regardless of whether it is ego dystonic or not) requiring psychiatric attention in a variety of coun-

---

[5]There is one notable exception to this rule. Posttraumatic stress disorder, characterized by psychiatric symptoms, is the only disorder that does not seem to stigmatize a person who has it. The diagnosis is taken as an honorable badge confirming that the bearer has gone through difficult times and that he or she deserves society's support and recognition of merit.

tries. In Japan, the previously used name for schizophrenia[6] has been changed to a term that is considerably less frightening—from "split mind disease" to "thought integration disorder"—and the description of the disease has been significantly changed. The positive effect of this change—for example, that doctors feel that it is easier to tell a patient his or her diagnosis and discuss treatment much more effectively—should make the developers of a classification system take the connotation of terms used in psychiatry into account, both in naming categories and in producing the criteria that will define them. This has not been done in the past: the growing power of patient and family organizations might be of major assistance in the search for terms that will not only be precisely defined but also acceptable to all those concerned.

To avoid stigmatization by a label of a mental illness, and the consequences of the stigma, patient and family organizations have sometimes taken extraordinary steps. For example, in France, an organization of families of people with mental illness lobbied and finally succeeded in reclassifying mental illness from a disease to an "invalidity." This classification change will allow families and patients to receive more support; however, this support comes at a cost of making the image of mental illness worse, effectively telling the general public that impairment related to mental illness is there to stay and that treatment of mental illness can do little to make people who have it recover and become valuable members of their communities.

Education of Health Workers

Over the past several decades, psychiatrists, proud of the significant increase in their knowledge, have continued to make the classification of mental disorders more and more complex. The number of categories has increased, and fixing their boundaries has required development of a complex system of inclusion and exclusion criteria. The detailed classification is usually not directly relevant to the choice of treatment. Thus, for example, the international classification of mental disorders now has some 60 categories for classification of various forms of depressive disorders, although treatment for all categories is similar.

A public classification, in Sir Aubrey Lewis's sense, should be simple, easy to remember, suitable for use in practice (e.g., provide some guidance about treatment) and epidemiological research, and

---

[6]In Japan (and some other countries in the Far East), diagnoses of mental illnesses are translated into the local language; in Europe, it is only Greece in which the word "schizophrenia" can be understood by people speaking Greek.

amenable to tests of reliability and clinical utility (i.e., give guidance for treatment or other care interventions). It also should have face validity in the sense that it allows the easy and reliable categorization of most diagnoses made in practice. The World Health Organization attempted to satisfy all users by producing three versions of the ICD-10 classification: 1) a version for research (this would be closer to a "private" classification in Sir Aubrey's sense); 2) a version for clinical work, suitable for use by specialists in psychiatry; and 3) a version for use in primary health care. The latter had 22 categories, chosen because they are frequently seen in primary health services, can be reliably diagnosed, and can be linked to specific advice about treatment. Thus, this third version also could serve as a teaching tool in the education of various categories of health workers who are not psychiatrists.

At present, unfortunately, most health workers are educated about psychiatry and the management of mental disorders on the basis of curricula with more complex classifications and by teachers oblivious of the consequences that presentation of such classifications will have for the care of mentally ill people both in the immediate future, when the health workers complete their training, and in the more remote future, when the students assume important decision-making positions in the health care system. What health workers learn in the course of their general training is rarely updated; therefore it is not surprising that decision makers the world over have an image of psychiatry (and of the best way to develop mental health programs), that is based on their training from many decades previous. They were taught psychiatry on the basis of a classification of mental disorders created in the late nineteenth and early twentieth centuries. That classification was created based on observations in mental hospitals at that time, and it served the purpose of reporting about mental illness in those institutions very well. The world, and our knowledge about mental illness as well as the practice of medicine, has changed meanwhile; yet decision makers trained decades ago think about the organization of mental health services, as well as about evaluation of these services, using theoretical constructs implied by the classification used in teaching psychiatry in schools of health personnel when they were students.

The delayed effect of teaching about psychiatry is not exceptional for psychiatry or other medical disciplines. It is therefore important to produce classifications of mental disorders that will take this delayed effect of medical school instruction into account. The "public" classification of mental disorders, with characteristics described earlier, might serve that purpose, and this remains a major challenge for the makers of international and national classifications of mental disorders.

The Abuse of Psychiatry

An international "public" classification that describes the categories of mental illnesses clearly could play an important role in preventing the abuse of psychiatry, which is sometimes supported by national classifications or classifications produced by a particular school of thought. The abuse of psychiatry for political purposes in the Soviet Union, for example, was supported by the existence of a classification that was developed in the United Soviet Socialist Republics and served to organize psychiatric care and treatment. This classification had categories with diagnoses that could be given to political dissidents and that led to the forced and harmful application of medication and other "treatment" measures. The universal acceptance of an international classification of mental disorders based on the best available knowledge could remove the legitimacy of such actions and help to make psychiatry a useful medical discipline, immune to abuse for political, financial, or other purposes.

The existence of such a classification also could serve to improve the quality of care offered to people with mental illness and to prevent abuse of psychiatry for other purposes. The introduction of new categories into such a classification, or any change of the classification, would have to be subjected to a serious examination of the evidence that underlies the reason for the change. At present, the process for doing this is not specified sufficiently. It is not at all clear how much, and what kind of, evidence would be necessary and sufficient in order to accept a proposal for a change of a category, for a change of criteria defining a category, or for a change of hierarchy of categories. Thus, commercial and personal motives may lead to the acceptance of changes that are not particularly well supported by evidence and that happen too rapidly; this means that it will not be possible to ensure that a single form of the classification is universally accepted and used.

Coda

Revisions of the classification of mental disorders are necessary when new knowledge becomes available and when there are significant changes in the health system that the classification is meant to serve. A revision of the classification is usually made by paying great attention to the formal features of the classification and congruence of the revision with the best available evidence and experience.

Thus, revisions of a classification produced in this sense can reflect current knowledge about a group of diseases and can satisfy epistemological strivings of its makers. However, a revision of a classification also has a number of remote effects that usually receive far too little attention in the process of revision. For example, a classification of mental disorders

- Affects the definition of psychiatry and the profession of psychiatrists.
- Influences and changes the nature of stigmatization that bears heavily on people with mental disorders and their families.
- Affects funding for mental health care and education of health care workers.
- Exerts a powerful effect on directions that research into the pathogenesis of mental disorders will take and on the relative importance of findings of such research.

Therefore, it is to be hoped that the process of revision of the ICD and important classifications such as DSM will include a way to consider these remote meta effects of a revision before their finalization and introduction as one of the basic elements of health services systems, research, and education related to psychiatry and to medicine, in general.

References

American Psychiatric Association: Diagnostic and Statistical Manual of Mental Disorders, 3rd Edition. Washington, DC, American Psychiatric Association, 1980

American Psychiatric Association: Diagnostic and Statistical Manual of Mental Disorders, 4th Edition. Washington, DC, American Psychiatric Association, 1994

American Psychiatric Association: Diagnostic and Statistical Manual of Mental Disorders, 4th Edition, Text Revision. Washington, DC, American Psychiatric Association, 2000

Fulford W, Sartorius N: The secret history of ICD and the hidden future of DSM, in Psychiatry as Cognitive Neuroscience: Philosophical Perspectives. Edited by Broome M, Bortolotti L. New York, Oxford University Press, 2009

Karkazis K, Feder EK: Naming the problem: disorders and their meanings. Lancet 372:2016–2017, 2008

Marneros A: Die Geburtsstunde der psychiatrischen Wissenschaft und Heilkunde in Deutschalnd. Die Psychiatrie 1:1–8, 2004

Sartorius N: Classification: an international perspective. Psychiatr Ann 6:22–35, 1976

Sartorius N: Diagnosis and classification: cross-cultural and international perspectives. Ment Health Soc 5:79–85, 1978

Sartorius N: International perspectives of psychiatric classification. Br J Psychiatry Suppl 152:9–14, 1988

Sartorius N: Understanding the ICD-10 Classification of Mental Disorders. London, Science Press, 1995

Sartorius N: Fighting for Mental Health: A Personal View. West Nyack, NY, Cambridge University Press, 2002

Sartorius N, Schulze H: Reducing the Stigma of Mental Illness. Cambridge, UK, Cambridge University Press, 2005

Stengel E: Classification of mental disorders. Bull World Health Organ 21:601–663, 1959

World Health Organization: International Classification of Diseases, 8th Revision. Geneva, World Health Organization, 1967

World Health Organization: The ICD-10 Classification of Mental and Behavioural Disorders: Clinical Descriptions and Diagnostic Guidelines. Geneva, World Health Organization, 1992

PART II

INTEGRATING DIMENSIONAL CONCEPTS
INTO A CATEGORICAL SYSTEM

CHAPTER 5

A Proposal for Incorporating Clinically Relevant Dimensions Into DSM-5

John E. Helzer, M.D.

Revisions to the illness definitions contained in DSM-IV (American Psychiatric Association 1994) and DSM-IV-TR (American Psychiatric Association 2000) can be disruptive to clinical practice, because such revisions require widespread changes and adjustments. It can be argued that, by making cross-study comparisons more difficult, revisions impede scientific progress as well. Clear exceptions were the original DSM (American Psychiatric Association 1952), which codified diagnostic labels and helped define the scope of psychiatric attention, and DSM-III (American Psychiatric Association 1980), which, by providing explicit illness definitions, was a major advance both clinically and scientifically. DSM-III definitions now have been revised twice, and although there are some areas (such as personality disorders) that warrant major restructuring, many psychiatrists question whether there is enough new evidence at this point for significant revisions to most of the illness definitions. There are three ways DSM-5 could effect major improvements in psychiatric taxonomy. A first way would be to accomplish a change that has been discussed with every revision but never attempted—that is, officially acknowledge the continuous nature of psychiatric disorder and provide a consistent method of quantifying illness severity. A second way would be to create a set of instruments for ascertainment of clinical data necessary for making the diagnoses. A third way would be to structure DSM-5 so that questions about the timing, content, and relative value of any contemplated future revision can be answered empirically. In this chapter, I address all three options.

Advantages of Adding a Dimensional (Quantitative) Approach to DSM-5

A more quantitative approach to DSM categorical diagnoses has been a topic of discussion for many years. There would be multiple clinical and research advantages to officially recognizing the obvious continuous nature of psychiatric disorder and reflecting this reality in the psychiatric taxonomy. Clinically, a judgment about illness severity is crucial to responsible clinical care. At present, without guidance from DSM-IV, quantification of severity is largely a subjective judgment by the clinician. However, the ability to objectively quantify illness severity in a way that is relatively consistent across patients, clinicians, and time—and based on straightforward criteria—would have significant advantages over a subjective, individualized approach. An assessment of illness severity is fundamental for most treatment decisions, but the ability to quantify individual diagnoses more precisely also would help us avoid other problems that sometimes occur when diagnostic assessment is strictly dichotomous. As a clinician, I realize we sometimes overvalue certain "cardinal" symptoms in making a diagnosis. For example, a prominent and unusual psychotic symptom, such as a bizarre delusion, is sometimes accepted as evidence of schizophrenia. However, even bizarre diagnostic symptoms can present cross-sectionally in other illnesses, such as schizoaffective or delusional disorder (Pope and Lipinski 1978). A "conversion symptom," such as pseudoparalysis, is often considered tantamount to a somatoform illness but can also occur in major depression. Self-mutilation, often considered indicative of borderline personality disorder, can occur in many other illnesses (Simeon and Hollander 2001)

A dimensional taxonomy also has clear research advantages. Statistical power is significantly reduced when we are constrained to use a categorical classification. In an effort to better understand illness causation and discover effective interventions, most nondiagnostic variables, such as illness risk factors, are measured quantitatively. However, much of the statistical advantage of that quantification is lost because we have to fall back on a categorical designation for the diagnosis. Statistically, patients who fall below the categorical threshold are treated as though they fall into the same group, no matter how close to the threshold they may be. Those who are at, or just exceed, the threshold are treated the same diagnostically as those who are positive on every possible symptom. Ironically, in the process of evaluating multiple symptoms and the severity of each, a standard part of making a psychiatric diagnosis, we actually ascertain the information necessary for a dimensional quantification. However, because DSM is designed as a categorical system, quantitative data that are gathered routinely are discarded once the diagnosis is decided on. Simply preserving and systematically using the quantitative information we have ascertained to make a diagnosis would greatly increase statistical power. As a consequence of the increased power, smaller research samples become informative, which in turn increases the likelihood of discovering important causal and other associations. Maximizing statistical power is especially important as we attempt to better understand subtle polygenic, neurochemical, and environmental risk factors for psychiatric illness.

Potential Drawbacks to a Dimensional Approach in DSM-5

There are potential drawbacks of moving to a quantitative approach to diagnosis in DSM-5. First, it would represent a significant change in a classification system that has been in place for more than 50 years. This could result in confusion and resistance. However, each revision of DSM requires users to adjust to new definitions and approaches. Such adjustment was most notable in 1980, with the move from descriptive illness definitions to the much more explicit definitions used in that edition, a change that was resisted by many people at the time. Each such change requires a period of adaptation, but evolution in illness definition is important to undertake when it is reflective of new knowledge or offers a more powerful taxonomic tool.

A more important potential drawback to adding a quantitative option to DSM is the risk that it would result in the creation of two relatively independent diagnostic systems, one categorical and one quantitative. Having two relatively independent systems would be unfortunate and clearly could create significant diagnostic confusion. Some differences in diagnostic options between a categorical and a dimensional approach may be inevitable; the distinction between alcohol abuse and alcohol dependence is an example. There is growing doubt about the distinction between abuse and dependence, as currently defined in DSM-IV, on the basis of available data (Hasin and Grant 1994; Martin et al. 1995). A quantitative approach to the taxonomy of the alcohol use disorders reveals that some of the symptoms now listed as part of the alcohol abuse definition actually have a more severe prognosis than some of the dependence symptoms, whereas some symptoms included in the dependence definition are at the mild end of the severity spectrum (Saha et al. 2006). Thus, from a quantitative standpoint, alcohol use disorder appears to be a single illness continuum rather than two discrete syndromes.

However, from a categorical standpoint, there might be early indicators of increased risk for alcohol dependence that are important to identify and label categorically for purposes of increased vigilance and prevention efforts. There also might be political pressure from the field for the separate identification of high-risk states versus confirmed diagnoses. Thus, there might be a desire to preserve a categorical distinction between alcohol abuse and dependence, even though, quantitatively, the syndrome is found to be clearly unidimensional. However, as long as the categorical diagnoses and the corresponding dimensional scale are based on the same set of symptoms, there is little risk of creating two entirely different diagnostic systems. Although subject to empirical confirmation, it is probable that patients with a categorical diagnosis of alcohol abuse will have a lower score on the corresponding quantitative diagnostic scale than will other patients who meet criteria for alcohol dependence. The correspondence between a given scale score and a particular categorical diagnosis may not be exact, but this is of little consequence. On the other hand, if the diagnostic scale is based on a different set, or even a subset, of symptoms—for example, those considered more quantifiable—then there is a significant risk of having two diagnostic systems that do not correspond.

A third potential drawback to a dimensional classification is often phrased as "emphasizing research needs at the expense of clinical utility." As both clinician and investigator, I would argue that this is not the case. Clinicians benefit from a dimensional system, just as investigators do. Categorical diagnoses are a convenience for communication, for rapid comprehension of a clinical situation, and for initial treatment planning. However, even at the clinical level, once a categorical diagnosis has been rendered, most decisions are based on dimensional concepts, such as illness severity, level of comorbidity, and degree of treatment response. On the other hand, investigators also benefit from the availability of categories. If an investigator is studying the efficacy of a new treatment for major depression, it would be counterproductive to enroll patients who do not meet the categorical criteria for major depression in the clinical trial. Because both categorical and dimensional approaches have utility, it is important that a dimensional diagnosis is not seen as a replacement for the categorical but rather as a complementary enhancement to be employed when useful.

One way of minimizing the perception that a categorical system is being replaced by a dimensional one would be to approach the creation of the latter in such a way that it builds on, and relates to, the categorical system in a clear and understandable way. Although the creation of a dimensional scale is likely to involve a statistical process, it is important that it not be a conceptual black box. Clinicians and investigators should be able to understand easily both the conceptual foundation and the general process by which the concept was realized. It also helps to realize that when it was published in 1980, DSM-III was considered a radical break with clinical practice and one that favored research at the expense of clinical utility. However, within a short time this perception changed, and DSM-III is now considered to have been an important innovative diagnostic paradigm that both greatly benefited clinicians and led to significant advances in psychiatric research. DSM-III has become such a standard part of the clinical diagnostic landscape that it is hard for those trained since 1980 to conceive of how chaotic clinical psychiatry was prior to its creation. However, after two major revisions, 30 years of work, and considerable new knowledge generated in part by the availability of explicit diagnostic criteria, it is now time for another "radical" new taxonomic paradigm.

Optimization of the Transition to a Dimensional Component in DSM-5

Given that there are both advantages and potential drawbacks to creating a dimensional component in DSM-5, it is important to consider ways of maximizing advantages and minimizing drawbacks. First, it is important to accept that the DSM developmental process, in place for at least 30 years, will continue largely unchanged in DSM-5. This process begins with the appointment of a group of experts for each diagnostic area (the diagnostic work groups), charged with creating (or revising) criteria for the various diagnostic entities that fall within the areas of expertise of group members. Although these members consult data, wherever possible, they also are called on to apply their clinical experience and best judgment to create the illness definitions. In the final analysis, this is an hierarchical, top-down approach as opposed to an empirically derived, bottom-up approach to classification. Many people who see the value of a more quantitative classification system also would argue that the original diagnostic definitions should be based solely on empirical analysis of clinical data rather than be created by expert decree. This point of view is worth serious consideration and is discussed later, but for DSM-5, the illness definitions will be created by committees of experts. In my view, in order to preserve uniformity in approach, it is crucial that any dimensional alternative in DSM-5 conform to the top-down, categorical definitions the work groups create for DSM-5.

Second, it is important for psychiatrists who are committed to viewing diagnosis as a continuous measure to recognize both the necessity of categorical distinctions for clinical decision making and the utility of these distinctions for clinical communication. Diagnosis is a convention that permits splitting the broad universe of psychopathology into more discrete units. The divisions can seem arbitrary, but longitudinal research for up to 30 years has demonstrated the predictive validity of categorical definitions (Coryell and Tsuang 1985; Coryell et al. 2009). Conversely, it is important for those psychiatrists who value a categorical approach to acknowledge the legitimacy, and to recognize the added power, of a dimensional classification and its utility for clinical decision making, just as it enhances research efforts.

Third, it is important to recognize that in order to avoid the Babel of competing definitions for the same diagnostic construct, there must be a clear and simple correspondence between categorical and dimensional approaches, and this correspondence must be consistent across all relevant diagnoses. The most straightforward way of achieving this correspondence would be to base the dimensional quantification strictly on symptoms contained in each DSM-5 categorical definition. There are many continuous and quantifiable features on which a dimension could be based, including duration of illness, severity, level of impairment, and use of services. However, if there is to be a clear correspondence between dimensional and categorical definitions, the most logical dimension would be the number of positive-symptom items in the DSM-5 definition that a patient reports and the reported severity of those symptoms. This dimension most closely reflects the process clinicians and investigators customarily use in assessing illness states. Therefore, the continuous, dimensional measure that corresponds to a given categorical definition could be as simple as the sum of the positive symptom items. For reasons discussed later, simply summing the number of positive symptom items without considering the severity or the salience of an individual item is not advisable, but a more sophisticated continuous measure, which is based solely on DSM-5-defined symptoms, would have many advantages: 1) it is conceptually straightforward for all diagnoses; 2) it has great clinical utility for both clinical and research efforts; and 3) it is consistent across diagnoses. Finally, a severity dimension is likely to correlate well with other possible dimensions, although this latter assumption would have to be tested empirically.

There is a history of meticulous efforts to create dimensions for major diagnoses that has been independent of the DSM revision process. One worthwhile example is that by Wanberg and Horn (1983) for alcohol use disorders. These efforts typically begin with an assessment of a wide array of symptoms, behaviors, and environmental measures that are used to create an empirically derived diagnostic definition. Such an effort has much to recommend it, as discussed later in the comparison of top-down and bottom-up approaches to taxonomy. However, as also noted, our dimensionalization task at this point in time is to create continuous measures for diagnoses defined in DSM-5. A head-to-head comparison of top-down and bottom-up approaches to illness definition should be an agenda item for a possible future revision, and the efforts by Wanberg and Horn, and others, might be quite useful when that time arrives.

Creation of Dimensional Equivalents for DSM-5 Diagnoses

In this proposal, the initial step is for the diagnostic work groups to proceed as they always have in creating the phenomenological definitions, including the signs and symptoms to be ascertained and the number and pattern of these items necessary for categorical diagnoses. The next step would be for the work groups to specify simple severity scales for each criterion item. In the past, a minimal-severity threshold often has been implied or defined for specific symptoms. The difference here would be to make this threshold more explicit by scoring each symptom on a simple dimension. As an example, Helzer et al. (2008a) proposed a three-point severity scale (0, 1, 2) for each of the substance use disorder criterion items, with 0=symptom not present, 1=mild to moderate, and 2=severe. Guidance by the appropriate diagnostic work group would be necessary to define the aspect of each symptom to be quantified and how the three-level scale should be scored in each case. Using DSM-IV alcohol dependence as an example, a three-point scale for the first dependence criterion (alcohol tolerance) might logically be based on the amount of alcohol needed to produce an effect, the second DSM criterion (withdrawal) might be based on the severity of withdrawal symptoms, and the third criterion (greater consumption than intended) might be based on the frequency of its occurrence. Conceptually, however, a three-point scale for individual symptom items is straightforward and could work for all diagnoses. There would be clear advantages for patients and clinicians alike if symptoms were scored in a simple and consistent manner across diagnoses. There may be persuasive reasons to deviate from such simple consistency in symptom rating, but in the interest of cross-diagnostic consistency, it would seem appropriate for a decision in this regard to rest with the DSM-5 Task Force rather than with each work group.

Although scoring symptom severity is not a necessary step, it is desirable for two reasons. First, because it is an additive process: even a simple, three-point specification of severity at the symptom level significantly enhances the range of dimensionality at the diagnostic level. Second, clinicians intuitively recognize the necessity of evaluating the severity of each symptom a patient reports during an examination and using this information in their clinical decision making. The suggestion here is to create measurement guidelines so as to provide greater uniformity to this currently intuitive process and provide a scoring mechanism so that this quantitative information is not discarded once a diagnosis is made. Future research also would benefit from documenting symptom severity, because, for example, gene expression in behavioral disorders may occur at the symptom level (van Praag 1990).

The next step would be to use an appropriate statistical tool, such as item response theory (Embretson and Reise 2000), to define a dimensional scale for each diagnosis based on the criterion items. Simply adding the number of criterion items a given patient endorses as positive is one method of scaling but might not be advisable. Often two or more symptoms are highly intercorrelated, and adding them could overemphasize the underlying construct they measure. Some symptoms might have greater salience or importance than others; adding them with equal weight would introduce "noise."

Once a dimensional scale for a diagnosis has been created statistically, the final step would be to use another statistical tool, such as receiver operating characteristics (ROC; Fawcett 2006), to identify the scale score that most closely corresponds to the defined categorical diagnostic threshold in terms of the number of identified cases. An estimate of the score that best relates to the categorical diagnosis would help orient clinicians and investigators and help ensure concordance between the categorical and dimensional options (Helzer et al. 2008b). Final selection of the appropriate statistical tool(s) for creating a dimensional scale and relating it back to a categorical definition requires special expertise (Kiernan et al. 2001; Kraemer 1992). As part of the DSM-5 process, steps are being taken to ensure that appropriate statistical consultation is available to the work groups.

Advantages of Simplicity of Proposed Approach

The principal advantages of the approach just described are its simplicity and clinical utility. It adheres strictly to the categorical definitions created by the work groups so as to ensure consistency between the categorical and dimensional approaches. It is conceptually straightforward; understanding the statistical tools necessary to create the diagnostic score is not essential to understanding the concept. In addition, this approach does not increase the effort burden for either examiners or patients, because the necessary clinical data already are part of any routine examination. Clinicians and investigators are equally comfortable thinking in terms of both symptom and illness severity. Severity is a quantitative or "dimensional" concept, and an assessment of severity has always been necessary for both clinicians and investigators. Although categorical diagnoses are convenient for communication, anyone who routinely encounters patients thinks in terms of severity and ascertains the information required to make that quantitative assessment. However, categorical criteria do tend to restrict our thinking to those patients who fall above the diagnostic threshold. The clinician first asks: Does the patient meet the categorical criteria for the diagnosis? Only if the answer to this question is positive does he or she then go on to ask: How severe is it? The same quantitative thinking can and should be applied also to those who fall short of meeting the full diagnostic definition: How close do they come? In conducting a diagnostic interview, clinicians routinely gather the quantitative information necessary to place a patient on this full-spectrum continuum. Acknowledging and incorporating a quantitative approach into the criteria does not increase the clinical workload, it merely enables consistency across patients, just as DSM-III and its successive revisions have enabled consistency in ascertaining the categorical definition.

In summary, this proposal suggests a method for creating dimensional scaling for each diagnosis that is simple, preserves the traditional DSM work group function, does not increase the ascertainment burden for physicians or the response burden for patients, and bears a clear relationship to the categorical definition at both the criterion and the diagnostic level. This scaling would be a significant step forward, would enhance both clinical and scientific progress in psychiatry, and would ensure that DSM remains a vibrant, cutting-edge tool for the future. The next section also offers a suggestion for structuring DSM-5 so that it anticipates possible needs for DSM-6.

Issues Not Addressed by This Proposal

The multiplicity of DSM diagnoses and coding options is growing. One observer has noted that the number of coding options (categories multiplied by specifiers) for mood disorders has increased with each DSM revision, from fewer than 10 in DSM-I to more than 2,000 in DSM-IV. The number of diagnoses, per se, has increased monotonically with each revision: 95 disorders in the original DSM, 130 in DSM-II, 188 in DSM-III, 215 in DSM-III-R (American Psychiatric Association 1987), and 283 in DSM-IV. It hardly seems defensible that all these diagnostic distinctions have been tested against the time-honored criteria for diagnostic validity, as proposed by Robins and Guze (1970). The task of creating quantitative scores for such a panoply would be overwhelming. It also strains credibility, because many of these putative distinctions may lie on the same dimensional continuum. One issue for the task force and work groups is whether dimensions should be created only for the major diagnoses or, perhaps, for some minimal subset of diagnoses. A possible approach to this dilemma is discussed later in the final section on anticipating future taxonomic questions.

A second issue remaining is whether the American Psychiatric Association should consider creating a set of diagnostic tools that corresponds to DSM-5 criteria and what form such a set of tools might take. From my epidemiological perspective, the need for consistency in assessment is as obvious as the need for uniform diagnostic criteria. Since the Epidemiologic Catchment Area (ECA) survey of the 1980s (Robins and Regier 1991), national prevalence surveys based on DSM criteria have become popular worldwide. The World Mental Health surveys are the latest example (Kessler 1999). This is an ongoing, coordinated set of household surveys in which diagnostic criteria, assessment instrument, and study design are held constant. Sampling design is sufficiently similar across the approximately 20 participating countries and cultures that comparative prevalence rates can be estimated. Such cross-site coordination proved quite useful in understanding cross-national comparisons of alcohol use disorders based on replication of ECA methodology (Helzer and Canino 1992). However, although the World Mental Health surveys purported to use the Composite International Diagnostic Interview (Robins et al. 1988), revisions were made in the interview that render the survey data, in the case of some disorders, not comparable with data from many other population surveys that also utilized that instrument. One particularly problematic example in the World Mental Health survey was the decision to ask questions about alcohol dependence only in those respondents who reported at least one symptom of alcohol abuse. From previous work, it is estimated that this revision resulted in an underestimate of as much as 30% of alcohol dependence. Furthermore, it vitiates any comparison of the cross-national diagnostic structure of dependence. It is hoped that an official American Psychiatric Association diagnostic interview, specifically constructed for DSM-5 diagnostic criteria, would mitigate against instrument revisions unique to specific studies. I am pleased to report that the American Psychiatric Association has appointed an instrument advisory group to consider creating such a set of instruments that could meet the needs of a wide array of users, including primary care providers with little training in psychiatric and behavioral illness, practicing psychiatrists, highly specialized investigators, taxonomists interested in diagnostic structure, and epidemiologists, who use nonclinician interviewers for general population surveys.

An instrument-advisory group will have to address a number of difficult questions. First is how to create a set of instruments that meets the varying needs of such a diverse group of users in a way that information ascertainment is coordinated to avoid the potential noncomparability of data described earlier. This requirement implies creating a set of tools that sufficiently addresses the various informational needs so that end-users do not feel instrument alteration is necessary.

Another question is how to capitalize on the growing variety and availability of electronic tools to facilitate clinical data collection, scoring of categorical and dimensional diagnoses, and even treatment planning. As noted, a dimensional component will almost certainly require that clinical data be statistically manipulated in order to create a quantitative score. Because an electronic tool would be required to do the statistical analysis, it might make sense to use such a tool to gather symptom data in the first place.

A third question, crucial to confront but likely to raise sensitivities, is the role of the clinical expert in gathering basic symptom information. There are several options for gathering the primary symptom data on which DSM diagnoses are based: a trained clinician asking questions in a free-form interview; a clinician using a symptom checklist or semistructured interview as a guide; a non-clinician interviewer using a fully structured interview; or a patient responding to a self-administered questionnaire. It is often assumed that an open-ended examination by an experienced psychiatrist is the gold standard for a valid psychiatric diagnosis, but there is evidence this is not necessarily the case. In fact, the considerable evidence, from studies in the 1970s and before, of unacceptably low diagnostic reliability between experienced psychiatrists (Helzer et al. 1977) led to the development of semi- and fully structured diagnostic interviews, such as the Schedule for Affective Disorders and Schizophrenia (Endicott and Spitzer 1979), Structured Clinical Interview for DSM Disorders (Spitzer et al. 1992), and DSM Checklist (Hudziak et al. 1993) to guide clinician assessments. Nor is it clear that use of a semistructured interview as a guide is an adequate gold standard either. One piece of evidence that challenges this assumption derives from the ECA survey (Robins and Regier 1991), for which the highly structured Diagnostic Interview Schedule (DIS) was created to enable nonclinician "lay" interviewers to gather symptom data necessary to make DSM-III diagnoses. In two of the ECA sites, St. Louis, Missouri, and Baltimore, Maryland, a psychiatrist reexamination of selected respondents was mounted in order to test agreement between psychiatrist and lay interviewer DIS-derived diagnoses. At both sites, psychiatrists used a semistructured interview to guide their examinations. In both sites, there were significant differences in the estimated prevalence rates of specific disorders based on the lay results compared with estimated prevalences based on the psychiatrist interviews. The problem was that the psychiatrists' results went in opposite directions in the two sites—higher than the lay results for a given diagnosis in one site, but lower in the other. Because Baltimore and St. Louis are two American cities of similar size and demography, the expectation is that prevalence estimates of illness would be reasonably concordant, across the two sites, when assessed using the same study design. This is what occurred when prevalence estimates were based on the lay DIS interview. In contrast, prevalence estimates based on the psychiatrists' assessments in the two sites were quite discrepant. The most discrepant cross-site prevalence estimate, based on the lay assessment, was still more consistent than the least discrepant psychiatrist difference (Robins 1985).

One possible conclusion from this finding is that interposing clinician judgment in the ascertainment of primary symptom data actually introduces error variance. An alternative approach would be to ascertain symptom data directly from respondents, without the interposition of a second party. Perhaps the best method of ascertaining symptom information is a patient self-administered interview. Many studies, dating as far back as the 1970s, indicate that symptom data reported by patients directly to a computer are accurate compared with a psychiatrist examination (Card et al. 1974) and that, for socially sensitive behaviors, patients are both more comfortable (Perlis et al. 2004) and more candid (Lucas et al. 1977) in reporting positive symptoms to a computer. Other studies have confirmed a much greater degree of candor in reporting to other automated devices such as Interactive Voice Response. For example, Kobak et al. (1997) found that respondents endorsed twice as much alcohol consumption when reporting to an Interactive Voice Response compared with either face-to-face or telephone interviews with a clinician. Using patient self-administered interviews as a basis for interview instruments that correspond to DSM-5 criteria is an option that should receive serious consideration by the Instrument Advisory Group.

Anticipation of Future Taxonomic Questions

As argued earlier, incorporation of a dimensional component into DSM-5 and development of uniform assessment tools offer a sufficient rationale for undertaking a revision to diagnostic criteria. Another major taxonomic issue might offer an important rationale for a future revision. As noted, the diagnostic criteria in DSM have always been created through a top-down approach. Groups of recognized authorities consult the literature and their clinical knowledge to create illness definitions. A top-down approach offers illness definitions that correspond with clinical observation; the salience of the definitions to clinical work is immediately obvious; this facilitates clinical communication and diagnostic reliability. The potential weakness is that, to the extent expert clinicians impose their preconceived ideas onto the diagnostic definitions, the top-down approach ceases to be an empirical process. Judgments about what constitutes core clinical criteria for a specific diagnosis differ even among experts. Furthermore, clinical experience tends to be biased, because those patients who come to clinical attention are generally the more seriously ill and not necessarily representative of the entire spectrum of a disorder (Allardyce et al. 2008). Explicit categorical definitions based on clinical observation tend to be reliable, but deviating from an empirical process by imposing preconceptions on nature may constrain validity.

An alternative approach would be to create definitions in a totally empirical way, using a so-called bottom-up approach. Rather than relying on expert authority, diagnostic definitions would be created by submitting large amounts of clinical data from various clinical and population samples to appropriate statistical testing in order to determine how symptoms cluster in nature. The Child Behavior Checklist (Achenbach 1999) is a well-known example of a dimensionally scored, bottom-up diagnostic system. Recent research has explored the relationships between DSM-IV diagnostic categories and comparable Child Behavior Checklist dimensions (Achenbach et al. 2005). An analysis of bottom-up checklist data from 39 cultures worldwide found dramatic uniformity of syndromal expression across groups that are highly dissimilar socially (Ivanova et al. 2007). The Spectrum Project (Cassano et al. 2004; Frank et al. 1998; Maser and Akiskal 2002; Maser and Patterson 2002) is an example of a bottom-up enhancement of DSM-IV, for adult diagnoses (see Chapter 3, this volume). Empirically derived definitions may correspond more closely to biologically and environmentally based etiologies. A bottom-up approach also permits a more complete probe of the underlying "latent" structure of disorders. This could be of importance in dealing with the diagnostic multiplicity problem mentioned earlier. A bottom-up approach also is likely to help address the issue of diagnostic proliferation mentioned earlier. There is an ongoing debate between diagnostic "lumpers" and "splitters" in psychiatric taxonomy. Experimentation with an empirically based bottom-up approach to diagnosis could help to clarify greatly where we should be drawing diagnostic lines.

Which of these approaches—top-down, bottom-up, or some combination of the two—would generate diagnostic definitions with the best construct and predictive diagnostic validity is an issue that should be explored prior to any further revision of DSM. Because such exploration would require several years to accomplish, DSM-5 assessment tools should be structured in a way that would make it possible to explore and compare top-down and bottom-up approaches so we can capitalize on what is learned and, it is hoped, improve diagnostic validity (Kendler 1990; Robins and Guze 1970). If a bottom-up approach could be shown to generate a significant increase in diagnostic validity, this would provide sufficient empirical justification for a DSM-6.

References

Achenbach TM: The Child Behavior Checklist and related instruments, in The Use of Psychological Testing for Treatment Planning and Outcomes Assessment, 2nd Edition. Edited by Maruish ME. Hillsdale, NJ, Erlbaum, 1999, pp 429–466

Achenbach TM, Bernstein A, Dumenci L: DSM-oriented scales and statistically based syndromes for ages 18 to 59: linking taxonomic paradigms to facilitate multitaxonomic approaches (see comment). J Pers Assess 84:49–63, 2005

Allardyce J, Suppes T, van Os J: Dimensions and the psychosis phenotype, in Dimensional Approaches in Diagnostic Classification: Refining the Research Agenda for DSM-V. Edited by Helzer J, Kraemer HC, Krueger RF, et al. Arlington, VA, American Psychiatric Association, 2008, pp 53–63

American Psychiatric Association: Diagnostic and Statistical Manual: Mental Disorders. Washington, DC, American Psychiatric Association, 1952

American Psychiatric Association: Diagnostic and Statistical Manual of Mental Disorders, 3rd Edition. Washington, DC, American Psychiatric Association, 1980

American Psychiatric Association: Diagnostic and Statistical Manual of Mental Disorders, 3rd Edition, Revised. Washington, DC, American Psychiatric Association, 1987

American Psychiatric Association: Diagnostic and Statistical Manual of Mental Disorders, 4th Edition. Washington, DC, American Psychiatric Association, 1994

American Psychiatric Association: Diagnostic and Statistical Manual of Mental Disorders, 4th Edition, Text Revision. Washington, DC, American Psychiatric Association, 2000

Card WI, Nicholson M, Crean GP, et al: A comparison of doctor and computer interrogation of patients. Int J Biomed Comput 5:175–187, 1974

Cassano GB, Rucci P, Frank E, et al: The mood spectrum in unipolar and bipolar disorder: arguments for a unitary approach. Am J Psychiatry 161:1264–1269, 2004

Coryell W, Tsuang MT: Major depression with mood-congruent or mood-incongruent psychotic features: outcome after 40 years. Am J Psychiatry 142:479–482, 1985

Coryell W, Solomon D, Leon A, et al: Does major depressive disorder change with age? Psychol Med 19:1–7, 2009

Embretson SE, Reise SP: Item Response Theory for Psychologists. Mahwah, NJ, Erlbaum, 2000

Endicott J, Spitzer RL: Use of the Research Diagnostic Criteria and the Schedule for Affective Disorders and Schizophrenia to study affective disorders. Am J Psychiatry 136:52–56, 1979

Fawcett T: An introduction to ROC analysis. Pattern Recognit Lett 27:861–874, 2006

Frank E, Cassano GB, Shear MK, et al: The spectrum model: a more coherent approach to the complexity of psychiatric symptomatology. CNS Spectr 3:23–34, 1998

Hasin DS, Grant B: Nosological comparisons of DSM-III-R and DSM-IV alcohol abuse and dependence in a clinical facility: comparison with the 1988 National Health Interview Survey results. Alcohol Clin Exp Res 18:272–279, 1994

Helzer JE, Canino GJ (eds): Alcoholism in North America, Europe, and Asia. New York, Oxford University Press, 1992

Helzer J, Robins LN, Taibleson M, et al: Reliability of psychiatric diagnosis, I: a methodological review. Arch Gen Psychiatry 34:129–133, 1977

Helzer JE, Bucholz KK, Gossop M: A dimensional option for the diagnosis of substance dependence in DSM-V, in Dimensional Approaches in Diagnostic Classification: Refining the Research Agenda for DSM-V. Edited by Helzer J, Kraemer HC, Krueger RF, et al. Washington, DC, American Psychiatric Publishing, 2008a, pp 19–34

Helzer JE, Wittchen HU, Krueger RF, et al: Dimensional options for DSM-V: the way forward, in Dimensional Approaches in Diagnostic Classification: Refining the Research Agenda for DSM-V. Edited by Helzer J, Kraemer HC, Krueger RF, et al. Washington, DC, American Psychiatric Publishing, 2008b, pp 115–127

Hudziak J, Helzer JE, Wetzel MW, et al: The use of the DSM-III-R Checklist for initial diagnostic assessments. Compr Psychiatry 34:375–383, 1993

Ivanova MY, Dobrean A, Dopfner M, et al: Testing the 8-syndrome structure of the child behavior checklist in 30 societies. J Clin Child Adolesc Psychol 36:405–417, 2007

Kendler KS: Toward a scientific psychiatric nosology: strengths and limitations. Arch Gen Psychiatry 47:969–973, 1990

Kessler RC: The World Health Organization International Consortium in Psychiatric Epidemiology (ICPE): initial work and future directions—the NAPE Lecture 1998. Nordic Association for Psychiatric Epidemiology. Acta Psychiatr Scand 99:2–9, 1999

Kiernan M, Kraemer HC, Winkleby MA, et al: Do logistic regression and signal detection identify different subgroups at risk? Implications for the design of tailored interventions. Psychol Methods 6:35–48, 2001

Kobak KA, Taylor LH, Dottl SL, et al: Computerized screening for psychiatric disorders in an outpatient community mental health clinic. Psychiatr Serv 48:1048–1057, 1997

Kraemer HC: Evaluating Medical Tests: Objective and Quantitative Guidelines. Newbury Park, CA, Sage, 1992

Lucas RW, Mullin PJ, Luna CB, et al: Psychiatrists and a computer as interrogators of patients with alcohol-related illnesses: a comparison. Br J Psychiatry 131:160–167, 1977

Martin CS, Kaczynski NA, Maisto SA, et al: Patterns of DSM-IV alcohol abuse and dependence symptoms in adolescent drinkers. J Stud Alcohol 56:672–680, 1995

Maser JD, Akiskal H: Spectrum concepts in major mental disorders. Psychiatr Clin North Am 25:xi–xiii, 2002

Maser JD, Patterson T: Spectrum and nosology: implications for DSM-V. Psychiatr Clin North Am 25:855–885, 2002

Perlis TE, Des Jarlais DC, Friedman SR, et al: Audio-computerized self-interviewing versus face-to-face interviewing for research data collection at drug abuse treatment programs. Addiction 99:885–896, 2004

Pope HG Jr, Lipinski JF Jr: Diagnosis in schizophrenia and manic-depressive illness: a reassessment of the specificity of "schizophrenic" symptoms in the light of current research. Arch Gen Psychiatry 35:811–828, 1978

Robins E, Guze SB: Establishment of diagnostic validity in psychiatric illness: its application to schizophrenia. Am J Psychiatry 126:983–987, 1970

Robins LN: Epidemiology: reflections on testing the validity of psychiatric interviews. Arch Gen Psychiatry 42:918–924, 1985

Robins LN, Regier DA (eds): Psychiatric Disorders in America. New York, Free Press, 1991

Robins LN, Wing J, Wittchen HU, et al: The Composite International Diagnostic Interview: an epidemiologic instrument suitable for use in conjunction with different diagnostic systems and in different cultures. Arch Gen Psychiatry 45:1069–1077, 1988

Saha TD, Chou SP, Grant BF: Toward an alcohol use disorder continuum using item response theory: results from the National Epidemiologic Survey on Alcohol and Related Conditions. Psychol Med 36:931–941, 2006

Simeon D, Hollander E (eds): Self-Injurious Behaviors: Assessment and Treatment. Washington, DC, American Psychiatric Press, 2001

Spitzer RL, Williams JB, Gibbon M, et al: The Structured Clinical Interview for DSM-III-R (SCID), I: history, rationale, and description. Arch Gen Psychiatry 49:624–629, 1992

van Praag HM: Two-tier diagnosing in psychiatry. Psychiatry Res 34:1–11, 1990

Wanberg KW, Horn JL: Assessment of alcohol use with multidimensional concepts and measures. Am Psychol 38:1055–1069, 1983

CHAPTER 6

Empirically Derived Personality Disorder Prototypes

Bridging Dimensions and Categories in DSM-5

Robert F. Krueger, Ph.D.
Nicholas R. Eaton, M.A.
Susan C. South, Ph.D.
Lee Anna Clark, Ph.D.
Leonard J. Simms, Ph.D.

The clinical relevance of personality has been acknowledged in modern editions of the *Diagnostic and Statistical Manual of Mental Disorders* (DSM)—that is, DSM-III through DSM-IV-TR (American Psychiatric Association 1980, 1987, 1994, 2000)—by the existence of Axis II. The creation of Axis II served as a key impetus to a flourishing of interest in personality disorders (Blashfield and Intoccia 2000). For any given patient, a clinician can record not only the current clinical diagnosis on Axis I but also personality disorder or relevant features on Axis II. Nevertheless, the conceptualization of personality disorder in modern editions of DSM, in terms of putatively categorical and categorically distinct disorders, has notable limitations. These limitations have been described at length elsewhere and include factors such as extensive comorbidity, symptom overlap, heterogeneous presentations, unreliability, and lack of validity or treatment utility for some personality disorders (Clark 2007; Jablensky 2002; Livesley 2003; Millon 2002; Tyrer 2007). As a result of these limitations, there is "notable dissatisfaction with the current conceptualization and definition of the DSM-IV-TR" (First et al. 2002, p. 124).

Two authors of this chapter, Drs. Krueger and Clark, are members of the DSM-5 Personality and Personality Disorders Work Group. This chapter represents some current thinking, on the part of these and the other authors of this contribution, about key directions to pursue as we work toward DSM-5. The chapter does not represent the official position of the DSM-5 Personality and Personality Disorders Work Group, nor can we predict with confidence the exact conceptualization of personality and personality disorder that will be included in DSM-5. Nevertheless, we describe here some ideas that have emerged in our recent collaborative research. Our hope is that these ideas may prove useful as we strive for an approach in DSM-5 that aims to overcome some of the limitations of DSM-IV.

Personality Prototypes as Configurations of Traits: Empirical Possibilities

Dimensional models of personality and personality disorder have been considered for previous editions of DSM but were not adopted, for a variety of reasons. Widiger et al. (2005) summarized proceedings of the December 2004 American Psychiatric Institute for Research and Education–sponsored pre-DSM-5 meeting on personality disorders, at which harmonization of various trait-classification systems was a major topic.

One major concern has been the plethora of trait-classification systems articulated. Fortunately, this concern has been addressed empirically. Specific traits and broad trait domains posited in various systems have been modeled together to see how these systems relate to one another. When this is done, various trait-classification systems line up fairly neatly and clearly, converging on broad domains of 1) emotional dysregulation/negative affect, 2) introversion, 3) antagonism, and 4) irresponsibility. Recent work, which augments existing personality disorder trait batteries with indices of DSM-IV Cluster A (e.g., schizotypal) personality disorder characteristics, has demonstrated that a complete system also should include a fifth domain of peculiarity/oddity (Harkness and McNulty 2006; Tackett et al. 2008; Watson et al. 2008).

Based on this literature, our view is that the field has progressed to the point where data now obviate concerns about "which dimensional model has empirical support" in terms of the broad, overarching domains of an empirically derived system. Also of note is the way in which these domains confer risk for development of multiple Axis I mental disorders: patterns of comorbidity among common mental disorders correspond closely with the underlying structure of personality-based risk for these conditions (Krueger and Markon 2006; Krueger and Tackett 2006).

However, a key clinical concern in implementing a dimensional system for personality in a diagnostic manual pertains to applying broad trait domains to specific patients. Broad domains, such as emotional dysregulation/negative affect, are critical organizational constructs, but they are somewhat abstract in terms of the conceptualization of a specific patient. Moving down to the level of specific facets (e.g., self-harming tendencies as a specific facet of emotional dysregulation/negative affect) enhances the richness and fidelity of case conceptualization for clinical application but increases the complexity of the system. A complex and detailed facet-level trait system, although psychologically richer, may prove to be prohibitive for routine clinical application.

In work described in this chapter, we have considered a potential empirical means of bridging the richness of a detailed system of trait description and the need to apply that system to specific patients. Research that converges on the aforementioned "abnormal five domains" focuses on ways in which variables are associated with one another when used as descriptors of people. This work is "variable-centered" (Block 1971), whereas newer statistical technologies allow rigorous modeling of how people tend to be distributed in a space delineated by a specific set of variables, thus allowing a "person-centered" approach to modeling personality data. The idea of studying personality in a person-centered way is by no means novel; a number of major personality theorists have explored this approach (e.g., Asendorpf 2006; Block 1971; Caspi 1998; Hart et al. 2003; Magnusson 1998; Pulkkinen 1996; Robins and Tracy 2003; van Leeuwen et al. 2004), including its utility for conceptualizing personality in clinical settings (Westen et al. 2006). Person-centered, model-based approaches also have utility in parsing heterogeneity within existing personality disorder constructs, such as borderline personality disorder (Lenzenweger et al. 2008).

A novel feature of the work presented here is the application of a person-centered, model-based approach to form a bridge between dimensional and categorical conceptualizations of normal and abnormal personality. Specifically, our modeling approach began with 15 fine-grained dimensions of an assessment instrument—the Schedule for Nonadaptive and Adaptive Personality (SNAP; Clark 1993)—that clearly delineate the major dimensions spanning normal and abnormal personality. We took a new approach to modeling the SNAP by applying model-based clustering (mixture modeling) to an extensive SNAP database. This approach allowed us to go beyond the modal structural question in the literature: "how are the variables delineated by an instrument or set of instruments (e.g., the SNAP) associated with each other?" Specifically, using model-based clustering we were able to ask: "How do people tend to be distributed in the space delineated by the SNAP dimensions? Can we identify meaningful and distinguishable groups of people? Could these groups serve as empirically derived, clinically applicable personality prototypes?"

Method

Participants

The total sample (N=8,690) of this study was composed of 24 subsamples of participants, all of whom had completed the SNAP previously. These subsamples included clinical patients (25% of total sample), college students (35.8%), community participants (9.3%), and military recruits (29.9%; see Table 6–1 for more detail and citations for component samples). The total sample was 52.9% female (gender data were missing for three participants). Participants self-identified as Caucasian (65.9%), African American (8.3%), and other (9.4%; ethnicity data were missing for 16.4% of participants). Participants ranged in age from 17 to 85 years (mean=26.7 years; SD=10.47; 1% missing).

Assessment

SNAP is a 375-item self-report personality questionnaire comprising 15 empirically derived facet-level dimensions of normal and pathological personality: 1) Negative Temperament, 2) Mistrust, 3) Manipulativeness, 4) Aggression, 5) Self-Harm, 6) Eccentric Perceptions, 7) Dependency, 8) Positive Temperament, 9) Exhibitionism, 10) Entitlement, 11) Detachment, 12) Disinhibition, 13) Impulsivity, 14) Propriety, and 15) Workaholism. The psychometric properties of the SNAP are strong and have been described previously (Clark 1993).

TABLE 6–1. Description of samples included in total data set ($N = 8{,}690$)

SAMPLE TYPE	N	SAMPLE DESCRIPTION	SOURCES
College	1,888	Undergraduates collected at Southern Methodist University and University of Iowa	Casillas and Clark 2002; Clark et al. 2009; Harlan and Clark 1999; Ready et al. 2000, 2001; Wu and Clark 2003
	1,223	Undergraduates collected at University of Virginia	Oltmanns and Turkheimer 2006
Military	2,026	Air Force cadets in basic training	Oltmanns and Turkheimer 2006
	572	Gulf War veterans	Simms et al. 2005
Community	173	Adoptees collected by Department of Psychiatry, University of Iowa	Cadoret and Langbehn, unpublished raw data
	636	Community adults collected in Dallas, TX, Minneapolis/St. Paul, MN, and Iowa City, IA	Clark et al. 2009; Vittengl et al. 1999
Patient	1,458	Mixed-patient samples collected in Dallas, TX, and Iowa City, IA	Casillas et al., manuscript under review; Clark et al. 2003; Clark et al. 2009; Ready and Clark 2002; Reynolds and Clark 2001; Vittengl et al. 1999
	714	Patients in Collaborative Longitudinal Personality Disorder Study	Morey et al. 2003

Data Analysis

We utilized finite-mixture modeling to determine whether participants fell into distinct clusters, defined by multivariate distributions of scores on the SNAP's 15 personality dimensions. The
MCLUST (Version 3) software package (Fraley and Raftery 2007)—in
the statistical language R—made it possible for us to conduct a model-
based cluster analysis. This type of analysis estimates the optimal
number of groups (i.e., clusters) of individuals necessary to account
for personality-scale data patterns in the total sample. In addition to
the *number* of clusters, this analysis allowed us to determine whether
these clusters have the same volume, shape, and orientation in geometric space. Finally, the mean vector and covariance matrix were
estimated for each of the 15 SNAP scales for each personality disorder
cluster identified.

We fit six models, each of which was computed with one to nine
clusters, to the data. The six models differed in the degree to which
they constrained the volumes, shapes, and orientations of the clusters. Table 6–2 gives cluster characteristics of each of these six models. For example, Table 6–2 shows that Model 1 constrains all clusters
to be spherical in shape and equal in volume. The volume of each
cluster corresponds with the size of the cluster in multivariate space
and indexes the heterogeneity of the cluster. That is, individuals in
a small cluster are all more similar to one another than are those
who are members of a larger cluster. The shape of each cluster relates
to the relative magnitudes of the covariance-matrix eigenvalues
within clusters and indexes the relative variability of individuals
along the variables that define the cluster. Thus, for example, in a
two-variable cluster, the more elongated the cluster shape, the more
widely individuals are dispersed on one variable compared with
their dispersal on the other. The orientation of each cluster relates
to the eigenvectors of the covariance matrix and indexes how the
cluster relates to the orienting axes.

Figure 6–1 provides a visual depiction of these characteristics for
a hypothetical analysis. In this example, participants' responses on
two variables (X and Y) have been cluster analyzed, yielding a four-
cluster solution (i.e., clusters A, B, C, and D). Cluster A, for example,
represents a highly homogeneous group of individuals who all have
low scores on variable X and high scores on variable Y. With regard
to volume, Cluster A has the smallest volume, Clusters B and D have
similar volumes, and Cluster C has the largest volume, meaning
that in terms of homogeneity of the clusters, A>B, B>C, and so on.
With regard to shape, Cluster A is circular, whereas Clusters B, C,
and D are elliptical, meaning that individuals are equally dispersed
along both of the traits in Cluster A but are more dispersed along
one trait than the other in the remaining three clusters. With regard
to orientation, Clusters C and D have similar orientations, which differ

TABLE 6–2. Bayesian information criterion (BIC) values for fitted models

	Cluster Characteristics			Number of Clusters								
Model	Shape	Volume	Orientation	1	2	3	4	5	6	7	8	9
1	Spherical	Equal	NA	−763,232	−737,715	−729,896	−724,941	−720,497	−716,794	−715,028	−713,091	−712,237
2	Spherical	Varies	NA	−763,232	−733,426	−726,854	−720,539	−716,358	−712,324	−710,752	−708,170	−707,048
3	Ellipsoidal	Equal	Equal	−694,125	−693,569	−690,178	−689,174	−689,151	−687,522	−687,309	−686,518	−686,729
4	Ellipsoidal	Equal	Varies	−694,125	−688,285	−687,911	−686,437	−686,608	−686,469	−686,072	−686,660	−686,242
5	Ellipsoidal	Varies	Varies	−694,125	−683,001	−681,091	−680,861	−679,687	−679,363	**−679,235**	−679,734	−679,579
6	Varies	Varies	Varies	−694,125	−681,877	−679,647	−679,496	—	—	—	—	—

Note. Numerical table entries represent BIC values; value indicating best model fit is in bold. The six models are ordered by parsimony, with Model 1 being most parsimonious. Models could involve clusters shaped either as spheres, ellipses, or a combination of both (i.e., "Varies"). Estimated volume of clusters could be either equal (i.e., all clusters have same volume) or variable across clusters. Orientation also could be equal or variable across clusters.

NA=orientation not estimated due to spherical cluster shape. Em dashes for Model 6 indicate that models with five or more clusters could not be estimated in this analysis. All BIC values were rounded to nearest whole number.

from that of Cluster B. Specifically, cluster members' scores on variables X and Y are positively correlated within Clusters C and D, negatively correlated in Cluster B, and uncorrelated in Cluster A, which, being circular, has no orientation. For additional information related to these characteristics, and the use of model-based cluster analysis in personality (psychopathy) in general, see, for example, Hicks et al. (2004).

The optimal properties of number, volume, shape, and orientation for personality disorder subtypes were determined by comparison of Bayesian information criteria (BIC) goodness-of-fit statistics. More favorable BIC values were assigned to models that 1) account better for the observed data and 2) minimize the number of estimated parameters (i.e., more parsimonious models). As each model tested yields a unique BIC value, the BIC values of all models can be compared simultaneously to determine which model is optimal. In MCLUST, BIC values that are less negative—in other words, BIC values closer to zero—indicate a better fit. A difference of 10 between two BIC values indicates the odds are 150:1 that the model with the BIC closer to zero is the better fitting of the two models (Raftery 1995). Once the optimal number and characteristics of clusters have been ascertained by model comparison, each participant is assigned membership to the most probable cluster based on his or her responses on the SNAP. A measure of uncertainty is calculated for each participant, which indicates the degree of confidence that the participant is a "true member" of the cluster to which he or she is assigned.

Results

BIC values resulting from the cluster analysis are presented numerically in Table 6–2 and graphically in Figure 6–2. The best-fitting model had a BIC value of –679,235 (shown in bold type in Table 6–2) and consisted of seven ellipsoidal clusters with variable volumes and orientations. The second-best-fitting model was similar but had one fewer cluster (BIC=–679,363). The magnitude of difference between these two BIC values indicated that the seven-cluster model was the optimal model, although the six-cluster model was slightly more parsimonious. Although a few BIC values for Model 6 could not be estimated in this analysis, several conclusions can be drawn from the results: 1) numerous subpopulations exist in these data; 2) seven clusters provide the best fit; and 3) these clusters are ellipsoidal and have different volumes and orientations in geometric space.

Once the optimal model was identified, posterior probabilities of membership in each of the seven clusters were calculated for every participant. Each participant was then assigned to the cluster with the

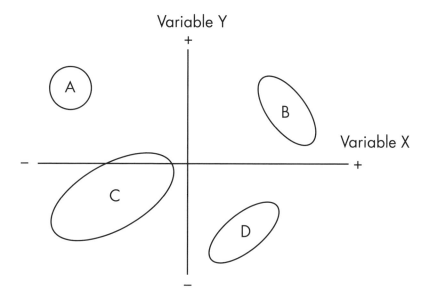

FIGURE 6–1. Hypothetical example of a four-cluster solution on two variables (X and Y).

highest posterior probability of membership for him or her. However, these cluster assignments were associated with varying degrees of uncertainty inversely related to the size of the posterior probabilities. For example, if an individual's posterior probability of membership in a particular cluster was near 1.0, the level of uncertainty associated with her assignment to this cluster was small (approaching zero). If an individual's posterior probabilities of membership in two clusters were both near 0.5, the level of uncertainty associated with her final assignment to a cluster was near 0.5 (i.e., the assignment to one cluster instead of the other was barely more certain than chance). The seven clusters were associated with somewhat varying levels of average assignment uncertainty, as can be seen in Table 6–3, which ranged from 0.127 (Cluster 6) to 0.227 (Cluster 7). These results indicate that although clusters differed somewhat in the average certainty with which their members were assigned, even the highest average assignment uncertainty was less than 25%.

The seven clusters that emerged from our analyses differed markedly in sizes and demographic compositions (see Table 6–4). The least populated cluster (Cluster 5; n=865) had nearly half as many members as the most populous cluster (Cluster 2; n=1,677). Clusters tended to be composed of slightly more females, with Cluster 5 having the highest percentage of female members (approximately 60%),

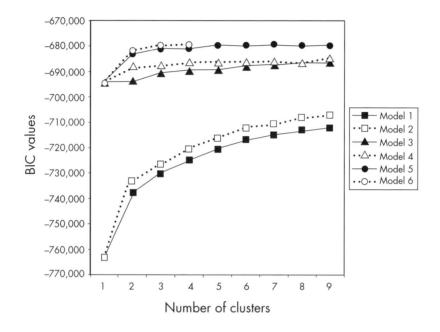

FIGURE 6–2.　Bayesian information criteria (BIC) values for the six fitted models with one to nine clusters.

TABLE 6–3.　Average assignment uncertainty for group members of each cluster

	UNCERTAINTY	
CLUSTER	MEAN	SD
1	0.210	0.177
2	0.149	0.169
3	0.208	0.173
4	0.190	0.176
5	0.181	0.165
6	0.127	0.156
7	0.227	0.174

and the average age of cluster members varied from 22 years (Cluster 3) to 29 years (Cluster 2).

Clusters also differed in the proportion of their members that came from patient, college, community, and military samples (Table 6–4). Clusters 2 and 5 were predominantly composed of patients, whereas Clusters 3, 4, and 6 had few patient members. College students made up the majority of members in Cluster 3; military recruits accounted for 61% of Cluster 4 and more than half of Cluster 6. Only Clusters 1 and 7 did not have a majority of members from a patient, college, community, or military sample. The largest subpopulation of Cluster 1 was college students (45.7%), whereas Cluster 7 showed a plurality of college students (37.9%) as well as notable percentages of military (27.8%) and patient (26.6%) members.

The seven clusters each had different configurations of SNAP-scale means. We transformed the SNAP scales for the total sample into T scores for the subsequent discussion. SNAP profiles for the clusters are presented in Figure 6–3; for ease of presentation, the clusters have been separated into three graphs with identical axes to facilitate comparison. Table 6–5 reports means and standard deviations for the clusters on each SNAP scale. Clusters differed markedly in their scale means and standard deviations as well as patterns of elevations across scales. To facilitate interpretation and comparison of these somewhat complex profiles, T scores that are one-half standard deviation greater than or less than the full sample mean of 50 (i.e., <45 or >55) are bolded in Table 6–5, and those >55 are bolded *and* underlined. Each cluster also was assigned an informal label to aid in conceptualizing its members.

Cluster 1 (*n*=1,374; 46% college students, 24% military recruits) showed no scales elevated above 55, but four scales fell below 45: Mistrust, Aggression, Self-Harm, and Eccentric Perceptions. Because most SNAP scales resulted in higher scores for increased pathology, these low scores indicate that Cluster 1 individuals showed *lower* levels of Mistrust, Aggression, Self-Harm, and Eccentric Perceptions, on average, than did individuals in the total sample. The relatively low standard deviations of these four scales also indicate that individuals in Cluster 1 tended not to vary much around this cluster's low scale averages. One might label this cluster as "normal or typical personality."

Individuals in Cluster 2 (*n*=1,677; 53% patients, 29% college students) showed increased levels of Negative Temperament, Self-Harm, Dependency, and Detachment and decreased levels of Positive Temperament. This cluster can be informally conceptualized as "distressed-dependent."

Individuals in Cluster 3 (*n*=1,196; 61% college students, 27% military recruits) reported high levels of Positive Temperament, Exhibitionism, and Entitlement coupled with low levels of Self-Harm and Detachment. Given the SNAP profile for this cluster, the young

TABLE 6–4. Demographic characteristics of clusters

Cluster	n	Females, %	Mean Age (SD)	Cluster members by sample type, %			
				Patient	College	Community	Military
1	1,374	51.1	26.9 (11.3)	14.1	45.7	16.2	23.9
2	1,677	54.7	29.2 (10.8)	52.5	29.4	5.8	12.3
3	1,196	52.8	22.1 (7.4)	5.0	60.6	7.5	26.8
4	1,288	52.0	25.8 (9.7)	7.6	21.8	9.5	61.0
5	865	59.9	28.8 (10.2)	59.3	26.6	3.8	10.3
6	961	52.2	27.6 (11.9)	7.7	26.0	14.6	51.7
7	1,329	49.0	26.1 (9.8)	26.6	37.9	7.8	27.8

TABLE 6–5. Schedule for Nonadaptive and Adaptive Personality (SNAP) scale means (and standard deviations) of each cluster

				CLUSTER			
SNAP SCALE MEASURE	1	2	3	4	5	6	7
Negative Temperament	45.2 (7.6)	**55.8** (6.9)	48.1 (8.5)	46.7 (7.6)	**65.0** (2.6)	**38.1** (3.9)	51.4 (8.2)
Mistrust	**41.8** (4.4)	53.0 (8.7)	47.0 (7.3)	51.9 (8.1)	**64.3** (6.7)	**40.0** (3.6)	53.5 (8.9)
Manipulativeness	45.6 (5.7)	54.0 (10.1)	54.4 (9.2)	43.6 (4.6)	**58.6** (11.3)	**41.0** (3.2)	52.7 (9.6)
Aggression	**44.4** (4.0)	53.4 (10.1)	50.6 (7.7)	**44.9** (4.2)	**60.0** (12.1)	**41.8** (2.2)	**55.3** (11.2)
Self-Harm	**44.3** (2.7)	**59.6** (9.6)	**44.4** (2.8)	**44.1** (2.6)	**64.8** (11.4)	**42.5** (1.2)	50.4 (6.1)
Eccentric Perceptions	**42.6** (4.4)	50.9 (9.5)	51.4 (8.7)	51.4 (9.0)	**59.7** (10.4)	**41.9** (4.2)	53.5 (10.4)
Dependency	49.5 (9.3)	**57.4** (10.5)	49.0 (8.3)	46.2 (6.0)	**58.9** (11.6)	**44.5** (5.6)	**44.0** (5.1)
Positive Temperament	48.4 (8.3)	**42.3** (10.0)	**58.1** (4.2)	**55.4** (5.9)	**43.2** (10.5)	**56.4** (4.9)	48.7 (9.6)
Exhibitionism	47.5 (8.4)	46.5 (9.5)	**59.2** (7.4)	49.7 (9.4)	47.2 (10.6)	51.1 (8.9)	50.0 (9.9)
Entitlement	47.0 (8.4)	46.7 (10.5)	**55.1** (8.9)	52.8 (8.9)	47.1 (11.5)	50.0 (8.0)	51.9 (10.0)
Detachment	46.8 (7.0)	**55.8** (9.8)	**42.2** (4.1)	48.9 (8.1)	**58.5** (10.2)	**41.3** (3.5)	54.9 (9.6)
Disinhibition	46.5 (7.0)	52.5 (9.6)	54.1 (9.1)	**43.3** (5.4)	**57.6** (10.4)	**41.8** (4.8)	54.3 (10.6)
Impulsivity	48.0 (8.0)	53.4 (9.9)	53.8 (9.8)	**42.7** (4.9)	**56.6** (10.0)	**41.8** (4.9)	53.0 (10.2)
Propriety	47.2 (9.8)	47.9 (9.8)	48.3 (9.3)	**58.1** (5.7)	49.6 (10.1)	53.9 (8.2)	46.8 (10.5)
Workaholism	46.4 (9.3)	49.0 (10.5)	48.2 (8.6)	**55.4** (8.4)	53.2 (11.3)	49.8 (8.3)	49.5 (10.2)

Note. Means that are more extreme than one-half standard deviation from *T* score mean (i.e., <45 or >55) are bolded; those bolded that are *T* score > 55 are also underlined.

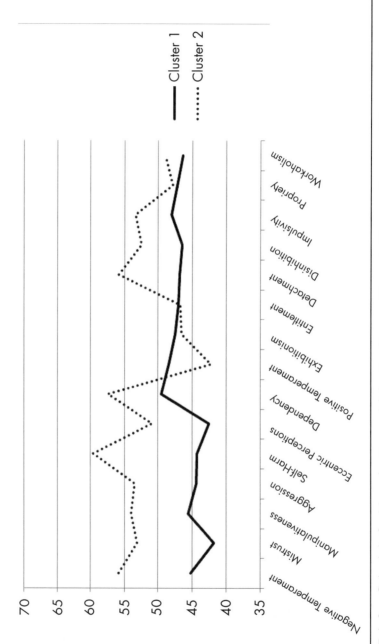

FIGURE 6–3.   Schedule for Nonadaptive and Adaptive Personality scale *T* scores for each of the seven clusters.

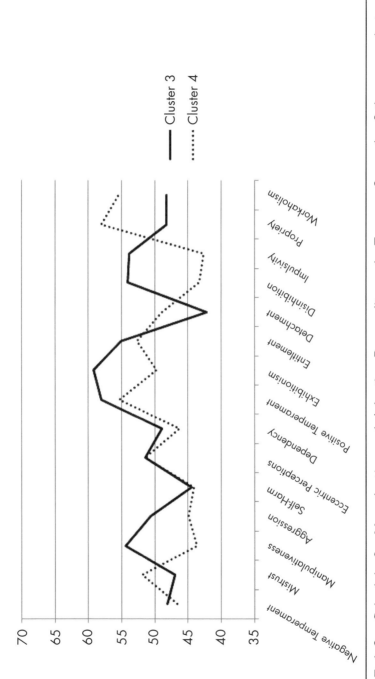

FIGURE 6–3.   Schedule for Nonadaptive and Adaptive Personality scale *T* scores for each of the seven clusters *(continued)*.

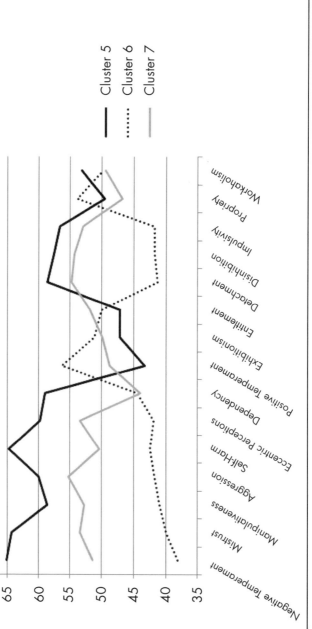

FIGURE 6–3. Schedule for Nonadaptive and Adaptive Personality scale *T* scores for each of the seven clusters *(continued)*.

average age (22.1 years) of its members, and its high percentage of college students, one might consider these individuals to be "wild-oat spreaders."

Cluster 4 ($n=1,288$; 61% military recruits, 22% college students) showed elevations for Positive Temperament, Propriety, and Workaholism and low levels of Aggression, Self-Harm, Disinhibition, and Impulsivity. Individuals in this cluster might be labeled "worker bees."

Cluster 5 ($n=865$; 59% patients, 27% college students) was composed of individuals who had higher-than-average Negative Temperament, Mistrust, Manipulativeness, Aggression, Self-Harm, Eccentric Perceptions, Dependency, Detachment, Disinhibition, and Impulsivity but also lower-than-average levels of Positive Temperament. These individuals had a broad array of pathological personality traits; this group might best be conceptualized as the "severe personality disorder" cluster.

Individuals in Cluster 6 ($n=961$; 52% military recruits, 26% college students) showed high Positive Temperament along with low levels of Negative Temperament, Mistrust, Manipulativeness, Aggression, Self-Harm, Eccentric Perceptions, Dependency, Detachment, Disinhibition, and Impulsivity. Individuals in this cluster showed a good deal of constraint and might be informally labeled "repressors."

Finally, Cluster 7 ($n=1,329$; 38% college students, 28% military recruits) showed high Aggression and low Dependency. This cluster might be labeled "rebels."

Discussion

We have presented preliminary evidence for the potential utility of a model-based, clustering/mixture-modeling approach to bridge finer-grained dimensions of personality and the need to apply those dimensions to specific patients via delineation of prototypes. We found evidence that SNAP dimensions delineate prototypical groups of people, as well as evidence that these groups had psychologically meaningful personality profiles.

A notable limitation of this work is the fact that the overall sample was composed of different groups—by virtue of the sampling scheme (assembling extensive available SNAP data)—as opposed to having been sampled systematically from a specific, well-defined population. A strength of our approach is that the sample has greater diversity when compared with a sample from a more restricted population (e.g., exclusively college students). A weakness is that various walks of life are represented in proportions that likely are not population representative. For this reason, the prototypes we describe should be conceptualized as contingent on the current sampling approach and should not be reified. We believe the approach that we undertook to deriving prototypes is methodologically sound and therefore holds promise for considering how dimensional traits may combine empirically into differentiable prototypes; however, sampling is likely to be a critical feature in person-centered modeling.

In this data set, for example, preliminary investigation into replicability of the prototypes suggested that they did *not* replicate well across subsamples of these data. This makes sense because the exercise we undertook involved mixing up people from different walks of life by assembling extensive available SNAP data. It is the contrast between these groups that might lead to potential "seams" in the data identified by mixture models. For example, Cluster 4 could be described as "conservative and restrained," and the modal sample of origin for persons in this cluster was the military. It is quite possible, however, that this cluster emerged here because military persons formed a major subsample of the current database. This is not to say that the typical person in the military might not have "conservative personality qualities" at a higher rate than, for example, the typical college student. Rather, these personalities might have blended more seamlessly if people were sampled continuously and smoothly, for instance, in a way that reflected the demographic proportions in the overall U.S. population.

Apparent discontinuities in personality distributions may be a function of sampling strategies (Tellegen 1981, as cited in Grove 1991); this is a key empirical question for future research on person-centered abnormal personality prototypes. It also is a highly challenging question because participants in research projects are often sampled from specific populations (e.g., clinical settings). Although it would be a major undertaking to measure personality in a highly detailed manner in a large sample from a well-defined population, these are exactly the data needed to contemplate the possibility of replicable personality prototypes that would generalize broadly. Such an endeavor also would be assisted by augmenting the variable space with more indicators of the peculiarity/oddity or Cluster A domain; the SNAP has only one scale covering this area (Eccentric Perceptions).

Nevertheless, we do believe that the current approach has potential utility in translating from variable-centered (dimensional) models to person-centered (prototype) models. Indeed, in large, representative samples from well-defined populations, this approach could test the idea of "thorough dimensionality" empirically. For example, one could use this strategy to accumulate evidence for the lack of meaningful cusps or seams in personality data (i.e., absence of compelling or replicable prototypes). Among the various possibilities: simpler models with fewer clusters might fit well; a sample might be well described in terms of one cluster, indicating that individuals' personalities are distributed continuously along multiple dimensions, following a specific distributional form; or a sample might be well described in terms of clusters that represent continuous gradations along multiple traits as opposed to unique combinations of traits. In these situations, the conclusion would be that personality distributions are "dimensional through and through" and that the complexity of human personality is not well captured by prototype schemes.

Even with an extensive, population-based data set in hand, however, additional methodological complexities deserve careful consideration—for example, the possibility that non-normality in multivariate distribution of traits contributes artifactually to evidence for putative prototypes (cf. Bauer and Curran 2003). These sorts of methodological complexities go well beyond the scope of this chapter, but the bottom line here is that sophisticated questions about nature of personality variation—at both the variable- and person-centered levels—are now amenable to empirical inquiry given the right data and the right models. We no longer have to rely on opinion or a priori preferences to arrive at a model of personality with a solid basis in data, for potential inclusion in DSM-5.

References

American Psychiatric Association: Diagnostic and Statistical Manual of Mental Disorders, 3rd Edition. Washington, DC, American Psychiatric Association, 1980

American Psychiatric Association: Diagnostic and Statistical Manual of Mental Disorders, 3rd Edition, Revised. Washington, DC, American Psychiatric Association, 1987

American Psychiatric Association: Diagnostic and Statistical Manual of Mental Disorders, 4th Edition. Washington, DC, American Psychiatric Association, 1994

American Psychiatric Association: Diagnostic and Statistical Manual of Mental Disorders, 4th Edition, Text Revision. Washington, DC, American Psychiatric Association, 2000

Asendorpf JB: Typeness of personality profiles: a continuous person-centered approach to personality data. Eur J Pers 20:83–106, 2006

Bauer DJ, Curran PJ: Distributional assumptions of growth mixture models: implications for over-extraction of latent trajectory classes. Psychol Methods 8:338–363, 2003

Blashfield RK, Intoccia V: Growth of the literature on the topic of personality disorders. Am J Psychiatry 157:472–473, 2000

Block J: Lives Through Time. Berkeley, CA, Bancroft Books, 1971

Casillas A, Clark LA: Dependency, impulsivity, and self-harm: traits hypothesized to underlie the association between Cluster B personality and substance abuse disorders. J Pers Disord 16:424–436, 2002

Casillas A, Clark LA, Sarrazin MS, et al: Personality predicts problem outcomes for substance abusers. Manuscript under review

Caspi A: Personality development across the life course, in Handbook of Child Psychology. Edited by Damon W. New York, Wiley, 1998, pp 311–388

Clark LA: Schedule for Nonadaptive and Adaptive Personality (SNAP): Manual for Administration, Scoring, and Interpretation. Minneapolis, University of Minnesota Press, 2003

Clark LA: Assessment and diagnosis of personality disorder: perennial issues and an emerging reconceptualization. Annu Rev Psychol 58:227–257, 2007

Clark LA, Vittengl J, Kraft D, et al: Separate personality traits from states to predict depression. J Pers Disord 17:152–172, 2003

Clark LA, Simms LJ, Wu KD, et al: Schedule for Nonadaptive and Adaptive Personality, 2nd Edition (SNAP-2). Minneapolis, University of Minnesota Press, 2009

First MB, Bell CB, Cuthbert B, et al: Personality disorders and relational disorders: a research agenda for addressing crucial gaps in DSM, in A Research Agenda for DSM-V. Edited by Kupfer DJ, First MB, Regier DA. Washington, DC, American Psychiatric Association, 2002, pp 123–199

Fraley C, Raftery A: MCLUST: Multivariate Normal Mixture Modeling and Model-Based Clustering, version 3.1–1. 2007. Available at: http://www.stat.washington.edu/mclust. Accessed June 29, 2009.

Grove WM: Performance of cluster analysis stopping rules as detectors of taxa, in Thinking Clearly About Psychology: Essays in Honor of Paul Everett Meehl, Vol II. Essays on Individual Differences. Edited by Grove WM, Cicchetti D. Minneapolis, University of Minnesota Press, 1991, pp 313–329

Harkness AR, McNulty JL: An overview of personality: the MMPI-2 personality psychopathology-five (PSY-5) scales, in MMPI-2: A Practitioner's Guide. Edited by Butcher JN. Washington, DC, American Psychological Association, 2006, pp 73–97

Harlan E, Clark LA: Short-forms of the Schedule for Nonadaptive and Adaptive Personality (SNAP) for self and collateral ratings: development, reliability, and validity. Assessment 6:131–146, 1999

Hart D, Atkins R, Fegley S: Personality and development in childhood: a person-centered approach. Monogr Soc Res Child Dev 68:i–vii, 1–109, 2003

Hicks BM, Markon KE, Patrick CJ, et al: Identifying psychopathy subtypes on the basis of personality structure. Psychol Assess 16:276–288, 2004

Jablensky A: The classification of personality disorders: critical review and need for rethinking. Psychopathology 35:112–116, 2002

Krueger RF, Markon KE: Understanding psychopathology: melding behavior genetics, personality, and quantitative psychology to develop an empirically based model. Curr Dir Psychol Sci 15:113–117, 2006

Krueger RF, Tackett JL (eds): Personality and Psychopathology. New York, Guilford, 2006

Lenzenweger MF, Clarkin JF, Yeomans FE, et al: Refining the borderline personality disorder phenotype through finite mixture modeling: implications for classification. J Pers Disord 22:313–331, 2008

Livesley WJ: Diagnostic dilemmas in classifying personality disorder, in Advancing DSM: Dilemmas in Psychiatric Diagnosis. Edited by Philips KA, First MB, Pincus HA. Arlington, VA, American Psychiatric Association, 2003, pp 153–190

Magnusson D: The logic and implications of a person-oriented approach, in Methods and Models for Studying the Individual. Edited by Cairns RB, Bergman LR, Kagan J. Thousand Oaks, CA, Sage, 1998, pp 33–64

Millon T: Assessment is not enough: the SPA should participate in constructing a comprehensive clinical science of personality. Society of Personality Assessment. J Pers Assess 78:209–218, 2002

Morey LC, Warner MB, Shea MT, et al: The representation of four personality disorders by the schedule for nonadaptive and adaptive personality dimensional model of personality. Psychol Assess 15:326–332, 2003

Oltmanns TF, Turkheimer E: Perceptions of self and others regarding pathological personality traits, in Personality and Psychopathology. Edited by Krueger RF, Tackett JL. New York, Guilford, 2006, pp 71–111

Pulkkinen L: Female and male personality styles: a typological and developmental analysis. J Pers Soc Psychol 70:1288–1306, 1996

Raftery AE: Bayesian model selection in social research. Sociol Methodol 25:111–163, 1995

Ready RE, Clark LA: Correspondence of psychiatric patient and informant ratings of personality traits, temperament, and interpersonal problems. Psychol Assess 14:39–49, 2002

Ready RE, Clark LA, Watson D, et al: Self- and peer-reported personality: agreement, trait ratability, and the "self-based heuristic." J Res Pers 34:208–244, 2000

Ready RE, Stierman L, Paulsen JS: Ecological validity of neuropsychological and personality measures of executive function. Clin Neuropsychol 15:314–323, 2001

Reynolds SK, Clark LA: Predicting personality disorder dimensions from domains and facets of the five-factor model. J Pers 69:199–222, 2001

Robins RW, Tracy JL: Setting an agenda for a person-centered approach to personality development: commentary. Monogr Soc Res Child Dev 68:110–122, 2003

Simms LJ, Casillas A, Clark LA, et al: Psychometric evaluation of the restructured clinical scales of the MMPI-2. Psychol Assess 17:345–358, 2005

Tackett J, Silberschmidt AL, Krueger RF, et al: A dimensional model of personality disorder: incorporating DSM Cluster A characteristics. J Abnorm Psychol 117:454–459, 2008

Tyrer P: Personality diatheses: a superior explanation than disorder. Psychol Med 37:1521–1525, 2007

van Leeuwen K, de Fruyt F, Mervielde I: A longitudinal study of the utility of the resilient, overcontrolled, and undercontrolled personality types as predictors of children's and adolescents' problem behavior. Int J Behav Dev 28:210–220, 2004

Vittengl JR, Clark LA, Owen-Salters E, et al: Diagnostic change and personality stability following functional restoration treatment in a chronic low back pain patient sample. Assessment 6:79–92, 1999

Watson D, Clark LA, Chmielewski M: Structures of personality and their relevance to psychopathology, II: further articulation of a comprehensive unified trait structure. J Pers 76:1545–1586, 2008

Westen D, Shedler J, Bradley R: A prototype approach to personality disorder diagnosis. Am J Psychiatry 163:846–856, 2006

Widiger TA, Simonsen E, Krueger R, et al: Personality disorder research agenda for the DSM-V. J Pers Disord 19:315–338, 2005

Wu KD, Clark LA: Relations between personality traits and self-reports of daily behavior. J Res Pers 37:231–256, 2003

CHAPTER 7

Options and Dilemmas of Dimensional Measures for DSM-5

Which Types of Measures Fare Best in Predicting Course and Outcome?

Hans-Ulrich Wittchen, Ph.D.
Michael Höfler, Ph.D.
Andrew T. Gloster, Ph.D.
Michelle G. Craske, Ph.D.
Katja Beesdo, Ph.D.

DSM-IV (American Psychiatric Association 1994) and ICD-10 (World Health Organization 1992) encourage clinicians and re-searchers to code all past and present mental disorders and syn-dromes based on categorically defined diagnostic criteria. As a result, multiple diagnoses have become the rule, with high rates of cross-sectional and lifetime comorbidity. This approach was closely linked to a set of basic principles by the designers of DSM-III through DSM-IV-TR (American Psychiatric Association 1980, 1987, 1994, 2000) and ICD-10. These principles aim to be 1) descriptive and comprehen-sive in the diagnostic assessment of patients, by specifying explicit categorical diagnostic criteria for all disorders; and 2) "atheoretical," by avoiding ambiguous terms and deleting—or at least specifying—hierarchical decisions, in the absence of clear empirical evidence from basic or clinical research.

Undoubtedly, these principles not only have resulted in improved reliability, consistency, and communication but also have fostered progress in basic, epidemiological, and clinical research as well as treatment. Indeed, there is substantial evidence that both the cross-sectional co-occurrence of symptoms and syndromes and the presence of prior and concurrent threshold categorical mental disorders have substantial impact on course, outcome, and treatment decisions (see, e.g., Beesdo et al. 2010; Bittner et al. 2004; Bruce et al. 2005; Howland et al. 2009; Lewinsohn et al. 2000; Shankman and Klein 2002; Wittchen et al. 2001; Woodward and Fergusson 2001).

However, given the lack of persuasive evidence of clear separation of DSM disorders, the descriptive approach and resultant high rates of comorbidity have been criticized from various perspectives (see Andrews et al. 2009; Regier et al. 2009). These critiques have been levied across multiple areas, such as symptomatology, treatment, course, genetics, and neurobiological and psychological measures and processes. Critical issues have been raised with regard to nosological considerations and particularly in terms of methodological problems (Wittchen et al. 1999, 2001, 2009a, 2009b). Lacking sufficiently detailed data, translation of these principles into explicit categorical criteria has led to the unfortunate situation in which many decisions about diagnostic criteria (e.g., thresholds for diagnostic presence) are based on clinical expert opinion rather than empirical evidence. It is fair to state that the designers of DSM-III, DSM-IV, and DSM-IV-TR were aware of these problems and called for comprehensive reevaluation of all threshold definitions, from the beginning. However, such systematic studies have been rare and fragmented.

Acknowledging these core problems, the designers and experts preparing the DSM-5 revision have decided to make a serious and systematic attempt to address them by considering—among other issues (see Regier et al. 2009)—the incorporation of "dimensional" measures and approaches on various levels as one potentially helpful strategy (Andrews et al. 2007; Helzer et al. 2007; Regier 2007; Shear et al. 2007). In this context, the term *categorical* is meant to describe binary decisions and measures, whereas *dimensional* covers any ordinal or interval scale with three or more ordered values. Dimensions therefore include three-point scales (i.e., none, some, many), a discrete score (e.g., symptom count), or a continuum (e.g., body mass index) that could be applied to either symptoms, criteria, diagnoses, or groups of disorders (Kraemer 2007). This approach takes into account the disadvantages of categorization (e.g., loss of power and precision, threshold problems; Smits et al. 2007) and the well-studied advantages of dimensional measures (e.g., enriched patient description; better reflection of the "true nature" of psychopathology for clinical and, in particular, research practice; potential to resolve threshold issues; and potential to reduce artificial comorbidity) while simultaneously retaining the advantages of the current descriptive categorical system (e.g., binary choices between case and non-case, ease of communication, and decision making). As a result of these considerations and the long-standing tradition of using dimensional approaches to supplement categorical diagnoses in research, the designers of DSM-5 have adopted a "mixed-categorical-dimensional" approach as a guiding principle.

Conceptual Challenges

The seemingly simple task of adding dimensions is related to a broad range of puzzling questions (Table 7–1). First, there are structural and pragmatic questions: what type (e.g., broad vs. narrow) of and how many dimensions are needed, and how complex should the dimensions be? Second, what should the dimensions target?: symptoms, course, constructs, and/or etiology? Third, on what scaling systems should dimensions be measured (e.g., are frequency and intensity scales sufficient)?

It seems reasonable to assume that such decisions can be made with relative ease for single disorders or within more homogeneous groups of disorders. The so-called supraordinate dimensions (Shear et al. 2007), for example, suggest a grid for anxiety disorders in which the most current categorical diagnostic criteria are conceptualized by dimensional measures, including intensity, frequency, and duration of the anxiety reaction, or the degree of avoidance behavior (Figure 7–1). Research findings offer several, partially well explored, options that range from single-domain scales (e.g., avoidance scales, such as the Mobility Inventory, to assess quantity and frequency of avoidance of different agoraphobic situations [Chambless et al. 1985]) through multidomain scales to measure fear/anxiety, avoidance, and interference, such as the Overall Anxiety Severity and Impairment Scale (Campbell-Sills et al. 2009), to multidomain interview approaches (e.g., Panic Disorder Severity Scale; Shear et al. 2001).

Considerably more complex challenges arise with regard to the construction and use of superordinate or cross-cutting dimensions that can be used as specifiers for all disorders. Examples are "distress" or "impairment" measures (Buist-Bouwman et al. 2008) and core psychopathological features such as a "dimensionally defined specifier" for panic attack. The challenges here are of conceptual (choosing most relevant core dimensions) and methodological (psychometric development, reliability, validity) natures.

TABLE 7–1. Core questions and potential targets for adding dimensional measures

QUESTIONS

Which dimensions should be chosen?
Broad ones ("superordinate," relevant to all disorders)?
Narrow ones ("supraordinate," relevant to one or several disorders [syndromatic])?
Cross-sectional, longitudinal, both?

How many dimensions are feasible?
For selected diagnoses and criteria?
For all criteria?

How complex and specific should dimensions be?
Uni- or multidimensional (one or various facets)?
Uni- or bipolar?
Simple or complex ratings?

Psychometric issues
Established scales?
New scales?

For whom?
Simple for clinical use versus complex for research?
Clinician versus patient-rated?

TARGETS

Symptoms
Types of signs and symptoms
Configurations of symptoms (syndromes)

Temporal/Time
Age at onset
Developmental
Acuity
Course (intermittent, chronic)
Duration
Outcome

Etiology
Dispositional (genetic, personality)
Neurobiological (neurobiological markers)
"Causal" trigger (event, substance, somatic, therapeutic)
Factors influencing course (social, psychological, therapeutic)

INTENSITY/FREQUENCY
For most dimensions above

DSM-IV anxiety diagnoses	Specific and shared evaluation domains[a] according to diagnostic criteria					
	Diagnosis-specific features	Anxiety reaction	Anticipatory anxiety	Avoidance behavior	Impairment disability	Distress/ Negative affect	Duration/ Persistence
Panic disorder						
Agoraphobia						
Generalized anxiety disorder						
Specific phobias						
Social phobia						
Obsessive-compulsive disorder						
Posttraumatic stress disorder						
Acute stress disorder						
Separation anxiety disorder						

Note. Severity/quantity/frequency measures referring to diagnostic criteria for DSM-IV anxiety diagnoses.
[a]Other possible domains may include etiological factors (e.g., neurobiological, developmental).

FIGURE 7–1. Targets for dimensions in anxiety disorders: the anxiety grid framework.

Source.   Shear MK, Bjelland I, Beesdo K, et al: "Supplementary Dimensional Assessment in Anxiety Disorders." *International Journal of Methods in Psychiatric Research* 16:S52–S64, 2007.

Procedural Challenges: Adding Dimensional Measures

The scope of options and possibilities regarding dimensional measures within a mixed categorical–dimensional system is incredibly large, yet currently available research evidence provides little guidance for answering the questions and deriving the best solutions. In addition, a strictly empirical, stringent test and psychometric exploration of options, which would involve sufficiently large national and international field trials, are not feasible. Thus, pragmatic considerations, careful consideration of the restricted range of available research evidence, and explorative reanalyses of existing data sets seem to be the only viable—although imperfect—way forward.

Pragmatic Criteria

Given that our clinical diagnostic classifications were developed primarily for routine care and administrative purposes, we have several general criteria (Table 7–2) for choosing among various dimensional approaches. An approach should be clinically useful, practical, easy to use, and time efficient, as well as be easy to learn and remember, and should simultaneously demonstrate appropriate levels of reliability and validity.

Sources and Research Evidence Providing Guidance

There is no doubt that treatment, psychological research, and neurobiological research have always been based predominantly on dimensional measures (Shear et al. 2007). In fact, most research studies have used a mixed categorical–dimensional approach. Unfortunately, such approaches are usually time consuming, thereby impeding their feasibility in routine care. Sources that may offer guidance for development of a mixed approach include the following:

1. *Clinical studies on efficacy of treatment* almost invariably use dimensional measures to examine effects of interventions, whether they be more or less simple, clinician-based rating scales such as the generic Clinical Global Impression scale (Guy 1976); the syndrome-specific Hamilton Anxiety Rating Scale (Hamilton 1959) or Depression Rating Scale (Hamilton 1960) in anxiety or mood disorders; or the Positive and Negative Syndrome Scale (Kay et al. 1987) in schizophrenia. Corresponding patient-rated instruments

---

TABLE 7–2. General criteria for selection of dimensional approaches

---

Ease of administration (practical)

No time burden (short)

Clinical utility (e.g., in terms of predicting outcome, choosing treatments, flagging risks, screening)

Reliability

Validity (psychometric and clinical)

Sensitivity and specificity

---

include the Beck Depression Inventory (Beck et al. 1961) and the Hospital Anxiety and Depression Scale (Zigmond and Snaith 1983). Thus, clinical trial data offer a broad and rich database that should, theoretically, offer considerable guidance. However, the value of these data might be quite restricted. First, many of these instruments and approaches are complex and time consuming in terms of administration and training required to obtain reliable results. Consequently, their standard use in routine care likely would be difficult and might result in diminished compliance. Second, information from such data might be misleading because of very restrictive inclusion and exclusion criteria typically used in clinical trials. Furthermore, it is likely that data from such studies would be influenced by selection bias, making it difficult to generalize findings to the respective total patient population.

2. *Multidimensional psychiatric ratings scales and platforms* are used in standard routine care and for documentation purposes. Older examples include the Inpatient Multidimensional Psychiatric Rating Scale (Lorr et al. 1963); the Brief Psychiatric Rating Scale (BPRS; Overall and Gorham 1988); and, in Europe, the AMDP system—Arbeitsgemeinschaft für Methodik und Dokumentation in der Psychiatrie (2007), or Association for Methodology and Documentation in Psychiatry. These types of dimensional approaches do not share the limitations discussed earlier for clinical studies. However, these approaches have the disadvantage of being based on earlier conceptual models for psychopathology and thus provide no conceptual link to DSM criteria or DSM diagnoses.

3. *Screening instruments* for either general caseness, such as the General Health Questionnaire (Goldberg and Blackwell 1970; Golderberg and Williams 1988), or derivates from the Composite International Diagnostic Screening approaches (Kessler et al. 2002, 2003; Wittchen and Pfister 1997) provide another source of information. Although screening approaches have a long and impressive record of psychometric exploration and are increasingly acceptable in routine care and research, their value as supraordi-

nate measures appears to be quite limited. The limitation lies in the fact that they were developed for caseness decisions, with considerations for optimal sensitivity and specificity, and not for reliable description of severity of a disorder.

4. *Epidemiological data* inherently include dimensional information. However, this source of data rarely has been considered and exploited, because of study limitations. Limitations include use of diagnostic screening questions; a restricted set of dimensional measures, lack of predefined outcomes, and lack of power with regard to targeted post hoc analyses. Such studies typically have been based on standardized and structured clinical interviews from which dimensional measures could be derived. Examples include the computation of symptomatic, subthreshold diagnostic conditions in addition to threshold conditions (e.g., Beesdo et al. 2009b; Wittchen et al. 2000), and the derivation of symptom counts as measures of severity of panic, anxiety reaction (e.g., Beesdo et al. 2007), mood (e.g., Beesdo et al. 2009a), and psychotic syndromes (Henquet et al. 2005). Also, interviews such as the Structured Clinical Interview for Panic-Agoraphobic Spectrum (Cassano et al. 1999), based on the spectrum disorder approach (Cassano et al. 1997; Frank et al. 1998), offer transdiagnostic data for a range of conditions.

To summarize, a wealth of data from various sources is available to provide at least some guidance with regard to some of the core questions in Table 7–1. Yet it is also evident that the knowledge is very fragmented, poorly integrated, and associated with a range of limitations and noteworthy deficits:

- Dimensional approaches that target symptoms and their intensities, frequencies, and associated distress have generally been well studied, whereas other targets listed in Table 7–1, such as duration, persistence, onset, and etiological factors, clearly have not been studied sufficiently.
- Most dimensional measures are exclusively cross-sectional and thus are relevant only for syndromal characterization, whereas most disorders demand a longitudinal, or even lifetime, assessment. Also, to our knowledge there are no established dimensional approaches that take into account nosological aspects. In particular, and unlike other areas in medicine, there have been no systematic attempts to introduce "staging" concepts as an ordinal proxy to a dimensional conceptualization of illness progression (Shear et al. 2007). This is despite the fact that such concepts exist for mental disorders such as panic attacks, panic disorder, agoraphobia (Fava et al. 2008; Klein 1981), and schizophrenic disorders (American Psychiatric Association 2000).

- Dimensional measures in psychopathological assessments would be preferable for a number of reasons (see earlier discussion). Yet because of a lack of research, it remains unclear which dimensional approaches and measures are viable for which forms of mental disorder. For example, with regard to improving the prediction of course and outcome of mental disorders, does it matter whether we use the BPRS, as a clinician-rated multidimensional characterization of the psychopathological spectrum, or do patient-rated scales such as the Symptom Checklist–90 (SCL-90; Derogatis 1977, 1992) fare better?

Do we need lengthy multi-item psychometric scales, or would a single-item rating do just as well? Are psychometric-factor analytically derived scales preferable over "dimensional" scores derived ad hoc from our current diagnostic criteria? Does it matter what type of diagnosis we are examining, or do findings differ substantially when different outcomes measures are considered?

Aims

Against this background, we discuss here results from a series of explorative analyses that used data from a phenotypical and longitudinal community sample in which a wide range of diagnostic issues were explored by means of dimensional, continuous, and categorical measures. We chose various baseline categorical and dimensional predictors, which we compared in their predictive value for various longitudinal outcomes. Analyses were focused on two groups of disorders, namely, DSM-IV anxiety and depressive disorders. Besides categorical DSM-IV diagnoses, various dimensional measures—ranging from simple ad hoc measures (e.g., number of panic attacks) to complex psychometric-scale measures—were used as putative predictors. Several domains were selected to reflect malignant longitudinal outcomes (i.e., global cumulative morbidity, disability, persistence, hospitalization, and suicide attempts).
Our core research questions were:

- To what degree do categorical DSM-IV diagnoses of anxiety and depressive disorders predict the long-term course and outcome?
- To what degree are additional dimensional measures able to improve prediction beyond the contribution of the categorical baseline diagnosis?
- Are there differential contributions of generic clinician-rated scale measures, patient-rated scale measures, and ad hoc measures (i.e., number or type of symptoms) derived from the diagnostic instrument?

- To what degree does predictive value differ by type of outcome measure considered?

Finally, to address a recent discussion about the most appropriate simple cross-cutting measure of anxiety for use in depressive disorders, as well as other non-anxiety disorders (Andrews et al. 2007), we present an example—related to the prediction of outcome of major depression—to examine whether simple anxiety measures are inferior to complex scales.

Methods

Sample

The Early Developmental Stages of Psychopathology Study (Lieb et al. 2000; Wittchen et al. 1998b) was a 10-year, prospective, longitudinal study involving a representative community sample of, originally, 3,021 adolescents and young adults ages 14–24 years at baseline (T0). Subjects were followed up prospectively over up to three waves (T1/T2/T3). Baseline response rate was 70.8%. Conditional subsequent response rates ranged between 88.0% (T1) and 73.2% (T3). For the purpose of this analysis, the total sample (N) was 2,716 subjects who had at least one recent follow-up (T2 [2.8–4.1 years after baseline] and/or T3 [7.3–10.6 years after baseline]).

Assessment

Individuals were assessed by trained clinical interviewers using the computer-assisted Munich-Composite International Diagnostic Interview (DIA-X/M-CIDI; Wittchen and Pfister 1997; Wittchen et al. 1998a). At baseline, the lifetime version of the DIA-X/M-CIDI was used; at each follow-up, the interval version for the respective length of the follow-up period was used. Diagnoses of mental disorders were computed with M-CIDI/DSM-IV algorithms.

Predictors

All measures reported here were assessed at baseline as part of the M-CIDI interview and the M-CIDI respondent booklet. Types of predictors used included the following:

- Categorical variables used as predictors were specific DSM-IV diagnoses of anxiety and depressive disorders and DSM-IV panic attack.

- Dimensional predictors chosen were the SCL-90 (Derogatis 1977), from which the total score, as well as the factor scores for anxiety and depression, was used despite questionable differential value, and the BPRS (Overall and Gorham 1988) total score.
- Ad hoc dimensional measures were derived from the M-CIDI, including number of DSM-IV panic symptoms during the worst panic attack at baseline, number of panic attacks in the follow-up period, number of somatoform symptoms, number of generalized anxiety disorder (GAD) symptoms, number of phobias, number of dysthymia symptoms, number of depression symptoms, and duration of episode (defined as number of months prior to baseline). These symptoms were categorized into low, middle, and high according to their distributions. The high and low groups were compared in the analysis.

Outcome Measures

Primary outcome measures, using T2 and T3 information, were as follows:

- Global Morbidity Scale score, which reflects the total psychopathological burden of each subject based on the number of all DSM-IV mental disorders during follow-up, taking subthreshold manifestations into account. This score has the following values: none (not even a subthreshold diagnosis); mild (at least subthreshold diagnosis but no threshold condition); moderate (at least one threshold mental disorder); severe (two or three diagnoses); and multimorbid-severe (four or more diagnoses).
- Persistence was operationalized as average diagnostic status (i.e., no disorder, symptoms only, subthreshold, full diagnosis) during follow-up (using age at onset and age of recency information), and then a median split was done.
- Disability was defined as total number of full (1) or partial (0.5) disability days due to mental or physical problems or drug use (maximum of reported T2 and T3 results).
- Suicide attempts during follow-up were documented.
- Hospitalization days during follow-up were recorded.

Statistical Analysis

Using categorical DSM-IV diagnostic status at baseline as the reference predictor for 10-year outcome, we modeled a series of logistic regressions to examine whether dimensional measures are superior or inferior in predictive value. Odds ratios, estimated from logistic regression, were adjusted for sex, age at last assessment, and follow-up duration. Dimensional predictors were calibrated to the distribution of the respective categorical predictor, allowing the estimation of incremental and nonincremental effects and direct comparisons among them by avoiding the power and scaling problems encountered when results from dimensional and categorical predictors are compared. The area under the curve (AUC), computed from receiver operating characteristic curves, was used to assess the degree of association between different baseline dimensional predictors and binary outcomes. AUC is the probability that a randomly selected outcome case will score higher in the predictor than a randomly selected outcome noncase. Stata Software package 10.1 (StataCorp 2009) was used for computing the robust variances, confidence intervals, and P values (by applying the Huber-White sandwich matrix) required when basing analyses on weighted data (Royall 1986).

Results

Conditional Probability of Benign and Malignant Global Diagnostic Outcome by Categorical Baseline Diagnostic Status

On the left side of Figure 7–2, the 10-year global morbidity outcome as a function of baseline anxiety and/or depression status (categorical: yes/no) is shown. To simplify presentation, only the proportion of respondents having a benign (none) or malignant (severe or multimorbid-severe) outcome is presented.

Having any threshold diagnosis, as compared with "no diagnosis" at baseline, was associated with lower proportions of benign global morbidity outcomes and higher proportions of malignant psychopathological outcomes 10 years later. Only 17.5% (panic attack) to 18.6% (GAD) of all subjects with a baseline anxiety disorder had no subsequent threshold mental disorders in the 10-year follow-up period. In contrast, 40.3% (panic attack) to 73.1% (panic disorder) had three or more mental disorders, defined by the global morbidity score as a "severe/multimorbid-severe" outcome. There was some noteworthy variation by type of diagnosis, particularly with regard to malignant outcomes. Baseline major depression was associated with less frequent malignant outcomes (33.2%) compared with baseline anxiety disorders (40.3%–73.1%). Number of diagnoses at baseline was associated with an increasing proportion of severe/multimorbid-severe outcome—that is, no baseline diagnosis (11.1%), one (24.5%), two (43.1%), or three or more (66.7%).

On the right side of Figure 7–2 is a graphical presentation of the association between comorbid anxiety and depression with a decreased

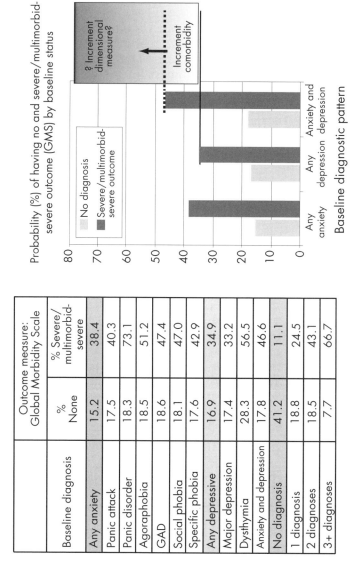

Baseline diagnosis	Outcome measure: Global Morbidity Scale	
	% None	% Severe/ multimorbid-severe
Any anxiety	15.2	38.4
Panic attack	17.5	40.3
Panic disorder	18.3	73.1
Agoraphobia	18.5	51.2
GAD	18.6	47.4
Social phobia	18.1	47.0
Specific phobia	17.6	42.9
Any depressive	16.9	34.9
Major depression	17.4	33.2
Dysthymia	28.3	56.5
Anxiety and depression	17.8	46.6
No diagnosis	41.2	11.1
1 diagnosis	18.8	24.5
2 diagnoses	18.5	43.1
3+ diagnoses	7.7	66.7

FIGURE 7–2. Conditional probability (%) of having no, versus a severe or multimorbid-severe, outcome over the 10-year follow-up period, by baseline diagnostic pattern. GMS=Global Morbidity Scale.

probability of no diagnosis in the follow-up period and increased probability of severe/multimorbid-severe ("malignant") course and outcome.

Calibrated Incremental Effects of Dimensional Measures

Most dimensional measures examined were associated with improved prediction of most outcome measures beyond the value of the categorical diagnosis, as expressed by significant odds ratios in Table 7–3A. Associations were strongest for the global morbidity score and somewhat weaker and less consistent for other outcome measures. This overall picture emerged for those patients with baseline anxiety as well as for those with depressive disorders. With regard to the global morbidity measure in the anxiety disorder subset, the highest odds ratios were found for numbers of dysthymia (7.7) and depressive symptoms (6.2), depression duration in months (5.5), and numbers of GAD and panic symptoms (4.9). It is noteworthy that the two lengthy psychometric scale measures were not superior to the simpler, ad hoc scales. Particularly weak associations were found for the clinician-rated BPRS.

Incremental values for baseline depression cases (Table 7–3B) were relatively similar, although it is noteworthy that the numbers of panic (OR= 6.0) and GAD (OR=6.9) symptoms were found to have a somewhat stronger association with malignant outcomes among baseline depression cases. Some differences between outcome measures should be noted. In comparison with other measures, prior depression duration and number of depressive symptoms appeared to be slightly superior to anxiety measures (where associations were moderate) in predicting suicide attempts. Hospitalization days were best predicted by number of depressive and dysthymic symptoms and depression duration. Number of GAD symptoms was the only significant anxiety measure. Number of disability days was best predicted by ad hoc measures of both anxiety and depression as well as by depression duration.

Incremental Effects by Specific Types of Diagnosis

Given the heterogeneity of anxiety disorders, we also examined associations for diagnostic subtypes, comparing the predictive values of the diagnoses with the scores calibrated to their respective distribution. Focusing on the two psychometric scale measures, with the global morbidity score as the outcome measure, Table 7–4 reveals that some categorical baseline diagnoses—namely, panic attack, panic disorder, and less impressively, GAD and dysthymia—were, in themselves, highly predictive of the morbidity score. In these disorders, the dimensional measure did not add significantly further predictive power. This was also the case for most of the other ad hoc developed quantitative measures derived from the Composite International Diagnostic Interview (data not shown), such as numbers of panic attack symptoms (OR=18.5), phobias (OR=6.2), or depression symptoms (OR=5.6). Despite being significant predictors, these measures do not have higher predictive value. In contrast, data in Table 7–4 also reveal that substantially higher odds ratios were found for diagnoses such as agoraphobia and social and specific phobias as well as for major depression. In these disorders, dimensional measures yielded higher odds ratios than the categorical diagnosis. Overall, and consistent with previous psychometric exploration (Table 7–3), the patient-rated SCL-90 total score yielded similar associations as the depression subscore, whereas the anxiety subscore faired worse in all comparisons. Also consistent with findings in Table 7–3, the clinician-rated BPRS score consistently was associated with the lowest odds ratios.

Prediction of Outcome of Major Depression: Effects of Various Anxiety Specifiers

We have shown that the predictive property of baseline depression diagnoses was only moderate, possibly because of the episodic nature of depression. Thus we explored whether the addition of anxiety specifiers improved prediction of global morbidity outcome. Table 7–5 reveals that all dimensional measures were significant. Consistent with previous findings, and as indicated in the *rescaled* AUC, simpler anxiety measures (numbers of panic symptoms, phobias, and anxiety disorders at baseline) fared almost as well as the much more complex and longer scale measures in predicting malignant outcomes.

It should be noted, however, that considerably different findings emerged when other outcomes were considered (not shown, data available on request). For example, suicide attempts were best predicted by number of anxiety diagnoses, in addition to the SCL-90 total and anxiety scores.

Conclusion

We explored to what degree various types of dimensional measures improved our predictions of various long-term courses and outcomes,

TABLE 7–3A. Calibrated incremental effects, in odds ratios (ORs), of dimensional measures, among subjects with baseline anxiety and depressive disorders

CALIBRATED PREDICTORS[a]	GMS[b]		SUICIDE ATTEMPTS		HOSPITALIZATION		DISABILITY DAYS	
	OR	95% CI	OR	95% CI	OR	95% CI	OR	95% CI
After adjustment for baseline anxiety								
SCL-90-Total	4.68	3.30 6.64	3.23	1.71 6.11	2.26	1.26 4.07	1.24	0.99 1.56
SCL-90-Anxiety	3.23	2.31 4.52	3.13	1.61 6.08	1.34	0.67 2.68	1.30	1.04 1.63
SCL-90-Depression	4.17	2.97 5.86	4.48	2.40 8.35	3.37	1.83 6.20	1.51	1.20 1.90
BPRS-Total	2.40	1.78 3.23	2.62	1.30 5.26	1.68	0.89 3.16	1.13	0.88 1.44
Number of somatoform symptoms	2.36	1.81 3.07	1.13	0.59 2.16	1.28	0.67 2.46	1.31	1.09 1.58
Number of panic anxiety symptoms	4.90	3.22 7.46	1.80	0.86 3.75	1.42	0.69 2.90	1.47	1.12 1.93
Number GAD symptoms	4.94	2.49 9.82	1.78	0.61 5.19	3.00	1.14 7.88	1.45	1.02 2.07
Number of phobias	3.38	2.38 4.81	2.70	1.30 5.64	0.98	0.45 2.12	1.28	0.98 1.67
Number of dysthymia symptoms	7.72	3.00 19.88	3.60	1.36 9.55	4.81	1.97 11.74	1.47	0.91 2.40
Number of depression symptoms	6.22	4.06 9.54	3.00	1.48 6.09	3.66	1.78 7.50	1.76	1.36 2.28
Duration of depression in months	5.45	3.58 8.29	4.14	1.88 9.11	3.02	1.50 6.08	1.69	1.30 2.20

Note.   All results are adjusted for sex, age at last assessment, and follow-up duration. BPRS=Brief Psychiatric Rating Scale; CI = confidence interval; GAD=generalized anxiety disorder; GMS=Global Morbidity Scale score; SCL-90= Symptom Checklist-90.
[a]Dichotomized to match frequency of those with any anxiety/depressive disorder, respectively. Some scales could not be well calibrated because of their distributions. [b]Severe/multimorbid-severe vs. none.

TABLE 7–3B. Calibrated incremental effects, in odds ratios (ORs), of dimensional measures, among subjects with baseline anxiety and depressive disorders

CALIBRATED PREDICTORS[a]	GMS[b]		SUICIDE ATTEMPTS		HOSPITALIZATION		DISABILITY DAYS	
	OR	95% CI	OR	95% CI	OR	95% CI	OR	95% CI
After adjustment for baseline depression								
SCL-90-Total	5.38	3.73 7.76	3.37	1.66 6.84	1.68	0.81 3.48	1.39	1.11 1.74
SCL-90-Anxiety	4.21	2.90 6.12	2.93	1.49 5.79	1.13	0.54 2.35	1.34	1.08 1.66
SCL-90-Depression	5.26	3.56 7.76	4.03	2.10 7.71	3.42	1.80 6.49	1.44	1.13 1.85
BPRS-Total	2.37	1.82 3.09	2.86	1.46 5.61	2.15	1.19 3.88	1.20	0.98 1.46
Number of somatoform symptoms	2.62	2.02 3.39	1.34	0.72 2.48	1.35	0.71 2.54	1.37	1.14 1.65
Number of panic anxiety symptoms	5.96	3.97 8.93	2.43	1.13 5.19	1.56	0.76 3.22	1.63	1.25 2.12
Number GAD symptoms	6.90	3.63 13.12	2.77	1.06 7.21	3.12	1.29 7.50	1.72	1.22 2.42
Number of phobias	4.20	2.80 6.32	1.94	0.93 4.06	0.57	0.21 1.61	1.59	1.20 2.11
Number of dysthymia symptoms	5.81	2.30 14.66	5.51	1.91 15.91	3.21	1.17 8.86	1.54	0.86 2.75
Number of depression symptoms	6.59	4.00 10.86	4.98	1.68 14.75	3.16	1.20 8.34	1.97	1.37 2.82
Duration of depression in months	5.95	3.81 9.29	5.51	2.49 12.18	2.44	0.95 6.26	1.90	1.39 2.60

Note. All results are adjusted for sex, age at last assessment, and follow-up duration. BPRS=Brief Psychiatric Rating Scale; CI = confidence interval; GAD=generalized anxiety disorder; GMS=Global Morbidity Scale score; SCL-90= Symptom Checklist–90.
[a]Dichotomized to match frequency of those with any anxiety/depressive disorder, respectively. Some scales could not be well calibrated because of their distributions. [b]Severe/multimorbid-severe vs. none.

TABLE 7–4. Syndrome-specific lack of incremental effects of selected scale measures on Global Morbidity Scale (GMS) outcome measure (total sample, $N = 2,719$)

		GMS OUTCOME MEASURE	
	PREDICTIVE ASSOCIATION OF CATEGORICAL DIAGNOSIS	CALIBRATED PREDICTIVE ASSOCIATION OF SCALE MEASURE	
BASELINE DIAGNOSIS	DIAGNOSIS, OR (95% CI)	SCL-90 TOTAL SCORE, OR (95% CI)	BPRS SCORE, OR (95% CI)
Panic attack	**28.8 (10.4–79.8)**	8.9 (4.3–18.5)	3.6 (2.1–6.0)
Panic	**18.6 (4.2–81.5)**	15.9 (5.1–49.1)	4.4 (2.0–9.8)
Agoraphobia	5.9 (2.3–15.3)	16.1 (6.3–41.1)	3.6 (1.8–7.1)
Social phobia	5.9 (3.2–11.1)	8.9 (4.3–18.5)	3.6 (2.1–6.0)
Generalized anxiety disorder	**12.2 (4.4–37.2)**	18.3 (6.7–50.1)	3.6 (5.1–24.4)
Major depressive disorder	2.9 (2.0–4.4)	6.5 (4.4–9.5)	3.4 (2.4–4.7)
Dysthymia	**11.1 (4.2–28.6)**	15.9 (6.3–40.4)	3.6 (1.8–7.1)

Note. Diagnoses with odds ratios shown in bold indicate conditions for which a categorical diagnosis itself is highly predictive (no, or only marginal, increase by dimensional measures).
BPRS=Brief Psychiatric Rating Scale; CI=confidence interval; OR=odds ratio; SCL-90=Symptom Checklist–90.

TABLE 7–5. Analysis of which baseline predictors predict Global Morbidity Scale score

BASELINE PREDICTOR	AUC	95% CI	AUC RESCALED[a]	95% CI
Number of panic symptoms	0.653	0.631–0.705	0.306	0.202–0.410
Number of phobias	0.605	0.524–0.686	0.209	0.048–0.371
Number of depressive symptoms	0.728	0.651–0.806	0.457	0.302–0.612
Number of DSM anxiety diagnoses	0.621	0.547–0.694	0.241	0.093–0.389
Brief Psychiatric Rating Scale anxiety (two items)	0.631	0.550–0.711	0.261	0.100–0.423
Symptom Checklist total	0.705	0.626–0.785	0.411	0.252–0.570
Symptom Checklist anxiety	0.676	0.594–0.759	0.353	0.187–0.518
Symptom Checklist depression	0.675	0.594–0.756	0.351	0.189–0.513

Note. N=305 subjects with depressive disorder at baseline. AUC=area under the curve; CI=confidence interval.
[a]AUC rescaled=(AUC−0.5) ÷ 2; maximum = 1.

beyond the effect of categorical baseline diagnoses. Overall, our analyses revealed an incremental value of dimensional measures, including simple ad hoc measures such as Composite International Diagnostic Interview–derived diagnostic counts, in predicting long-term outcomes—including global morbidity, suicide attempts, hospital days, and disability days—above and beyond effects of baseline anxiety disorders or baseline depressive disorders.

However, results varied substantially as a function of baseline diagnosis and outcome measure. For example, using our dimensional scale measures revealed no higher predictive value for the global outcome for panic attack and panic disorder and comparatively little value for GAD and dysthymia. The presence of panic attacks/panic disorder was a particularly powerful predictor by itself. In these cases, using dimensional measures did not improve prediction; in fact, it might actually have blurred the picture.

For other anxiety disorders, as well as depressive disorders, patient-rated dimensional measures, derived from the SCL-90, and ad hoc–derived dimensional measures from the diagnostic interview were associated with considerably improved predictions for at least some outcomes considered. Interestingly, clinician-rated measures from the BPRS, whether total score or single-domain scores for anxiety and depression (data available on request), contributed less than patient-rated measures.

Another noteworthy observation is that longer psychometric scales, with many items, did not necessarily perform better than shorter and simpler measures. For example, single BPRS items for anxiety were not inferior to the BPRS total score in prediction of global outcome (additional analyses not presented here). Also, crude and clearly imperfect ad hoc continuous measures, such as symptom counts, were almost as predictive as complex scaled measures. Yet this preliminary observation needs further testing and replication. In this respect, the high predictive power of chronic and long-lasting dysthymia symptoms, as well as illness duration before baseline, underlines the well-known clinical observation that previous course best predicts future course.

As expected, there was some variation in predictive value, depending on what outcome was considered. Smaller effects and fewer significant effects were observed for the outcome measures "number of disability days" and "hospitalization" in the follow-up period. Largest effects were observed for the global outcome measure and less consistently for suicide attempts. This suggests that the measures we considered might have considerably different values for other less severe or more global outcomes, such as general health and functioning.

In the prediction of depression, additional anxiety specifiers, whether long and complex, such as the SCL-90 Anxiety subscale, or shorter simple measures, such as numbers of panic symptoms, phobias, or anxiety diagnoses at baseline, partially contributed to the substantial incremental prediction of long-term course and outcome. However, it also should be noted that measures that address aspects of the previous course of illness at baseline, such as prior duration and number of dysthymia symptoms (2+ years' duration), seem to be superior in predicting malignant-outcome patterns. The prediction of suicide was associated with both baseline severity of depression and number of anxiety disorders (the SCL total and anxiety scores, respectively).

Overall, our findings confirm previous evidence that dimensional measures of various types are a useful addition to categorical diagnoses for some diagnoses more than others. The finding that improved prognostic value was achieved almost equally well with short and brief measures and indices is encouraging with regard to the feasibility of this approach. It should be taken into account, however, that our findings are restricted by the validity of the dimensional scales incorporated herein. Yet our findings do not signal that uni- or multidimensional psychometric scales with more items are not necessarily better than simpler ad hoc measures derived from the diagnostic assessment itself. This finding—if confirmed—might be seen as encouragement to use such simpler approaches in the upcoming DSM-5 field trials.

However, the considerable variability in our findings, by diagnosis and outcome domain considered, suggests that it might be a complex and difficult task to derive measures that work equally well across all diagnoses and outcome domains. Given the heterogeneity of findings in anxiety disorders, the identification of one single, comprehensive, quantitative anxiety measure for use as cross-cutting specifier in all diagnoses might be more challenging than the search for a cross-cutting depression measure. This, indirectly, also suggests that development of new measures and concurrent validity studies might be particularly instructive in anxiety disorders.

These conclusions should be interpreted against a number of limitations and caveats. Our analyses and findings should be seen as explorative. Neither the choice of measures nor the study design was meant, originally, to address the question of the relative value of dimensional measures as opposed to categorical measures. We also were bound to use a quite restrictive set of predictors and outcomes, because potentially more appropriate measures (such as avoidance behavior) either were not available or could not be presented here because of space limitations. For the current analyses, we favored mostly malignant outcomes and might have neglected potentially important signals for less severe types of outcome measures. Furthermore, our statistical analyses were not comprehensive; we considered only a restricted set of diagnoses and outcomes and did not test, with rigor, all possible measures and combinations. Finally, results are partially confounded by the mode and method of assessment. That is, predictor variables, derived from ad hoc diagnostic information from the Composite International Diagnostic Interview, are more similar to some of the outcome variables, with potentially overlapping variance, than are nondiagnostic interviews (BPRS) and questionnaires (SCL).

To conclude, systematic studies are needed to develop an optimal set of anxiety-related measures that explore the value of a global anxiety index versus measures of specific features, including anxiety, panic, worry, and avoidance (compare Shear et al. 2007). In comparison with this task, derivation of depression measures seems to be easier, as reflected by the consistency of our findings and the effect sizes. The upcoming DSM-5 field trials might be one option to examine acceptance, feasibility, and utility of both simpler and more complex dimensional measures as well as the utility of these measures as cross-cutting specifiers, in particular.

References

American Psychiatric Association: Diagnostic and Statistical Manual of Mental Disorders, 3rd Edition. Washington, DC, American Psychiatric Press, 1980

American Psychiatric Association: Diagnostic and Statistical Manual of Mental Disorders, 3rd Edition, Revised. Washington, DC, American Psychiatric Press, 1987

American Psychiatric Association: Diagnostic and Statistical Manual of Mental Disorders, 4th Edition. Washington, DC, American Psychiatric Press, 1994

American Psychiatric Association: Diagnostic and Statistical Manual of Mental Disorders, 4th Edition, Text Revision. Washington, DC, American Psychiatric Press, 2000

Andrews G, Brugha T, Thase M, et al: Dimensionality and the category of major depressive episode. Int J Methods Psychiatr Res 16:S41–S51, 2007

Andrews G, Goldberg DP, Krueger RF Jr, et al: Exploring the feasibility of a meta-structure for DSM-V and ICD-11: could it improve utility and validity? Psychol Med 39:1993–2000, 2009

Arbeitsgemeinschaft für Methodik und Dokumentation in der Psychiatrie: Das AMDP-System: Manual zur Dokumentation psychiatrischer Befunde. Göttingen, Germany, Hogrefe, 2007

Beck AT, Ward CH, Mendelsohn M, et al: An inventory for measuring depression. Arch Gen Psychiatry 4:561–571, 1961

Beesdo K, Bittner A, Pine DS, et al: Incidence of social anxiety disorder and the consistent risk for secondary depression in the first three decades of life. Arch Gen Psychiatry 64:903–912, 2007

Beesdo K, Höfler M, Leibenluft E, et al: Mood episodes and mood disorders: patterns of incidence and conversion in the first three decades of life. Bipolar Disord 11:637–649, 2009a

Beesdo K, Hoyer J, Jacobi F, et al: Association between generalized anxiety levels and pain in a community sample: evidence for diagnostic specificity. J Anxiety Disord 23:684–693, 2009b

Beesdo K, Pine DS, Lieb R, et al: Incidence and risk patterns of anxiety and depressive disorders and categorization of generalized anxiety disorder. Arch Gen Psychiatry 67:47–57, 2010

Bittner A, Goodwin RD, Wittchen H-U, et al: What characteristics of primary anxiety disorders predict subsequent major depressive disorder? J Clin Psychiatry 65:618–626, 2004

Bruce SE, Yonkers KA, Otto MW, et al: Influence of psychiatric comorbidity on recovery and recurrence in generalized anxiety disorder, social phobia, and panic disorder: a 12-year prospective study. Am J Psychiatry 162:1179–1187, 2005

Buist-Bouwman MA, Ormel J, De Graaf R, et al: Psychometric properties of the World Health Organization Disability Assessment Schedule used in the European Study of the Epidemiology of Mental Disorders. Int J Methods Psychiatr Res 17:185–197, 2008

Campbell-Sills L, Norman SB, Craske MG, et al: Validation of a brief measure of anxiety-related severity and impairment: the Overall Anxiety Severity and Impairment Scale (OASIS). J Affect Disord 112:92–101, 2009

Cassano GB, Michelini S, Shear MK, et al: The panic-agoraphobic spectrum: a descriptive approach to the assessment and treatment of subtle symptoms. Am J Psychiatry 154:27–38, 1997

Cassano G, Banti S, Mauri M, et al: Internal consistency and discriminant validity of the Structured Clinical Interview for Panic-Agoraphobic Spectrum (SCI-PAS). Int J Methods Psychiatr Res 8:138–145, 1999

Chambless D, Caputo G, Hasin F, et al: The mobility inventory for agoraphobia. Behav Res Ther 23:35–44, 1985

Derogatis LR: SCL-90-R: Administration, Scoring and Procedures Manual for the Revised Version. Baltimore, MD, John Hopkins University School of Medicine, Clinical Psychometrics Research Unit, 1977

Derogatis LR: SCL-90-R, Administration, Scoring and Procedures Manual-II. Towson, MD, Clinical Psychometric Research, 1992

Fava GA, Rafanelli C, Tossani E, et al: Agoraphobia is a disease: a tribute to Sir Martin Roth. Psychother Psychosom 77:133–138, 2008

Frank E, Cassano G, Shear M, et al: The spectrum model: a more coherent approach to the complexity of psychiatric symptomatology. CNS Spectr 3:23–34, 1998

Goldberg DP, Blackwell B: Psychiatric illness in general practice. a detailed study using a new method of case identification. Br Med J 1:439–443, 1970

Golderberg D, Williams P: A User's Guide to the General Health Questionnaire. Windsor, UK, NFER-Nelson, 1988

Guy W: ECDEU Assessment Manual for Psychopharmacology (Publ No ADM-76-338). Rockville, MD, U.S. Department of Health, Education, and Welfare, 1976

Hamilton M: The assessment of anxiety-states by rating. Br J Med Psychol 32:50–55, 1959

Hamilton M: A rating scale for depression. J Neurol Neurosurg Psychiatry 23:56–62, 1960

Helzer J, Bucholz K, Gossop M: A dimensional option for the diagnosis of substance dependence in DSM-V. Int J Methods Psychiatr Res 16:S24–S33, 2007

Henquet C, Krabbendam L, Spauwen J, et al: Prospective cohort study of cannabis use, predisposition for psychosis, and psychotic symptoms in young people. Br Med Bull 330:1–4, 2005

Howland RH, Rush AJ, Wisniewski SR, et al: Concurrent anxiety and substance use disorders among outpatients with major depression: clinical features and effect on treatment outcome. Drug Alcohol Depend 99:248–260, 2009

Kay SR, Fiszbein A, Opler LA: The positive and negative syndrome scale (PANSS) for schizophrenia. Schizophr Bull 13:261–276, 1987

Kessler RC, Andrews G, Colpe LJ, et al: Short screening scales to monitor population prevalences and trends in nonspecific psychological distress. Psychol Med 32:959–976, 2002

Kessler RC, Barker PR, Colpe LJ, et al: Screening for serious mental illness in the general population. Arch Gen Psychiatry 60:184–189, 2003

Klein DF: Anxiety reconceptualized, in Anxiety: New Research and Changing Concepts. Edited by Klein DF, Rabkin JG. New York, Raven, 1981, pp 235–263

Kraemer CH: DSM categories and dimensions in clinical and research contexts. Int J Methods Psychiatr Res 16:S8–S15, 2007

Lewinsohn PM, Rohde P, Seeley JR, et al: Natural course of adolescent major depressive disorder in a community sample: predictors of recurrence in young adults. Am J Psychiatry 157:1584–1591, 2000

Lieb R, Isensee B, von Sydow K, et al: The Early Developmental Stages of Psychopathology Study (EDSP): a methodological update. Eur Addict Res 6:170–182, 2000

Lorr M, Klett CJ, McNair DM, et al: Manual: Inpatient Multidimensional Psychiatric Scale. Palo Alto, CA, Consulting Psychologists Press, 1963

Overall J, Gorham D: The Brief Psychiatric Rating Scale (BPRS): recent developments in ascertainment and scaling. Psychopharmacol Bull 24:97–99, 1988

Regier DA: Dimensional approaches to psychiatric classification: refining the research agenda for DSM-V: an introduction. Int J Methods Psychiatr Res 16:S1–S5, 2007

Regier DA, Narrow WE, Kuhl EA, et al: The conceptual development of DSM-V. Am J Psychiatry 166:645–650, 2009

Royall RM: Model robust confidence intervals using maximum likelihood estimators. Int Stat Rev 54:221–226, 1986

Shankman SA, Klein DN: The impact of comorbid anxiety disorders on the course of dysthymic disorder: a 5-year prospective longitudinal study. J Affect Disord 70:211–217, 2002

Shear MK, Rucci P, Williams J, et al: Reliability and validity of the Panic Disorder Severity Scale: replication and extension. J Psychiatr Res 35:293–296, 2001

Shear MK, Bjelland I, Beesdo K, et al: Supplementary dimensional assessment in anxiety disorders. Int J Methods Psychiatr Res 16:S52–S64, 2007

Smits N, Smit F, Cuijpers P, et al: Using decision theory to derive optimal cut-off scores of screening instruments: an illustration explicating costs and benefits of mental health screening. Int J Methods Psychiatr Res 16:219–229, 2007

StataCorp LP: Stata Statistical Software: Release 10.1. College Station, TX, Stata Corporation, 2009

Wittchen H-U, Pfister H: DIA-X-Interviews: Manual für Screening-Verfahren und Interview; Interviewheft Längsschnittuntersuchung (DIA-X-Lifetime); Ergänzungsheft (DIA-X-Lifetime); Interviewheft Querschnittuntersuchung (DIA-X-12 Monate); Ergänzungsheft (DIA-X-12Monate); PC-Programm zur Durchführung des Interviews (Längs- und Querschnittuntersuchung); Auswertungsprogramm. Frankfurt, Germany, Swets & Zeitlinger, 1997

Wittchen H-U, Lachner G, Wunderlich U, et al: Test-retest reliability of the computerized DSM-IV version of the Munich-Composite International Diagnostic Interview (M-CIDI). Soc Psychiatry Psychiatr Epidemiol 33:568–578, 1998a

Wittchen HU, Perkonigg A, Lachner G, et al: Early Developmental Stages of Psychopathology Study (EDSP): objectives and design. Eur Addict Res 4:18–27, 1998b

Wittchen H-U, Höfler M, Merikangas KR: Toward the identification of core psychopathological processes? Arch Gen Psychiatry 56:929–931, 1999

Wittchen H-U, Lieb R, Pfister H, et al: The waxing and waning of mental disorders: evaluating the stability of syndromes of mental disorders in the population. Compr Psychiatry 41:122–132, 2000

Wittchen H-U, Schuster P, Lieb R: Comorbidity and mixed anxiety-depressive disorder: clinical curiosity or pathophysiological need? Hum Psychopharmacol 16:S21–S30, 2001

Wittchen H-U, Beesdo K, Gloster AT: A new meta-structure of mental disorders: helpful step in the future or harmful step back to the past? Psychol Med 39:2083–2089, 2009a

Wittchen H-U, Beesdo K, Gloster AT: The position of anxiety disorders in structural models of mental disorders. Psychiatr Clin North Am 32:465–481, 2009b

Woodward LJ, Fergusson DM: Life course outcomes of young people with anxiety disorders in adolescence. J Am Acad Child Adolesc Psychiatry 40:1086–1093, 2001

World Health Organization: International Statistical Classification of Diseases and Related Health Problems, 10th Revision. Geneva, Switzerland, World Health Organization, 1992

Zigmond AS, Snaith RP: The hospital anxiety and depression scale. Acta Psychiatr Scand 67:361–370, 1983

PART III

ASSESSING FUNCTIONAL IMPAIRMENT FOR CLINICAL SIGNIFICANCE AND DISABILITY

CHAPTER 8

Clinical Significance and Disorder Thresholds in DSM-5

The Role of Disability and Distress

William E. Narrow, M.D., M.P.H.
Emily A. Kuhl, Ph.D.

The *Diagnostic and Statistical Manual of Mental Disorders* (DSM) is the de facto reference for defining mental disorders. As such, it is used by clinicians in specialty and nonspecialty settings as well as researchers, government agencies, policymakers and legislatures, the insurance industry, the legal system, and the general public. Although the introductory chapter of DSM-IV-TR (American Psychiatric Association 2000) clearly states that the manual should only be

The authors wish to acknowledge the members of and advisors to the DSM-5 Impairment and Disability Assessment Study Group, whose continuing efforts and contributions helped make this chapter possible. Those individuals include Jane S. Paulsen, Ph.D. (Chair); Gavin Andrews, M.D.; Glorisa Canino, Ph.D.; Lee Anna Clark, Ph.D.; Michelle G. Craske, Ph.D.; Hans Wijbrand Hoek, M.D., Ph.D.; Helena C. Kraemer, Ph.D.; David Shaffer, M.D., F.R.C.P.; Cille Kennedy, Ph.D. (advisor); Martin Prince, M.D., M.Sc., M.R.C.Psych. (advisor); and Michael R. Von Korff, Sc.D. (advisor).

used by "individuals with appropriate clinical training and experience in diagnosis" and "the specific diagnostic criteria included in DSM-IV-TR are meant to serve as guidelines to be informed by clinical judgment and are not meant to be used in a cookbook fashion" (American Psychiatric Association 2000, p. xxxii), the multiple contexts in which the manual is used virtually guarantees that nonclinicians will be interpreting its diagnostic criteria.

One of the hallmarks of the most common psychiatric symptoms is their continuity with normal personality variations and responses to stress. Some of these normal states, such as depressed mood or anxiety, are so common as to be considered a part of normal life experience. Even perceptual aberrations, such as hallucinations, are surprisingly common experiences in people who do not have mental disorders (Van Os et al. 2000). Traits such as shyness or a need for orderliness are well understood as normal variants of personality. The question, then, is how to draw a threshold that distinguishes normal traits and emotional states from experiences that are indicative of pathology.

Such a threshold is important for many reasons. A clear diagnostic threshold serves to protect a pathological condition from being trivialized as "medicalization of the normal." It indicates that a condition is one that is outside the realm of common experience and also does not represent something transient or self-limiting. An individual with such a condition, in theory, would need treatment or attention of some sort. It is likely that in specialty mental health settings, the clinician is not often called on to determine whether an individual has a disorder, given the stigma and access problems associated with seeking mental health treatment. In other words, the barriers to seeking and receiving care are so great that most individuals presenting for treatment do indeed have a mental disorder of some kind (Narrow et al. 1993; Regier et al. 1993). The decisions in such settings are thus likely to involve deciding which disorder the individual presenting for treatment has and which treatment is indicated.

However, in some settings, such as general medical practice or community-based household survey research, deciding whether the individual has a disorder may be a more frequent dilemma. In general medical settings, diagnoses of mental disorders are often not made in patients who meet criteria for a mental disorder. In the case of major depressive disorder, for example, this may be due to physician factors (e.g., unfamiliarity or discomfort with diagnosis and treatment of mental disorders) (Gallo et al. 2002) or to threshold factors: depressed patients in primary care settings often have symptoms that are subthreshold for disorder or barely meet criteria (Jackson et al. 2007). Problems with diagnostic thresholds in community surveys can complicate population-level estimation of need for mental health services; community surveys are discussed further later in the chapter.

DSM-III and DSM-III-R

The developers of DSM-III (American Psychiatric Association 1980) revolutionized psychiatric diagnosis by providing specific operational diagnostic criteria for mental disorders. They also developed a definition of a mental disorder that has been maintained through all subsequent editions of the manual. This definition states that

> each of the mental disorders is conceptualized as a clinically significant behavioral or psychological syndrome or pattern that occurs in an individual and that is associated with present distress (e.g., a painful symptom) or disability (i.e., impairment in one or more important areas of functioning) or with a significantly increased risk of suffering death, pain, disability or an important loss of freedom. In addition, this syndrome or pattern must not be merely an expectable or culturally sanctioned response to a particular event, for example, the death of a loved one. Whatever its original cause, it must currently be considered a manifestation of a behavioral, psychological, or biological dysfunction in the individual. Neither deviant behavior (e.g., political, religious, or sexual) nor conflicts that are primarily between the individual and society are mental disorders unless the deviance or conflict is a symptom of a dysfunction in the individual, as described above. (pp. xxi–xxii)

For the purposes of this chapter it should be noted that the term *clinically significant* is attached to the behavioral syndrome and that the boundaries of disability and functioning are not specified.

The basic DSM-III disorder criteria listed required symptoms, duration, and exclusions. It was thought at the time that the explicit and rigorous specification of these criteria would define a pathological syndrome that minimized false-positive and false-negative diagnoses (Spitzer and Wakefield 1999). Few explicit criteria for clinical significance, distress, or impairment were placed in the diagnostic criteria for DSM-III or DSM-III-R (American Psychiatric Association 1987). However, a global assessment of functioning was a recommended part of the diagnostic assessment in both volumes (Highest Level of Adaptive Functioning in Past Year in DSM-III and the Global Assessment of Functioning scale in DSM-III-R) and was placed on Axis V of the multiaxial diagnostic scheme. Because of a paucity of relevant research evidence in psychiatry at the time, DSM-III was developed largely through a consensus process based on the clinical experiences of its developers. Little was known about the epidemiology of mental disorders in community populations, including differences in the characteristics of mental disorders seen in clinical settings compared with those identified in the community.

Epidemiologic Catchment Area and National Comorbidity Survey Prevalence Estimates

DSM-III stimulated a wealth of new research based on its operationalized diagnostic criteria. Notably, the Diagnostic Interview Schedule (DIS), a lay interview for epidemiological surveys based on DSM-III criteria, was developed for use in the National Institute of Mental Health Epidemiologic Catchment Area (ECA) program. The results of the ECA program were surprising in many ways. High rates of several disorders previously thought to be rare, such as obsessive-compulsive disorder, were found, as were high rates of co-occurrence between mental disorders. The overall rate of mental disorders was also higher than expected, particularly when based on the respondents' retrospective reports of symptoms occurring over their lifetimes (Robins and Regier 1991). The National Comorbidity Survey (NCS), a nationally representative survey of mental disorders based on DSM-III-R criteria, found even higher rates of disorders, with an overall lifetime rate of mental disorders approaching 50% (Kessler et al. 1994). The discrepancies in reported rates of mental disorders between the ECA and the NCS, which were conducted only 10 years apart, raised many questions about the surveys' methodologies, the DSM diagnostic criteria, and the assessment instruments used to operationalize these criteria (Regier et al. 1998). Several factors were found to have potential significance in the reported prevalence rate discrepancies. Among them were changes in diagnostic criteria between DSM-III and DSM-III-R, changes in the assessment instruments (the DIS in the ECA and the University of Michigan version of the Composite International Diagnostic Interview [CIDI] for the NCS), and discrepancies in the use of the "clinical significance questions" contained in both diagnostic assessment instruments.

The clinical significance questions were placed in the DIS and the CIDI to ensure that a symptom or a syndrome endorsed by the respondent was of sufficient severity to be clinically important. The questions asked whether the respondent had mentioned the symptom/syndrome to a clinician, whether he or she had taken medication more than once for the symptom/syndrome, and whether the symptom/syndrome had interfered with the respondent's life or activities. The developers of the DIS believed that such a distinction was particularly important for anxiety symptoms, which were thought to be commonplace in the population, often self-limiting or nondistressing, and thus not of clinical import. Consequently, the clinical significance questions for anxiety disorders were asked for each endorsed symptom, and a symptom was counted as positive only if the respondent endorsed one of the clinical significance questions. For the remainder of disorders in the DIS, and for all of the disorders in the University of Michigan CIDI, if clinical significance questions were asked, they were asked at the syndrome level—that is, for a cluster of endorsed disorder symptoms. It is important to note that these clinical significance questions were developed well before the publication of DSM-IV (American Psychiatric Association 1994) and its "clinical significance criterion" (discussed later) and thus do not map directly onto the concepts contained in this criterion.

A reanalysis of the ECA and NCS data (Narrow et al. 2002) revealed that, except for anxiety disorders in the ECA, the clinical significance questions were asked but not used for prevalence estimates in either survey. As expected, when these questions were put into the diagnostic algorithms for each survey, prevalence rates declined. The decline in rates was larger for the NCS than for the ECA, which had the effect of bringing the prevalence estimates closer together. The populations with "clinically significant" disorders also had higher service use rates and higher levels of clinical severity as assessed by the limited measures available in the surveys. Thus, adding clinical significance data to the disorders identified a population more likely needing attention from mental health service planners and policymakers. Similar findings have been published from an Australian data set (Slade and Andrews 2002).

More recently, analyses of the prevalence of posttraumatic stress disorder in two population studies found that inclusion of the clinical significance criterion decreased the conditional lifetime prevalence of posttraumatic stress disorder by 28% in one sample and by 37% in the second sample (Breslau and Alvarado 2007). However, application of the criterion failed to differentiate between patients with functional impairment as measured by presence versus absence of work-loss/distress days (Breslau and Alvarado 2007). Others have questioned whether the criterion is effective in improving validity when applied using diagnostic interviews administered by lay persons and nonclinical professionals, who are commonly employed in epidemiological surveys (Beals et al. 2004).

It is clear that the clinical significance questions used in the DIS and the University of Michigan CIDI were not sufficient to define a threshold for mental disorders. Little attention was given in the ECA study and the NCS, beyond the rudimentary clinical significance questions, to symptom severity or to distress and limitations in social and occupational functioning, which would have been needed to adequately address the open questions of diagnostic thresholds.

DSM-IV: The Clinical Significance Criterion and Its Problems

The developers of DSM-IV attempted to address concerns about over-inclusion by adding the clinical significance criterion to many more diagnoses compared with DSM-III-R. More than 70% of all DSM-IV diagnostic criteria sets contain the criterion (Lehman et al. 2002). Wording of the criterion throughout DSM-IV varies somewhat but is generally as follows: "The disturbance causes clinically significant distress or impairment in social, occupational, or other important areas of functioning." This criterion differs from the DSM definition of mental disorder by requiring clinical significance of the individual's distress or impairment in social, occupational, or other areas of functioning rather than clinical significance of the "behavioral or psychological syndrome or pattern," as in the definition of mental disorder.

Spitzer and Wakefield (1999) have been among the most prominent critics of the clinical significance criterion, dismissing its addition to DSM-IV as "strictly conceptual" (p. 1857) rather than empirical. The vagueness and subjectivity of the criterion terminology are considered particularly problematic and result in a circular definition: a disorder is defined by clinically significant distress or impairment, which is distress or impairment significant enough to be considered a disorder. The criterion addresses the definition's requirement that a mental disorder be "associated with present distress (e.g., a painful symptom) or disability (i.e., impairment in one or more important areas of functioning)," but it does not address the alternative option that the syndrome be associated "with a significantly increased risk of suffering death, pain, disability or an important loss of freedom." This may then lead to increased false-negative assessments. The term "clinically significant" is not defined or operationalized, and in fact, DSM-IV concedes that "assessing if this criterion is met...is an inherently difficult judgment" (p. 7), but the clinician is given no guidance on how to address this difficulty. The difficulty in operationalizing clinical significance is compounded by potential cultural and ethnic differences. Coyne and Marcus (2006) reported that use of the clinical significance criterion resulted in a reduction in prevalence of major depressive disorder among African Americans, whereas no such pattern was found among white patients.

The criterion may result in false-negatives in cases for which the diagnostic criteria make it redundant. For some disorders (e.g., conduct disorder, selective mutism, dissociative fugue, male erectile disorder, substance dependence), the symptoms themselves might be considered inherently distressing or impairing. Not only, then, is inclusion of the criterion unnecessary, but it may result in patients being disqualified from a diagnosis if they do not report significant distress or impairment (Spitzer and Wakefield 1999; Wakefield and First 2003). A "high-functioning" heavy alcohol user who denies social problems from drinking may otherwise meet the criteria for alcohol dependence but evade diagnosis because this requirement is not met.

Use of the clinical significance criterion does not coincide with the perspective of general medicine that distress or functional impairment is generally not required to make a diagnosis (Üstün and Kennedy 2009). Indeed, many asymptomatic conditions in general medicine are diagnosed based on knowledge of their progression or increased risk for a poor outcome (e.g., early malignancies or HIV infection, hypertension). To suggest that such disorders do not exist until they cause distress or disability would be unthinkable. On the other hand, some accepted medical disorders are rarely if ever considered clinically significant (e.g., male pattern baldness, renal glycosuria), in that they do not require treatment (cosmetic considerations notwithstanding for baldness) or even watchful monitoring. Mental disorders in DSM-IV are held to a different standard. Ongoing stigmatization of mental disorders in society may play a role in setting this standard by encouraging those in the mental health field to "prove" that mental disorders are real, disabling, and treatable. The use of the clinical significance criterion adds strength to this argument but, as noted earlier, distances this group of disorders from the rest of medicine.

Although the criterion was developed out of a need for threshold clarification, its inclusion with diagnostic criteria, conflating disability with the disorders' symptomatology, may actually hinder attempts to find underlying causes of disorders and treatments. In community studies, some subjects meet full symptom criteria for a disorder but deny any significant life interference as a result of these symptoms. It is likely that these individuals represent a heterogeneous group: some will likely go on to develop limitations in activities in the future, whereas others will experience a diminution of their symptoms or disorder remission without ever developing disabilities. The implications for prevention and treatment are clear in the first group but not the second. Conversely, those with symptoms not meeting the threshold for disorder status can express significant life interference as a result of those symptoms, and there is emerging evidence of effective treatments for subthreshold depressive symptoms (Judd et al. 2004; Oxman et al. 2008). Other studies have shown different rates of recovery from DSM symptoms as opposed to improvements in social functioning, with social functioning lagging behind improvements in symptomatology (Hirschfeld et al. 2002; Vittengl et al. 2004). It is likely that the risk and protective factors for the development of disability are not the same factors that lead to the development of the symptom syndromes of mental disorders (Clayer et al. 1998; Kessler et al. 2003b; Merikangas et al. 2007; Scott et al. 2009; Stein et al. 2008). Some studies have shown that specific symptoms are associated with specific disabilities (e.g., psychosis symptoms and impaired social cognition [Penn et al. 2008; Toomey et al. 2002]), suggesting that a focus on the relationship between specific symptoms and their impact on skills needed for adequate social functioning is needed, rather than focusing on full symptom syndromes.

Whither Distress?

Distress is not defined in DSM, and it is unclear what the concept is intended to mean. Some of the writings about the clinical significance criterion indicate that "distress" could be understood in its more general, colloquial meaning—that is, emotional upset, discomfort, or pain (Spitzer and Wakefield 1999). There is also a large base of research in which distress is characterized on the basis of combinations of more highly defined concepts of depression, anxiety, and sometimes somatic symptoms (e.g., Kessler et al. 2002, 2003a). The former conceptualization is problematic in that it has little empirical evidence to support its definition and use. If the latter conceptualization is used, there is a high risk of confounding distress with symptomatology, particularly for depression, anxiety, and somatoform disorders, but also with many other disorders in which these symptoms play a prominent role (West et al. 2009). Deciding at what level distress becomes clinically significant is also problematic because empirically established thresholds are based on symptom severity.

The clinical significance criterion, by requiring distress "or" functional impairment for the diagnosis of a mental disorder, may also have the effect of reducing attention to functional impairment in clinical settings. Because distress, as demonstrated by some investigators (Evangelia et al. 2010; Mond et al. 2009; Rickwood and Braithwaite 1994; Sareen et al. 2005), is tied to seeking services, it might be hypothesized that most patients seen by clinicians will initially be distressed, thus satisfying the criterion and removing the need to assess functional impairment. If distress is attributed to persons other than the patient (e.g., parents of children, caretakers of dementia patients), then even more patients would meet this criterion. Finally, distress can be caused by external factors, such as societal disapproval, which is, arguably, not a reason to pathologize a behavior.

Beyond the Clinical Significance Criterion: Symptom Severity and Disability

As noted, one of the goals of the operationalized symptom criteria of the DSM system was to specify a group of symptoms that were in aggregate severe enough to cross a threshold separating psychopathology from normal psychological reactions to stressors and transient, self-limiting states. Thus, it follows that one should be able to diagnose a disorder on the basis of its symptom severity without regard for its impact on activities. One of the methods used to quantify severity, particularly for polythetic criteria sets, is *symptom counts,* for example, for major depressive disorder; after a minimum number of symptoms is specified as the threshold for disorder, mild disorders are characterized as being at the symptom threshold or with few symptoms beyond the threshold, severe disorders are characterized by having all or almost all symptoms specified for the disorder, and moderate disorders fall in between mild and severe. However, even though the symptom sets appeared on their face to delineate definite disorders, experience in community surveys, as described earlier, showed that they did have problems, particularly around the mild end of the severity dimension.

Some of these problems may stem from insufficient severity specifications of the symptoms themselves. (Antipsychiatry groups have long criticized DSM by pulling symptoms from the criteria sets that by themselves could be seen as normal behavior.) It is true that some symptoms are based on extremes of normal behavior and use vague frequency specifiers, such as "often," that do not give much guidance as to threshold. It is unclear whether an accumulation of symptoms, which by themselves may not be pathological, can specify a disorder, or whether each symptom must rise to a severity level to count as a symptom. Other symptoms, particularly for children and adolescents, are judged against an unspecified normative developmental trajectory.

Finally, some symptoms, especially those for substance abuse and for "externalizing" disorders such as antisocial personality disorder and attention-deficit/hyperactivity disorder, are confounded with the consequences of the disorders, also known as *impairments in functioning.* Similar confounding is exhibited in Axis V's Global Assessment of Functioning scale, which was intended to assess overall functioning by operationalizing social, occupational, and relational limitations. The scale has been criticized, however, for including symptom specifiers in its descriptions, for example, level of suicidal ideation, delusions and hallucinations, and flat affect. Not surprisingly, several studies have found that Axis V significantly correlates with symptoms, and in some studies even more so than functioning (Goldman et al. 1992; Hilsenroth et al. 2000; Roy-Byrne et al. 1996; Skodol et al. 1988).

The World Health Organization Conceptualizations of Disorder and Functioning

The World Health Organization (WHO) has developed a "family of International Classifications" which includes the *International Classification of Diseases,* 10th Revision (ICD-10; World Health Organization 1992), the *International Classification of Functioning, Disability, and Health* (ICF; World Health Organization 2001), and the *International Classification of Health Interventions* (ICHI, under development). The ICD-10 mental disorders are presented in two versions, "clinical guidelines" and "criteria for research," with the latter being in close harmony with DSM-IV symptom criteria. In contrast to the approach taken by DSM-IV, however, the diagnostic guidelines and criteria contained in the mental disorders chapter of ICD-10 do not contain a requirement for clinically significant distress or impairment in social functioning.

The ICF terminology is considerably different from that commonly used in U.S. health care settings, but parallels can be easily drawn. The ICF contains descriptions of three different levels of human *functioning:* body structures and functions, activities (tasks or actions of the individual), and participation in society. ICF "body functions" closely associated with mental disorders include consciousness, orientation, intellect, temperament and personality, energy and drive, insight, regulation of emotion, and sleep. ICF "activities and participation" include learning and applying knowledge, carrying out general tasks and demands, communication, mobility, self-care, participation in domestic life, engagement in interpersonal interactions, and involvement in major life activities (e.g., education, occupational, economic, community, social, and civic endeavors). Environmental factors, a fourth domain that affects all three levels of function, are also included in the ICF, and personal factors such as gender, age, education, and social status are also recognized as important, although they are not listed. Activities and participation are recognized as having potentially overlapping aspects; they are listed together in the ICF, and considerable latitude is given to the users of the ICF as to whether a specific domain is to be considered an activity or participation construct.

Disability in ICF refers to impairments, activity limitations, and participation restrictions. Limitations in body structure and functions are called *impairments;* impairments of ICF mental functions are often similar to DSM-IV symptoms. *Activity limitations* are similar to DSM-IV "impairments in social, occupational, and other areas of functioning," although some DSM-IV symptoms would qualify as activity limitations in ICF. *Participation restrictions* refer to problems with interacting in society at large (e.g., physical barriers, stigma, discrimination). A coding system was developed as a part of the ICF, allowing documentation of specific impairments, activity limitations, and participation restrictions at different levels of specificity.

For activity limitations and participation restrictions, there are two possible qualifiers, describing *performance* and *capacity.* The performance qualifier describes "what an individual does in his or her current environment." The capacity qualifier describes an individual's ability to execute a task or an action, indicating "the highest probable level of functioning of a person in a given domain at a given moment." Although the performance qualifier takes personal assistance or the use of assistive devices into account, the capacity qualifier attempts to describe the person's ability in a standardized, "environmentally adjusted" environment, without the use of personal assistance or assistive devices.

As the preceding explanation indicates, the ICF is a detailed and complex framework for describing disability. It has not been used widely in the United States, with the possible exception of rehabilitation settings. Several countries have started the process of streamlining the ICF for use in health standards and legislation. Development of ICF-based indicators and reporting systems for use in rehabilitation, disability evaluation, and elder care have been started in various countries including Australia, Canada, Italy, India, Japan, and Mexico.

In the United States, the National Center for Vital and Health Statistics studied the ICF for 18 months and in 2001 sent a report to then U.S. Department of Health and Human Services Secretary Tommy Thompson. The report acknowledged broad agreement on the importance of collecting functional status information for clinical care, public health practice, policy, and administration and recommended the selection of a code set for functional status data in standardized records and selection and testing of a code set for these purposes. It also recognized important practical issues to be addressed before widespread reporting of functional status begins, such as finding a method for incorporating functional status information into standardized records and determining the feasibility and costs of collecting these data. The potential value of the ICF was acknowledged, but endorsement as an official code set was not given.

The WHO has designated the U.S. Department of Health and Human Services as the North American Collaborating Center to advance the use of ICF. Work is also being done by the American Speech, Language and Hearing Association, the American Occupational Therapy Association, and the American Psychological Association. All of these organizations worked together to develop a standard functional assessment procedure manual based on the ICF, and a wide range of educational, training, and pilot-testing efforts were planned; results of these efforts have not been published.

Conclusion and Recommendations

As development of DSM-5 moves closer to fruition, addressing the limitations of diagnostic assessment in DSM-IV and DSM-IV-TR becomes increasingly imperative and can strengthen the way diagnostic syndromes and disability are represented in the future. The adoption of a common language and better-defined terminology should be encouraged. The terms *impairment, functioning, disability*, and *distress* are used by U.S. mental health professionals in ways that are more often than not ill defined and confusing to those who use the WHO's ICD and ICF terminology and classification systems. The goal of harmonization between DSM-5 and ICD-11 will be made easier if DSM-5 makes an attempt to harmonize its approach to its specification of disability as well as its symptom criteria. Although the ICF system provides a well thought out framework for defining and naming the consequences of disorders, it is virtually totally unfamiliar to U.S. psychiatrists, and the problems in disseminating an unfamiliar classification and terminology to a new audience must be considered and addressed.

Of note, development of the ICF was made possible by a cooperative agreement (U01MH035883) that provided funding to the WHO from the National Institute of Mental Health, National Institute on Alcohol Abuse and Alcoholism, and National Institute on Drug Abuse over a period of 19 years (1983–2001). The WHO/Alcohol, Drug Abuse, and Mental Health Administration Joint Project on Diagnosis and Classification, later named the WHO/National Institutes of Health (NIH) Joint Project on the Assessment of Disablement, first supported the development of WHO instruments for the assessment, diagnosis, and classification of disorders related to substance abuse and mental or neurological illness, and then the development of the ICF classification of disabilities. Several current and former members of the NIH staff who worked on the development of the ICF include the author (W.E.N.), Cille Kennedy, Ph.D.; Darrel A. Regier, M.D., M.P.H.; Wilson Compton, M.D., M.P.E.; and Bridget F. Grant, Ph.D., all of whom are members of the DSM-5 Task Force, Work Groups, or Adviser Groups. Furthermore, the WHO Disability Schedule II, which was developed alongside the ICF with grant funding from NIH, may serve as a candidate measure in DSM-5 for assessing disability and impairment within the context of the ICF framework.

The multiple uses of DSM diagnoses should be acknowledged and dealt with in terms of the role of symptoms and their consequences. One of the most important distinctions that should be made is the use of diagnoses for clinical purposes versus research purposes. Assessment of clinical significance is an important part of determining need for treatment, both at the level of the individual clinical encounter and for setting policy for mental health services. Ideally, clinical significance would be inherent in the symptom presentations of each DSM disorder through clear specification of the mental functions that underlie the disorders, methods to accurately measure these functions, and the severity and duration of the symptoms. However, it is unlikely, given the state of the science, that mental disorder syndromes can be sufficiently defined to achieve this goal at this time. Therefore, for the time being, the use of distress and activity limitations will retain its usefulness in determining clinical significance for clinical, policy, and reimbursement purposes. For the reasons elucidated in earlier sections of this chapter, research into the causes of mental disorders could well be confounded by the required use of these clinical significance specifiers, and investigators should be aware of the potential problems in using them to define their study groups.

Disability (activity limitations) should be separated from symptom criteria as much as possible. Separating symptoms from disability would need to occur at two levels: the symptom criteria and the clinical significance criterion. The separation of symptoms from activity limitations will highlight the need to assess both areas in a diagnostic evaluations and treatment follow-ups and, as noted earlier, may enhance research into the causes of mental disorders.

Distress should be dropped as a criterion for a diagnosis of mental disorder. In its place, symptom criteria should be examined with an eye toward clarifying terms and, when possible, strengthening their face validity for designating psychopathology. Strengthening the symptom criteria and allowing dimensional assessment of the commonly understood psychological components of distress, such as depression, anxiety, and somatization, across all disorders should greatly reduce the need to consider the currently ill-defined DSM concept of distress. Dropping the distress requirement will also serve to focus attention on activity limitations. However, removing this requirement may be easier for some disorders than for others.

More research should be conducted on the consequences of mental disorders. Because mental disorders and disabilities appear to have separate trajectories, precise but separate assessments of each will likely advance research into the etiology of disabilities related to mental disorders. Investigations at the level of individual symptoms associated with a disorder may be more likely to yield explanations for resulting disabilities than are investigations at the level of the disorder. Assessments of comorbid symptoms outside the diagnostic criteria of a particular disorder, as are being proposed for DSM-5, are also likely to yield useful information. However, it can be expected that explanations of activity limitations will be complex, involving symptoms as well as personal characteristics (e.g., demographic factors, personality traits, culture) and environmental risk and protective factors.

References

American Psychiatric Association: Diagnostic and Statistical Manual of Mental Disorders, 3rd Edition. Washington, DC, American Psychiatric Association, 1980

American Psychiatric Association: Diagnostic and Statistical Manual of Mental Disorders, 3rd Edition, Revised. Washington, DC, American Psychiatric Association, 1987

American Psychiatric Association: Diagnostic and Statistical Manual of Mental Disorders, 4th Edition. Washington, DC, American Psychiatric Association, 1994

American Psychiatric Association: Diagnostic and Statistical Manual of Mental Disorders, 4th Edition, Text Revision. Washington, DC, American Psychiatric Association, 2000

Beals J, Novins DK, Spicer P, et al: Challenges in operationalizing the DSM-IV clinical significance criterion. Arch Gen Psychiatry 61:1197–1207, 2004

Breslau N, Alvarado GF: The clinical significance criterion in DSM-IV posttraumatic stress disorder. Psychol Med 37:1437–1444, 2007

Clayer J, Bookless C, Air T, et al: Psychiatric disorder and disability in a rural community. Soc Psychiatry Psychiatr Epidemiol 33:269–273, 1998

Coyne JC, Marcus SC: Health disparities in care for depression possibly obscured by the clinical significance criterion. Am J Psychiatry 163:1577–1579, 2006

Evangelia N, Kirana PS, Chiu G, et al: Level of bother and treatment-seeking predictors among male and female in-patients with sexual problems: a hospital-based study. J Sex Med 7 (2 Pt 1):700–711, 2010

Gallo JJ, Meredith LS, Gonzales J, et al: Do family physicians and internists differ in knowledge, attitudes, and self-reported approaches for depression? Int J Psychiatry Med 32:1–20, 2002

Goldman HH, Skodol AE, Lave TR: Revising Axis V for DSM-IV: a review of measures of social functioning. Am J Psychiatry 149:1148–1156, 1992

Hilsenroth MJ, Ackerman SJ, Blagys MD, et al: Reliability and validity of DSM-IV axis V. Am J Psychiatry 157:1858–1863, 2000

Hirschfeld R, Dunner D, Keitner G, et al: Does psychosocial functioning improve independent of depressive symptoms? A comparison of nefazodone, psychotherapy, and their combination. Biol Psychiatry 51:123–133, 2002

Jackson JL, Passamonti M, Kroenke K: Outcome and impact of mental disorders in primary care at 5 years. Psychosom Med 69:270–276, 2007

Judd LL, Rapaport MH, Yonkers KA, et al: Randomized, placebo-controlled trial of fluoxetine for acute treatment of minor depressive disorder. Am J Psychiatry 161:1864–1871, 2004

Kessler RC, McGonagle KA, Zhao S, et al: Lifetime and 12-month prevalence of DSM-III-R psychiatric disorders in the United States: results from the National Comorbidity Survey. Arch Gen Psychiatry 51:8–19, 1994

Kessler RC, Andrews G, Colpe LJ, et al: Short screening scales to monitor population prevalences and trends in non-specific psychological distress. Psychol Med 32:959–976, 2002

Kessler RC, Barker PR, Colpe LJ, et al: Screening for serious mental illness in the general population. Arch Gen Psychiatry 60:184–189, 2003a

Kessler RC, Ormel J, Demler O, et al: Comorbid mental disorders account for the role impairment of commonly occurring chronic physical disorders: results from the National Comorbidity Survey. J Occup Environ Med 45:1257–1266, 2003b

Lehman AF, Alexopoulos GS, Goldman H, et al: Mental disorders and disability: time to reevaluate the relationship?, in A Research Agenda for DSM-V. Edited by Kupfer DJ, First MB, Regier DA. Washington, DC, American Psychiatric Publishing, 2002, pp 201–218

Merikangas KR, Ames M, Cui L, et al: The impact of comorbidity of mental and physical conditions on role disability in the US adult household population. Arch Gen Psychiatry 64:1180–1188, 2007

Mond JM, Hay PJ, Darby A, et al: Women with bulimic eating disorders: when do they receive treatment for an eating problem? J Consult Clin Psychol 77:835–844, 2009

Narrow WE, Regier DA, Rae DS, et al: Use of services by persons with mental and addictive disorders: findings from the National Institute of Mental Health Epidemiologic Catchment Area Program. Arch Gen Psychiatry 50:95–107, 1993

Narrow WE, Rae DS, Robins LN, et al: Revised prevalence estimates of mental disorders in the United States: using a clinical significance criterion to reconcile 2 surveys' estimates. Arch Gen Psychiatry 59:115–123, 2002

Oxman TE, Hegel MT, Hull JG, et al: Problem-solving treatment and coping styles in primary care minor depression. J Consult Clin Psychol 76:933–943, 2008

Penn DL, Sanna LJ, Roberts DL: Social cognition in schizophrenia: an overview. Schizophr Bull 34:408–411, 2008

Regier DA, Narrow WE, Rae DS, et al: The de facto US mental and addictive disorders service system: epidemiologic catchment area prospective 1-year prevalence rates of disorders and services. Arch Gen Psychiatry 50:85–94, 1993

Regier DA, Kaelber CT, Rae DS, et al: Limitations of diagnostic criteria and assessment instruments for mental disorders Implications for research and policy. Arch Gen Psychiatry 55:109–115, 1998

Rickwood DJ, Braithwaite VA: Social-psychological factors affecting help-seeking for emotional problems. Soc Sci Med 39:563–572, 1994

Robins LN, Regier DA (eds): Psychiatric Disorders in America: The Epidemiologic Catchment Area Study. New York, The Free Press, 1991

Roy-Byrne P, Dagadakis C, Unutzer J, et al: Evidence for limited validity of the revised global assessment of functioning scale. Psychiatr Serv 47:864–866, 1996

Sareen J, Cox BJ, Afifi TO, et al: Perceived need for mental health treatment in a nationally representative Canadian sample. Can J Psychiatry 50:643–651, 2005

Scott KM, Von Korff M, Alonso J, et al: Mental-physical comorbidity and its relationship with disability: results from the World Mental Health Surveys. Psychol Med 39:33–43, 2009

Skodol AE, Link BG, Shrout PE, et al: The revision of axis V in DSM-III-R: should symptoms have been included? Am J Psychiatry 145:825–829, 1988

Slade TB, Andrews GA: Empirical impact of DSM-IV diagnostic criterion for clinical significance. J Nerv Ment Dis 190:334–337, 2002

Spitzer RL, Wakefield JC: DSM-IV diagnostic criterion for clinical significance: does it help solve the false positives problem? Am J Psychiatry 156:1856–1864, 1999

Stein MB, Belik SL, Jacobi F, et al: Impairment associated with sleep problems in the community: relationship to physical and mental health comorbidity. Psychosom Med 70:913–919, 2008

Toomey R, Schuldberg D, Corrigan P, et al: Nonverbal social perception and symptomatology in schizophrenia. Schizophr Res 53:83–91, 2002

Üstün B, Kennedy C: What is "functional impairment"? Disentangling disability from clinical significance World Psychiatry 8:82–85, 2009

Van Os J, Hanssen M, Bijl RV, et al: Strauss (1969) revisited: a psychosis continuum in the general population? Schizophr Res 45:11–20, 2000

Vittengl JR, Clark LA, Jarrett RB: Improvement in social-interpersonal functioning after cognitive therapy for recurrent depression. Psychol Med 34:643–658, 2004

Wakefield JC, First MB: Clarifying the distinction between disorder and non-disorder: confronting the overdiagnosis (false positives) problem in DSM-V, in Advancing DSM: Dilemmas in Psychiatric Diagnosis. Edited by Phillips KA, First MB, Pincus HA. Arlington, VA, American Psychiatric Association, 2003, pp 23–56

West JC, Narrow WE, Stipec MR, et al: Dimensional assessment of psychopathology among patients treated by psychiatrists. Poster presentation at the 99th annual meeting of the American Psychopathological Association, New York City, March 2009

World Health Organization: International Statistical Classification of Diseases and Related Health Problems, 10th Revision. Geneva, World Health Organization, 1992

World Health Organization: International Classification of Functioning, Disability and Health (ICF). Geneva, World Health Organization, 2001

CHAPTER 9

Assessing Activity Limitations and Disability Among Adults

Michael Von Korff, Sc.D.
Gavin Andrews, M.D.
Madeleine Delves

In this chapter, we survey the assessment of activity limitations and disability in adult populations and propose ways to improve the assessment processes. Specifically, we

- Summarize the World Health Organization's framework for assessing activity limitations and disability, which was articulated in the 2001 *International Classification of Functioning, Disability and Health* (ICF; World Health Organization 2001).
- Review evidence relevant to psychometric properties of such assessment with the World Health Organization Disability Assessment Schedule II (WHODAS II), a questionnaire based on the ICF (Rehm et al. 1999).
- Review key evidence regarding measurement properties of assessment, based on clinician ratings, drawing on research concerning the Global Assessment of Functioning (GAF; Spitzer and Forman 1979; Startup et al. 2002).
- Identify limitations and unresolved shortcomings of available methods of assessment through self-report scales and clinician ratings.
- Propose next steps, which take advantage of strengths of existing assessment methods; consider their limitations; and provide approaches that might eventually overcome shortcomings that currently are unresolved.

We do not attempt here a comprehensive review of prior work on self-report and clinician-rating measures of activity limitation and disability; the sheer number of available disability measures precludes such an undertaking. An unpublished review of disability measures, undertaken during development of the WHODAS II, identified more than 70 scales that measure global and specific disabilities, exclusive of a much larger number of disease-specific questionnaires (T.B. Ustun and M. Lofty, unpublished manuscript).

ICF Framework for Assessment of Disability

The ICF distinguishes impairments from activity limitations and participation restrictions. *Impairment* is a deviation from population norms for physical or mental abilities or function. Thus, inadequate ability to metabolize glucose, high blood pressure, and degenerative changes in joints are all impairments. Psychological symptoms (depression, anxiety), cognitive deficits, hallucinations and delusions, and physical pains are also impairments. *Activity limitations* are difficulties an individual has in executing life activities. *Function* is a global term that encompasses both impairments and life activities. *Disability* refers to decrements in function, which are known at the body level as impairments, at the person level as activity limitations, and at the societal level as participation restrictions (see Figure 9–1). Based on substantial empirical evidence concerning determinants of activity limitations and disabilities, the ICF views impairments, activity limitations, and participation restrictions as being influenced by contextual factors, including personal factors (e.g., age, education, motivation) and environmental factors (e.g., cultural norms, public accommodations, family supports), as depicted in Figure 9–2. Thus, activity limitations and disabilities are determined by impairments of human organisms (physical, psychophysical, and psychological) and by contextual factors that influence adaptation to impairments.

Drawing on the ICF framework, we focus here on what is known about assessment of activity limitations and person-level disabilities. Typically, impairment can be assessed as part of the assessment of a specific disease or condition. For example, the presence of major depression is defined by the number and duration of depressive symptoms that are considered impairments by the ICF. In contrast, activity limitations and participation restrictions necessarily are defined at the level of the whole person. It is practically and conceptually difficult to ascribe activity limitations and disabil-

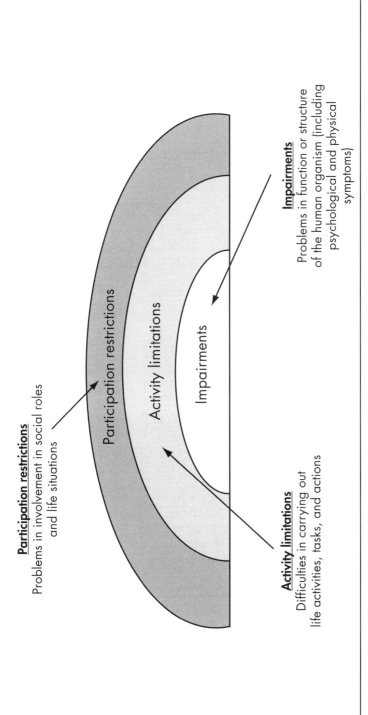

FIGURE 9–1. World Health Organization International Classification of Functioning, Disability and Health perspectives on disability.

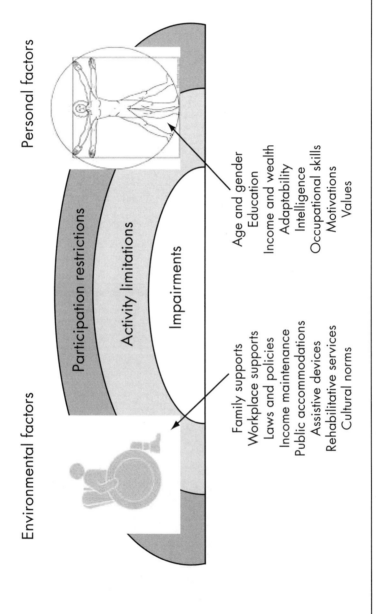

FIGURE 9–2.   Contextual factors that influence disability.

ity to a specific mental or physical disorder, for two reasons: 1) activity limitations are strongly affected by the presence of comorbid conditions (Scott et al. 2009); and 2) limitations are influenced by contextual factors (personal and environmental), distinct from disease-specific impairments. For these reasons, the ICF views activity limitations and disability as phenomena to be assessed intrinsically for the whole person rather than ascribing the limitations and disability to a specific disorder or impairment.

Assessment of Disability by Patient Self-Report: WHO Disability Assessment Schedule II

The WHODAS II is a 36-item self-report questionnaire that assesses activity limitations and participation restrictions for adults during the prior month; there is also a 12-item version (Rehm et al. 1999). Both the 36-item and 12-item versions assess six different adult functional roles: 1) understanding and communication; 2) self-care; 3) mobility (getting around); 4) interpersonal relationships (getting along with others); 5) work and household roles (life activities); and 6) community and civic roles (participation). The 36-item WHODAS II has six items within each of the six functional roles, whereas the 12-item version has two items within each functional role.

As depicted in Figure 9–3, initial psychometric evaluation of the WHODAS II supported the hypothesis that each of the six functional roles was strongly correlated with an underlying *global disability* latent variable. WHODAS II scores overall, and for each of the functional roles, usually are estimated by dividing the sum score by the highest possible score and multiplying by 100; thus, higher scores denote greater disability.

Both versions of the WHODAS II are supplemented by items that ask about the number of days in the prior month during which difficulties with activity limitations were present; the number of days the respondent was totally unable to carry out usual activities; and the number of days the respondent had to cut back on or reduce usual activities due to any health condition.

The WHODAS II was developed to assess difficulties due to health conditions, including diseases, illnesses, or injuries as well as mental or emotional problems and problems with alcohol or drugs. In reviewing what has been learned about the measurement properties of the WHODAS II, general issues in the assessment of activity limitations and person-level disabilities are considered.

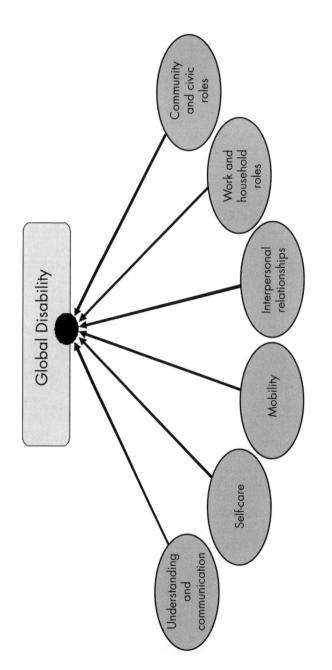

FIGURE 9–3. Global disability and functional roles.

Global Disability

Psychometric evaluation of WHODAS II items has consistently replicated an observation, generally found in prior research, concerning measurement of activity limitations with self-report items. A global disability factor explains a large share of the variance of items across seemingly distinct domains of disability (e.g., self-care, mobility, social interaction, work role). Rehm et al. (1999) found that a global disability latent variable explained 50%–95% of variance in individual items in the 12-item version of the WHODAS II. In a factor analysis of a large set of measures of psychosocial functioning, including the WHODAS II, Ro and Clark (2009) found that a general factor explained 65% of common variance. In analyses of general population samples from four countries, Von Korff et al. (2008) found that functional role scores for a modified version of the WHODAS II had factor loadings on a global disability factor that averaged 0.50 for understanding and communication, 0.63 for self-care, 0.76 for mobility, 0.49 for interpersonal relationships, and 0.69 for work and household role, across all four countries.

Two important implications of the large common variance are explained by the global disability factor: 1) it is possible to measure reliably the severity of activity limitations with relatively brief self-report scales; and 2) although it is often stated that disability is multidimensional, it has been observed generally that scales that measure seemingly distinct domains of disability are highly correlated with one another. Although it is true that factor analysis usually extracts multiple factors, when applied to a large set of items that assess activity limitations, no consensus on the underlying dimensions of disability has emerged from decades of psychometric research on disability assessment. Although the six functional roles assessed by the WHODAS II are clinically relevant, and have been found to show profile differences across disorders, there is not yet robust empirical validation of the six functional roles or agreement that defining them as subdomains of global disability is the most parsimonious way of describing the variance in the WHODAS II item set.

Internal Consistency

Research has found that—in common with many other self-report disability measures—the internal consistency of the WHODAS II, and of each of the functional role subscales, is generally high. Across studies that have reported Cronbach's α for the WHODAS II, the average estimate of coefficient α for the total WHODAS II score was 0.94 (Baron et al. 2008; Chisolm et al. 2005; Chwastiak and Von Korff 2003; McKibbin et al. 2004; Pösl et al. 2007; Ro and Clark 2009). The ranges and means for estimates of coefficient reported in these studies, for each of the six WHODAS II scales that measure functional roles, are shown in Table 9–1. The overall understanding and communication, mobility, work/household role, and community/civic role scale scores were consistently found to have high internal consistency. The self-care and interpersonal relationship scale scores were less reliable but achieved acceptable levels of internal consistency across studies.

Test-Retest Reliability

Research also has provided strong support for the test-retest reliability of the WHODAS II. McKibbin et al. (2004) found the intraclass correlation of WHODAS II scores was 0.89 among older persons with schizophrenia when assessed on two occasions 12 weeks apart. Chopra et al. (2008) studied persons with arthritis and Chisolm et al. (2005) studied adults with acquired hearing loss, and both groups also found high test-retest reliability for each of the WHODAS II subscales (see Table 9–2). The high test-retest reliability estimates not only reflect well on the reliability of the WHODAS II and each of the scales measuring functional roles, but also suggest that WHODAS II scores tend to be stable over time—up to 12 weeks among persons with diverse chronic conditions (schizophrenia, arthritis, acquired hearing loss).

Concurrent Validity

There now is a large literature assessing the validity of the WHODAS II in a wide range of populations. In summarizing these results, we refer to correlations of the WHODAS II with other measures as strong (0.50 or greater), moderate (from 0.40 to 0.49), and modest (from 0.20 to 0.39). Table 9–3 summarizes the results of these studies. In brief, moderate-to-strong correlations have been found between WHODAS II scores and validating measures of activity limitations, including disease-specific measures, among persons with arthritis (Baron et al. 2008); depression and back pain (Chwastiak and Von Korff 2003); ankylosing spondylitis (van Tubergen et al. 2003); HIV/AIDS (Kemmler et al. 2003); schizophrenia (Ertugrul and Ulug 2002; McKibbin et al. 2004); acquired hearing loss (Chisolm et al. 2005); or systemic sclerosis (Hudson et al. 2008a, 2008b) as well as rehabilitation patients (Pösl et al. 2007) and in general population samples in diverse countries and cultures (Kim et al. 2005; Von Korff et al. 2008).

It is not particularly surprising that evaluation of concurrent validity of the WHODAS II, relative to other self-report disability measures, has provided strong support for its validity. Typically, moderate-to-strong correlations among different scales that seemingly measure different facets of activity limitation and disability have been observed because the test items for different scales generally measure the same global disability latent variable. That said, the

TABLE 9–1. Summary of studies that have estimated internal consistency (Cronbach α) for World Health Organization Disability Assessment Schedule II (WHODAS II) scores

	RANGE	MEAN
Understanding and communication	0.80–0.87	0.85
Self-care	0.65–0.92	0.76
Mobility (getting around)	0.75–0.95	0.87
Interpersonal relationships (getting along)	0.68–0.86	0.75
Work and household role (life activities)	0.91–0.97	0.93
Community and civic role (participation)	0.77–0.89	0.85
Overall WHODAS II score	0.89–0.96	0.94

Source. Baron et al. 2008; Chisolm et al. 2005; Chwastiak and Von Korff 2003; McKibbin et al. 2004; Pösl et al. 2007; Ro and Clark 2009.

accumulated evidence, across diseases and across countries, that the WHODAS II shows moderate-to-strong correlation with other widely used measures of disability and activity limitation supports its continued use, particularly given its grounding in the conceptual framework of the ICF.

Responsiveness to Change

Before-after effect size is used widely as a measure of responsiveness to change. In before-after comparisons, an effect size of 0.20–0.49 is considered small, 0.50–0.79 moderate, and 0.80 or greater large. In general, large effect sizes are more likely to be observed for changes in impairment-specific measures than for changes in measures of activity limitation and disability. Studies that have estimated responsiveness to change of the WHODAS II, relative to other measures of functioning, are shown in Table 9–4. Among patients with trauma, depression, and back pain, WHODAS II scores were found to have effect sizes in the moderate range. Among patients with ankylosing spondylitis, acquired hearing loss (subsequent to provision of a hearing aid), and panic/agoraphobia (subsequent to treatment), WHODAS II effect sizes were in the small range. Across four studies in which the WHODAS II was compared with the subscales of the Short Form–36 (SF-36) that assess disability, the WHODAS II had a larger effect size for 13 comparisons and a smaller one for 3 comparisons. WHODAS II effect size exceeded the SF-36 subscales by greater than 0.10 for ten of these comparisons, whereas an SF-36 subscale score exceeded the effect size of the WHODAS II by greater than 0.10 for one comparison.

TABLE 9–2.　Summary of studies that have assessed test-retest reliability (intraclass correlation) of the World Health Organization Disability Assessment Schedule II (WHODAS II)

	ARTHRITIS	HEARING LOSS	
	1-WEEK INTERVAL	2-WEEK INTERVAL	10-WEEK INTERVAL
Understanding and communication	0.85	0.85	0.81
Self-care	0.82	0.91	0.81
Mobility	0.96	0.91	0.85
Interpersonal relationships	0.91	0.81	0.71
Work and household role		0.82	0.75
Work	0.96	—	—
Household	0.91	—	—
Community and civic role	0.83	0.91	0.87
Overall WHODAS II score	0.96	0.93	0.87

Source.　Arthritis data adapted from Chopra et al. 2008; hearing loss data adapted from Chisolm et al. 2005.

Although the WHODAS II effect size for depressed primary care patients was in the moderate range, WHODAS II effect sizes for patients treated for anxiety disorders were smaller (0.26 for panic/agoraphobia, 0.13 for social phobia). In this study (Perini et al. 2006), the available disability measures ("Days Out of Role" and "Days Cut Back") had similar effect sizes to those for the WHODAS II. It is not clear whether the changes in activity limitation for these patients were small or if the available disability measures were not sensitive to improvements in activity limitation. A symptom-severity scale (the K-10) had effect sizes in the moderate range (see Table 9–4), and the Social Interaction Anxiety Scale for social phobia and the Depression Anxiety Stress Scale for panic/agoraphobia had effect sizes that exceeded 0.90. However, the WHODAS II had much larger effect sizes when used to compare patients who had improved clinically with those who had not.

Cross-National Applicability

A considerable number of research findings suggest that self-report disability measures have similar performance properties in diverse countries and languages, including both developed and developing

TABLE 9–3. Summary of studies that have assessed concurrent validity of the World Health Organization Disability Assessment Schedule II (WHODAS II)

POPULATION	MAIN RESULTS	STUDY
Arthritis	Moderate-to-strong correlations with disease activity, disease-specific function, and physician-rated disease severity	Baron et al. 2008
Back pain and depression	Moderate-to-strong correlations with disease-specific function (back pain), SF-36 disability subscales, and Work Limitation Questionnaire scales	Chwastiak and Von Korff 2003
Ankylosing spondylitis	Strong correlations with SF-36 disability scales and disease-specific function scales	van Tubergen et al. 2003
HIV/AIDS	Moderate-to-strong correlations with disease-specific function scales	Kemmler et al. 2003
Schizophrenia (older patients)	Moderate-to-strong correlation with quality of well-being scale; inconsistent and (when present) modest correlation with positive and negative symptoms of schizophrenia; not correlated with role-playing tasks that simulate everyday function or cognitive deficits	McKibbin et al. 2004
Schizophrenia	Strongly correlated with positive and negative symptoms of schizophrenia; not correlated with performance on neuropsychological tests of cognitive deficit	Ertugrul and Ulug 2002

TABLE 9–3. Summary of studies that have assessed concurrent validity of the World Health Organization Disability Assessment Schedule II (WHODAS II) *(continued)*

POPULATION	MAIN RESULTS	STUDY
Acquired hearing loss	Strongly correlated with SF-36 subscales that assess disability; modest-to-moderate correlations with hearing-loss severity scores	Chisolm et al. 2005
Systemic sclerosis	Moderate-to-strong correlations with SF-36 subscales that measure disability; moderate correlation with patient global rating of disease severity; strong association with disease-specific measure of function	Hudson et al. 2008a, 2008b
Rehabilitation patients (musculoskeletal disorders, internal conditions, stroke, breast cancer)	Moderate-to-strong correlations with SF-36 subscales that measure disability	Pösl et al. 2007
General population sample, Korea	Strong correlation with numbers of physical illness, depression, and Mini-Mental State Examination score	Kim et al. 2005
General population samples, six European countries	Strong correlation with SF-12 physical function score; modest and variable correlations with Sheehan Disability ratings across 17 developed/developing countries (modified version of WHODAS II with filter items that caused measurement problems)	Von Korff et al. 2008

Note.   SF=Short Form.

countries (Kim et al. 2005; Scott et al. 2009; Von Korff et al. 1996, 2008). However, there also is evidence that disability levels and disability cutpoints, across countries, cannot be used to compare disability levels or prevalence rates across countries (Von Korff et al. 2008). This circumstance is not unique to cross-national comparisons of disability, because a similar circumstance is encountered in comparisons of prevalence rates of mental disorders and cognitive impairment across countries.

Limitations and Unresolved Shortcomings

Although WHODAS II appears to provide reliable and valid self-report assessment of disability, it has several limitations and unresolved shortcomings:

1. Despite many decades of research on self-report disability measures, uncertainty remains about what these measures capture and what they miss. There is no gold standard for assessment of disability in functional roles.
2. The reliability and validity of WHODAS II are likely to be greater in assessing global disability than in assessing activity limitations in specific functional roles.
3. There is no standard way of incorporating information about unemployment due to health problems, or activity limitation days due to health problems, into WHODAS II scores. The 36-item version of WHODAS II includes a supplementary question about employment status, which asks about inability to work due to health problems. The 12-item version of WHODAS II includes questions about activity limitation days. However, these items are not integrated into either the subscale scores or the overall score of WHODAS II.
4. Patients who cannot provide valid information on a self-report questionnaire, either self-administered or administered by interview, will yield invalid data with WHODAS II. Patients for whom self-report data may be invalid include developmentally disabled persons who do not understand the questions, persons with dementia or severe cognitive impairments, persons in the acute phase of psychotic disorders, and persons who may not be motivated to provide accurate information.
5. It is unclear whether self-report disability measures are able to detect decrements in performance that might occur among persons whose premorbid performance was at high levels. Self-report questions that specifically ask respondents to compare their current and past performances in work/household roles, interpersonal relationships, and community/civic roles should be developed and tested to address this shortcoming.

TABLE 9–4. Summary of studies that have assessed responsiveness to change (effect size) of the World Health Organization Disability Assessment Schedule II (WHODAS II)

POPULATION	EFFECT-SIZE ESTIMATE		STUDY
Trauma patients assessed 7 weeks after injury and 1 year later	WHODAS II	0.65	Soberg et al. 2007
	SF-36 Physical Function	0.48	
	SF-36 Social Function	0.45	
	SF-36 Role Physical	0.49	
	SF-36 Role Emotional	0.28	
Depressed patients assessed 2–4 weeks after primary care visit and 3 months later	WHODAS II	0.60	Chwastiak and Von Korff 2003
	SF-36 Physical Function	0.43	
	SF-36 Social Function	0.64	
	SF-36 Role Physical	0.53	
	SF-36 Role Emotional	0.22	
	Roland Bodily Pain Disability Scale	0.48	
Back pain patients assessed 2–4 weeks after primary care visit and 3 months later	WHODAS II	0.65	Chwastiak and Von Korff 2003
	SF-36 Physical Function	0.03	
	SF-36 Social Function	0.81	
	SF-36 Role Physical	0.10	
	SF-36 Role Emotional	0.66	
Social phobia patients pre- to posttreatment	WHODAS II	0.13	Perini et al. 2006
	Days Out of Role	0.13	
	Days Cut Back	0.21	
	K-10 (symptom severity)	0.69	
Panic/agoraphobia patients pre- to posttreatment	WHODAS II	0.26	Perini et al. 2006
	Days Out of Role	0.26	
	Days Cut Back	0.31	
	K-10 (symptom severity)	0.53	

TABLE 9–4. Summary of studies that have assessed responsiveness to change (effect size) of the World Health Organization Disability Assessment Schedule II (WHODAS II) *(continued)*

POPULATION	EFFECT-SIZE ESTIMATE		STUDY
Ankylosing spondylitis patients assessed before and 3 weeks after spa treatment	WHODAS II	0.39	van Tubergen et al. 2003
	SF-36 Physical Function	0.26	
	SF-36 Social Function	0.32	
	SF-36 Role Physical	0.32	
	SF-36 Role Emotional	0.13	
	Bath Ankylosing Spondylitis Functional Index	0.37	
	Dougados Functional Index	0.33	
	Health Assess Questionnaire for Ankylosing Spondylitis	0.26	
	Ankylosing Spondylitis Quality of Life Index	0.22	
Acquired hearing loss patients assessed before and 10 weeks after provision of hearing aids	WHODAS II	0.20	McArdle et al. 2005
	Communication	0.52	
	Communication/Civic role	0.13	
	Abbreviated Profile Hearing Aid Benefit	2.19	
	Hearing Aid Handicap Inventory	0.74	

Note. SF=Short Form.

Clinician Ratings

Andrews et al. (World Health Organization 2000) have developed a clinician-rated proxy version of the WHODAS II, employing the same 1-month time frame. This version assesses the same six functional roles; elicits information on how many days activity limitations were present; and asks the same questions regarding activity limitation days as the 12-item version. (A copy of this form is provided in the appendix to this chapter.)

The reliability and validity of this ICF-based clinician rating form has not been assessed yet, but it is based on the ICF conceptual framework that differentiates activity limitations and disability from symptoms/impairments. Using this clinician rating form in tandem with the self-rated 12- (or 36-) item version of the WHODAS II could dramatically advance the assessment of disability, in both research and clinical practice. An important first step in making the clinician-rated proxy version of the WHODAS II available for field testing and research would be to develop a Web-based program that 1) trains users in the underlying concepts of assessing activity limitations; 2) demonstrates its use in several video interviews with transparent ratings; and 3) provides vignettes or interviews that are rated by the trainee, with provision for checking and correcting ratings.

The clinician-rated proxy version of WHODAS II also does not provide for detecting decrements from premorbid high levels of functioning. Like the self-report version, the clinician-rated version should be modified to test ratings that specifically assess such decrements in performance.

Summary

Available research supports the following conclusions regarding the WHODAS II:

- It is well grounded in the ICF framework, measuring global disability and activity limitations defined within functional roles.
- The internal consistency and test-retest reliability of the overall WHODAS II score are both high, suggesting potential utility in assessment of individual patients as well as assessment of group differences.
- The internal consistency of WHODAS II subscales that assess functional roles are also generally high but may not be sufficient to support reliable assessment of individual patients. The subscales that assess understanding and communication, mobility, work and household role, and community and civic role have high internal consistency, whereas the subscales that assess self-care and interpersonal relationships have somewhat lower internal consistency.

A growing body of research supports the concurrent validity of the WHODAS II—in comparison with other widely used disability measures—in a wide range of patient populations and general population samples and across different countries and languages of administration. Evaluation of responsiveness to change has indicated that the WHODAS II performs at least as well as, and perhaps better than, the SF-36 subscales that assess disability across a wide range of chronic conditions. However, self-report measures of activity limitation generally have been found to have no more than moderate responsiveness to change in assessment of improvement in global disability. This may be because global disability shows less marked improvement than do specific impairments. Alternatively, future research may develop more sensitive measures of activity limitation that show larger effect sizes in detecting change in disability levels. With these caveats in mind, the WHODAS II was found in several studies to be as responsive to change as disease-specific functional measures.

Clinical Assessment of Disability: Global Assessment of Functioning

A possible strategy to enhance assessment of disability might be to use parallel self-report and clinician-disability ratings in tandem. This approach not only would yield two perspectives on disability but also would provide a means of understanding agreements and discrepancies between the two assessments and, ultimately, of improving the reliability and validity of both types of ratings. At present, the most widely used clinician rating of disability is the GAF, and we review research here that has assessed measurement of disability with that instrument. The GAF was not developed within the ICF framework; it neither assesses activity limitations in specific functional roles nor distinguishes person-level disability and activity limitations from disorder-specific impairments.

The GAF is a 100-point scale that measures psychological, social, and occupational functioning. It is assessed by a mental health practitioner, and scores vary from 1–10 (persistent danger of hurting self or others OR persistent inability to maintain minimum personal hygiene OR serious suicidal act with clear expectation of death) to 91–100 (superior functioning in a wide range of activities; life's problems never seem to get out of hand; is sought by others because of his or her many positive qualities; no symptoms) (American Psychiatric Association 2000).

First introduced in 1980 for DSM-III (American Psychiatric Association 1980), the GAF was intended to measure "psychological, social, and occupational functioning" in patients and replaced a previous "simple measure of adaptive functioning" with a 90-point scale (Goldman et al. 1997). The GAF was modified in 1987 for DSM-III-R (American Psychiatric Association 1987), with the experimental inclusion of further scales: the Social and Occupational Functioning Assessment, Global Assessment of Relational Functioning, and Defensive Functioning scales (American Psychiatric Association 2000; Goldman et al. 1997; Schorre and Vandvik 2004). In 1994, the GAF scale was altered from 0–90 to 0–100, allowing for differentiation of high-functioning individuals (American Psychiatric Association 1994).

Reliability

Initial testing of the GAF found interrater reliabilities of between 0.69 and 0.80 in field trials (Spitzer and Forman 1979). Independent follow-up trials observed less favorable and more variable interrater reliability coefficients ranging from 0.49 to 0.61 (Fernando et al. 1986; Goldman et al. 1997; Mezzich et al. 1985; Rey et al. 1988; Russell et al. 1979). After the changes for DSM-III-R were introduced, more recent reliability studies have estimated intraclass correlation coefficients across raters of 0.33–0.96 (Greenberg and Rosenheck 2005; Hall 1995; Karterud et al. 2003; Oliver et al. 2003; Roy-Byrne et al. 1996; Söderberg et al. 2005; Tungström et al. 2005; Vatnaland et al. 2007). This suggests that high reliability is possible but that differences in rater training and performance may be critically important in achieving high levels of reliability.

In fact, research has shown that training and performance of a rater are fundamental to the reliability of GAF results (Bodlund et al. 1994; Jones et al. 1995; Loevdahl and Friis 1996; Oliver et al. 2003; Pedersen et al. 2007; Piersma and Boes 1997; Roy-Byrne et al. 1996; Schorre and Vandvik 2004; Söderberg et al. 2005; Vatnaland et al. 2007). Raters less interested in clinical functioning, relevant to clinical decisions, may rate more realistically, as shown by Piersma and Boes (1997) and Roy-Byrne et al. (1996). Studies by Schorre and Vandvik (2004), Vatnaland et al. (2007), Pederson et al. (2007), and Loevdahl and Friis (1996) all found higher reliability in raters with more experience or training. Attitude and motivation of a rater also can affect reliability (Söderberg et al. 2005). For example, Vatnaland et al. (2007) found that the GAF was unreliable in clinical situations but that it was highly reliable when used by researchers. Increased precision also was found when the number of raters was increased, with two raters providing the optimum evaluation (Pedersen et al. 2007).

Validity

The GAF has been shown by several studies to correlate closely with symptom levels, but several studies also have found that GAF correlates better with symptoms than with disability levels (Moos et al. 2002; Niv et al. 2007; Pedersen et al. 2007; Roy-Byrne et al. 1996; Tungström et al. 2005). Although research also has demonstrated a close association between GAF scores and clinical outcome (Fowler et al. 2004; Greenberg and Rosenheck 2005; Hay et al. 2003; Karterud et al. 2003; Moos et al. 2002; Niv et al. 2007; Roy-Byrne et al. 1996; Tungström et al. 2005), the question remains as to whether this is due more to association with symptom levels or to disability outcomes. Patterson and Lee (1995) found that six predictors accounted for 52% of variation in GAF scores. Of these, access to and ability to use transportation was the best predictor, and GAF scores were independent of patients' Axis I or II disorders.

In contrast, Karterud et al. (2003), in a Norwegian study of patients with panic disorder, found patients had lower GAF scores than control subjects and higher GAF scores than patients with schizotypal or schizoid tendencies. Moos et al. (2002) found that clinical diagnoses and symptoms were stronger predictors of global functioning than was social or occupational functioning. This group also found that the only social or occupational factor that independently predicted global functioning was employment status, which accounted for less than 1% of variance.

Greenberg and Rosenheck (2005) found that veterans with schizophrenia, Alzheimer's disease, drug abuse/dependence, personality disorders, and posttraumatic stress disorder all had lower GAF scores than did control subjects, but this study did not assess the extent to which this was explained by greater disability of the patient populations. Tungström et al. (2005), in a study in Sweden, found that 17% of variance in GAF scores was due to diagnostic differences in DSM Axis I. Although few individual disorders have been specifically examined, the GAF has been shown to be invalid among pediatric patients with learning disabilities (Oliver et al. 2003) and among adults with schizophrenia during acute psychosis (Tungström et al. 2005). Overall, the available literature indicates that, rather than being a pure reflection of social and occupational disability and activity limitations, the GAF scale is influenced by the severity and nature of a patient's mental disorder. Indeed, the anchors for GAF ratings suggest consideration of psychopathology, along with disability levels, in making GAF ratings.

Summary

Research on the GAF suggests that clinician ratings provide a potentially reliable and valid approach to assessing activity limitations and disability. However, for clinician disability ratings to be reliable and valid, the rating form and supporting instructions need to be structured and to differentiate activity limitations clearly from psychiatric symptoms (which GAF does not). In addition, a practical means of training raters would be needed to increase interrater reliability of clinician disability ratings. Ongoing attention to the calibration and motivation of clinicians trained to make structured disability ratings also might be helpful.

Practical Approaches for Improvement of Disability Assessment

On the basis of our review, we recommend the following steps to improve disability assessment in clinical practice and research:

1. Methods of assessment of activity limitations and disability should be developed within the ICF framework. Specifically, methods should assess activity limitations and disability, not impairments (including psychiatric symptoms).
2. Development of improved methods for assessment of disability and activity limitations should build from the extensive methodological work already completed for the WHODAS II, work which has established its reliability, validity, and responsiveness to change in assessment of a wide range of disorders and its usefulness in diverse countries and languages.
3. Given limitations of both self-report and clinician-rated assessments, the self-report and clinician-rated proxy versions of the WHODAS II should be used in tandem in both clinical practice and research.
4. The WHODAS II should be augmented with items that determine whether a patient is unable to work because of health problems. Existing items that assess activity limitation days in the prior month should be retained. This information might be incorporated into the scoring of the WHODAS II.
5. Both the self-report and the clinician-rated proxy versions should be enhanced with items developed to assess decrements in functioning from previously high levels of performance.
6. Country-specific normative data for the WHODAS II should be published from available World Health Organization surveys, including means scores, standard deviations, and WHODAS II scores at key percentiles of the population distributions (e.g., fifth,

tenth, fifteenth, twenty-fifth, fiftieth, seventy-fifth, eighty-fifth, ninetieth, and ninety-fifth percentiles). As distributional data become available on clinician-rated versions of the WHODAS II, these also should be published.

In conclusion, development of the ICF framework and extensive work in development and testing of the WHODAS II in the assessment of disability, within the ICF framework, provide a strong foundation for future development of brief, reliable, and valid methods of assessment of activity limitations in clinical practice and research. By using self-report and clinician-rated proxy versions of this instrument in tandem, it is likely that significant advances could be made in assessment of activity limitations and disability.

References

American Psychiatric Association: Diagnostic and Statistical Manual of Mental Disorders, 3rd Edition. Washington, DC, American Psychiatric Association, 1980

American Psychiatric Association: Diagnostic and Statistical Manual of Mental Disorders, 3rd Edition, Revised. Washington, DC, American Psychiatric Association, 1987

American Psychiatric Association: Diagnostic and Statistical Manual of Mental Disorders, 4th Edition. Washington, DC, American Psychiatric Association, 1994

American Psychiatric Association: Diagnostic and Statistical Manual of Mental Disorders, 4th Edition, Text Revision. Washington, DC, American Psychiatric Association, 2000

Baron M, Schier O, Hudson M, et al: The clinimetric properties of the World Health Organization Disability Assessment Schedule II in early inflammatory arthritis. Arthritis Rheum 59:382–390, 2008

Bodlund O, Kullgren G, Ekselius L, et al: Axis V–Global assessment of functioning scale: evaluation of a self-report version. Acta Psychiatr Scand 90:342–347, 1994

Chisolm TH, Abrams HB, McArdle R, et al: The WHO-DAS II: psychometric properties in the measurement of functional health status in adults with acquired hearing loss. Trends Amplif 9:111–126, 2005

Chopra P, Herrman H, Kennedy G: Comparison of disability and quality of life measures in patients with long-term psychotic disorders and patients with multiple sclerosis: an application of the WHO Disability Assessment Schedule II and WHO Quality of Life-BREF. Int J Rehabil Res 31:141–149, 2008

Chwastiak LA, Von Korff M: Disability in depression and back pain: evaluation of the World Health Organization Disability Assessment Schedule (WHO DAS II) in a primary care setting. J Clin Epidemiol 56:507–514, 2003

Ertugrul A, Ulug B: The influence of neurocognitive deficits and symptoms on disability in schizophrenia. Acta Psychiatr Scand 105:196–201, 2002

Fernando T, Mellsop G, Nelson K, et al: The reliability of axis V of DSM-III. Am J Psychiatry 143:752–755, 1986

Fowler JC, Ackerman SJ, Speanburg S, et al: Personality and symptom change in treatment-refractory inpatients: evaluation of the phase model of change using Rorschach, TAT, and DSM-IV Axis V. J Pers Assess 83:306–322, 2004

Goldman HH, Skodol AE, Lave TR: Revising Axis V for DSM-IV: a review of measures of social functioning, in DSM-IV Sourcebook. Edited by Widiger TA, Frances AJ, Pincus HA, et al. Washington, DC, American Psychiatric Association, 1997, pp 439–459

Greenberg GA, Rosenheck RA: Using the GAF as a national mental health outcome measure in the Department of Veterans Affairs. Psychiatr Serv 56:420–426, 2005

Hall RC: Global assessment of functioning: a modified scale. Psychosomatics 36:267–275, 1995

Hay P, Katsikitis M, Begg J, et al: A two-year follow-up study and prospective evaluation of the DSM-IV axis V. Psychiatr Serv 54:1028–1030, 2003

Hudson M, Steele R, Taillefer S: Quality of life in systemic sclerosis: psychometric properties of the World Health Organization Disability Assessment Schedule II. Arthritis Rheum 59:270–278, 2008a

Hudson M, Thombs BD, Steele R, et al: Clinical correlates of quality of life in systemic sclerosis measured with the World Health Organization Disability Assessment Schedule II. Arthritis Rheum 59:279–284, 2008b

Jones SH, Thornicroft G, Coffey M, et al: A brief mental health outcome scale: reliability and validity of the Global Assessment of Functioning (GAF). Br J Psychiatry 166:654–659, 1995

Karterud S, Pedersen G, Bjordal E, et al: Day treatment of patients with personality disorders: experiences from a Norwegian treatment research network. J Pers Disord 17:243–262, 2003

Kemmler G, Schmied B, Shetty-Lee A, et al: Quality of life of HIV-infected patients: psychometric properties and validation of the German version of the HQOL-HIV. Qual Life Res 12:1037–1050, 2003

Kim JM, Stewart R, Glozier N, et al: Physical health, depression and cognitive function as correlates of disability in an older Korean population. Int J Geriatr Psychiatry 20:160–167, 2005

Loevdahl H, Friis S: Routine evaluation of mental health: reliable information or worthless "guesstimates"? Acta Psychiatr Scand 93:125–128, 1996

McArdle R, Chisolm TH, Abrams HB, et al: The WHO-DAS II: measuring outcomes of hearing aid intervention for adults. Trends Amplif 9:127–143, 2005

McKibbin C, Patterson TL, Jeste DV: Assessing disability in older patients with schizophrenia: results from the WHODAS-II. J Nerv Ment Dis 192:405–413, 2004

Mezzich AC, Mezzich JE, Coffman GA: Reliability of DSM-III vs. DSM-II in child psychopathology. J Am Acad Child Psychiatry 24:273–280, 1985

Moos RH, Nichol AC, Moos BS: Global Assessment of Functioning ratings and the allocation and outcomes of mental health services. Psychiatr Serv 53:730–737, 2002

Niv N, Cohen AN, Sullivan G, et al: The MIRECC version of the Global Assessment of Functioning scale: reliability and validity. Psychiatr Serv 58:529–535, 2007

Oliver P, Cooray S, Tyrer P, et al: Use of the Global Assessment of Function scale in learning disability. Br J Psychiatry Suppl 44:S32–S35, 2003

Patterson DA, Lee MS: Field trial of the Global Assessment of Functioning Scale-Modified. Am J Psychiatry 152:1386–1388, 1995

Pedersen G, Hagtvet KA, Karterud S: Generalizability studies of the Global Assessment of Functioning–Split version. Compr Psychiatry 48:88–94, 2007

Perini SJ, Slade T, Andrews G: Generic effectiveness measures: sensitivity to symptom change in anxiety disorders. J Affect Disord 90:123–130, 2006

Piersma HL, Boes JL: The GAF and psychiatric outcome: a descriptive report. Community Ment Health J 33:35–41, 1997

Pösl M, Cieza A, Stucki G: Psychometric properties of the WHODAS II in rehabilitation patients. Qual Life Res 16:1521–1531, 2007

Rehm J, Ustun TB, Saxena S, et al: On the development and psychometric testing of the WHO screening instrument to assess disablement in the general population. Int J Methods Psychiatr Res 8:110–122, 1999

Rey JM, Stewart GW, Plapp JM, et al: Validity of Axis V of DSM-III and other measures of adaptive functioning. Acta Psychiatr Scand 77:535–542, 1988

Ro E, Clark LA: Psychosocial functioning in the context of diagnosis: assessment and theoretical issues. Psychol Assess 21:313–324, 2009

Roy-Byrne P, Dagadakis C, Unutzer J, et al: Evidence for limited validity of the revised global assessment of functioning scale. Psychiatr Serv 47:864–866, 1996

Russell AT, Cantwell DP, Mattison R, et al: A comparison of DSM-II and DSM-III in the diagnosis of childhood psychiatric disorders, III: multiaxial features. Arch Gen Psychiatry 36:1223–1226, 1979

Schorre BE, Vandvik IH: Global assessment of psychosocial functioning in child and adolescent psychiatry: a review of three unidimensional scales (CGAS, GAF, GAPD). Eur Child Adolesc Psychiatry 13:273–286, 2004

Scott KM, Von Korff M, Alonso J, et al: Mental-physical co-morbidity and its relationship with disability: results from the World Mental Health Surveys. Psychol Med 39:33–43, 2009

Soberg HL, Bautz-Holter E, Roise O, et al: Long-term multidimensional functional consequences of severe multiple injuries two years after trauma: a prospective longitudinal cohort study. J Trauma 62:461–470, 2007

Söderberg P, Tungström S, Armelius BA: Reliability of global assessment of functioning ratings made by clinical psychiatric staff. Psychiatr Serv 56:434–438, 2005

Spitzer RL, Forman JB: DSM-III field trials, II: initial experience with the multiaxial system. Am J Psychiatry 136:818–820, 1979

Startup M, Jackson MC, Bendix S: The concurrent validity of the Global Assessment of Functioning (GAF). Br J Clin Psychol 41:417–422, 2002

Tungström S, Söderberg P, Armelius BA: Relationship between the Global Assessment of Functioning and other DSM axes in routine clinical work. Psychiatr Serv 56:439–443, 2005 van Tubergen A, Landewe R, Heuft-Dorenbosch L, et al: Assessment of disability with the World Health Organization Disability Assessment Schedule II in patients with ankylosing spondylitis. Ann Rheum Dis 62:140–145, 2003

Vatnaland T, Vatnaland J, Friis S, et al: Are GAF scores reliable in routine clinical use? Acta Psychiatr Scand 115:326–330, 2007

Von Korff M, Ustun TB, Ormel J, et al: Self-report disability in an international primary care study of psychological illness. J Clin Epidemiol 49:297–303, 1996

Von Korff M, Crane PK, Alonso J, et al: Modified WHODAS-II provides valid measure of global disability but filter items increased skewness. J Clin Epidemiol 61:1132–1143, 2008

World Health Organization: WHO DAS II Disability Assessment Schedule Training Manual: A Guide to Administration. Geneva, World Health Organization, 2000

World Health Organization: International Classification of Functioning, Disability and Health. Geneva, World Health Organization, 2001. Available at: http://www.who.int/classifications/icf/en/. Accessed July 13, 2009.

Appendix: Clinician-Rated Proxy Version of WHO Disability Assessment Schedule II

World Health Organization
Disability Assessment Schedule II

Phase 2 Field Trials – Health Services Research
6-Item Clinician Proxy Version

For Office Use Only:

__ __ __ - __ __ __ - __
Center#   Subject # - Time #

__ __/ __ __ / __ __
Day / Month / Year

Pop: Dwelling:
❑   Gen   ☐ Independent
❑   Drg   ☐ Assisted
❑   Alc   ☐ Hospitalized
❑   Mnh
❑   Phys
❑   Other

This questionnaire asks about <u>difficulties due to health conditions</u>. Health conditions include diseases or illnesses, other health problems that may be short or long lasting, injuries, mental or emotional problems, and problems with alcohol or drugs.

Think back over the <u>last 30 days</u> and, to the best of your knowledge, answer these questions thinking about how much difficulty your <u>patient</u> had while doing the following activities. For each question, please circle only <u>one</u> response.

H1	How do you rate your patient's <u>overall health in the past 30 days</u>?	Very good	Good	Moderate	Bad	Very Bad

In the last 30 days, <u>how much difficulty</u> did your patient have in…						
CS1	<u>Understanding and communicating</u>. • Concentrating or remembering • Finding solutions to problems • Learning something new • Generally understanding and communicating with people	None	Mild	Moderate	Severe	Extreme/ Cannot Do
CS2	<u>Getting around</u>. • Standing for long periods • Standing up from sitting down • Moving around inside the home • Getting out of the home • Difficulty with walking a long distance such as a kilometer	None	Mild	Moderate	Severe	Extreme/ Cannot Do
CS3	<u>Self care</u>. • Washing his/her whole body • Getting dressed • Eating • Staying alone for a few days	None	Mild	Moderate	Severe	Extreme/ Cannot Do
CS4	<u>Getting along with people</u>. • Dealing with people who are strangers • Maintaining a friendship • Getting along with people who are close • Controlling feelings	None	Mild	Moderate	Severe	Extreme/ Cannot Do
CS5	<u>Household activities or work or school activities</u>. • Getting these activities done • Doing these activities well • Doing them as quickly as needed	None	Mild	Moderate	Severe	Extreme/ Cannot Do

Please continue to the next page …

In the last 30 days, <u>how much difficulty</u> did your patient have in…		None	Mild	Moderate	Severe	Extreme/ Cannot Do
CS6	<u>Participation in society.</u> • The world and other people creating problems • Discrimination • Problems in living with dignity • Problems joining in community activities	None	Mild	Moderate	Severe	Extreme/ Cannot Do

H2	Overall, how much did all of these difficulties interfere with your patient's life?	Not at all	Mildly	Moderately	Severely	Extremely
H3	Overall, in the past 30 days, <u>how many days</u> were these difficulties present?	RECORD NUMBER OF DAYS ___/___				
H4	In the past 30 days, for how many days was your patient <u>totally unable</u> to carry out his/her usual activities or work because of any health condition?	RECORD NUMBER OF DAYS ___/___				
H5	In the past 30 days, not counting the days that your patient was totally unable, for how many days did your patient <u>cut back</u> or <u>reduce</u> his/her usual activities or work because of any health condition?	RECORD NUMBER OF DAYS ___/___				
H6	In the past 30 days, how many days have you seen or spoken with your patient?	RECORD NUMBER OF DAYS ___/___				

This completes the questionnaire. Thank you.

CHAPTER 10

Measuring Disability Across Physical, Mental, and Cognitive Disorders

Martin Prince, M.D.
Nick Glozier, Ph.D.
Renata Sousa, Ph.D.
Michael Dewey, Ph.D.

The 10/66 Dementia Research Group's research has been funded by the Wellcome Trust Health Consequences of Population Change Program (GR066133 Prevalence phase in Cuba and Brazil; GR08002 Incidence phase in Peru, Mexico, Argentina, Cuba, Dominican Republic, Venezuela, and China), the World Health Organization (India, Dominican Republic, and China), the United States Alzheimer's Association (IIRG 04 1286 Peru, Mexico, and Argentina), and FONACIT/CDCH/UCV (Venezuela). Principal Investigators for the 10/66 centers are Professor Juan Llibre Rodriguez (Cuba), Dr. Daisy Acosta (Dominican Republic), Dr. Mariella Guerra (Peru), Dr. Aquiles Salas (Venezuela), Dr. Ana Luisa Sosa (Mexico), Dr. Joseph Williams (Chennai, India), Professor K.S. Jacob (Vellore, India), and Professor Yueqin Huang (China). The Rockefeller Foundation supported our dissemination meeting at their Bellagio Center. Alzheimer's Disease International has provided support for networking and infrastructure. Dr. Nick Glozier was supported by a Wellcome Trust entry-level fellowship when he conducted the study on responsiveness.

Measurement of disability is important for both population and health services research. Description of health states—at the level of diagnoses, impairments, and symptom severity—cannot capture the impact of disease at an individual and societal level, much of which is quite context dependent. For population research, measures of disability can be used to track the health of a population over time, compare the relative health of different populations or subgroups, and, as one index of disease impact, determine the allocation of finite health care resources between different types of disorders. As a consequence of demographic and health transitions, the incidence and prevalence of chronic diseases are increasing in all world regions (Fuster and Voûte 2005). The Global Burden of Disease (GBD) report uses disability, together with mortality, as twin indicators of the relative burden of different health conditions and indicates that years lived with disability contribute significantly to overall disease burden to an increasing extent in low- and middle- as well as high-income countries (Murray and Lopez 1996; World Health Organization 2006). For health services research, including randomized controlled trials, disability and quality of life are routinely included as patient-reported outcomes. In principle, generic disability measures can capture the effects of comorbidity (particularly important for older people) and can allow meaningful comparisons to be made, both of severity of disability between different physical, mental, and cognitive disorders and of relative effectiveness of interventions applied to the disorders.

A major conceptual advance in this area has been the World Health Organization's (WHO) formulation of the consequences of health conditions, the *International Classification of Impairments, Disabilities and Handicaps* (ICIDH; World Health Organization 1980), now revised as the *International Classification of Functioning, Disability and Health* (ICF; World Health Organization 2001). In ICF, *disability* is defined as "the negative aspects of the interaction between an individual (with a health condition) and that individual's contextual factors (personal and environmental factors)." Interactions include impairments (affecting the body), activity limitations (affecting actions or behavior), and participation restrictions (affecting experience of life). The structure and content of ICIDH/ICF is reflected in many disability instruments, in that they assess the consequence of disease at one or, in some cases, several of these levels. Different approaches include

- *Self-identification as disabled.* This is widely used in national censuses and surveys and involves variations on the question "Do you have a limiting disability?" This approach tends to yield the lowest prevalence in surveys and is thought to be associated with considerable underreporting, particularly in low- and middle-income countries (Mont 2007a). The term *disability* may not be widely understood and/or may be thought of as pertaining only to severe limitation. The term is often stigmatized, particularly with respect to disabilities associated with mental disorder. Furthermore, in many developed countries, the term is applied to those in receipt of certain social benefits, eligibility and uptake of which is subject to a host of external political and economic factors (Organisation for Economic Co-operation and Development 2003). Finally, there is a strong normative element to this type of assessment, in that the comparator (what constitutes disability and nondisability) will tend to vary between individuals according to, for example, age, education, and culture (Mont 2007a).

- *List of common chronic disease diagnoses or impairments.* The main limitation of this approach is that most diagnoses do not relate in any linear or predictable way to disability and dependency. One of the weaknesses of the GBD approach, acknowledged by its authors, is that levels of disability typically associated with particular conditions were estimated in a consensus exercise involving clinicians and other key informants (Murray and Lopez 1996). Furthermore, self-report of diagnoses requires awareness, which may depend on availability of health care; therefore, underreporting will be a problem, particularly in low- and middle-income countries (Mont 2007b). Self-reported impairment, for example, in breathing, seeing, or limb function may arise from a variety of diagnoses, and self-report is less likely to be biased by awareness. The number of organ systems impaired is a simple and parsimonious approach for rating overall illness severity (Burvill et al. 1990; Lindesay 1990) that has been shown to correlate highly with disability (Burvill et al. 1990) and handicap and fully mediates associations between numbers of diagnoses and these outcomes (Harwood et al. 1998).

- *Activities of daily living (ADL) assessments.* These comprise self-reports of difficulties in carrying out core tasks essential to daily life and typically include self-care (washing, feeding, dressing, toileting), mobility, and sometimes social interactions (conversing or relating with others). Many such measures have desirable hierarchical scale properties (Prince 1998). However, ADL measures tend to be biased toward detection of consequences of physical disorders and may not detect mild degrees of disability. These limitations may be addressed through inclusion of instrumental ADL— more complex higher-level activities such as shopping, or managing finances. However, instrumental ADL, much more than ADL, are likely to be culturally and contextually dependent.

- *Health status.* Some generic measures combine items that assess symptoms, impairments, activity limitations, and participation restrictions into composite scales. One example is the Health of the Nation Outcome Scales, a mandated mental health outcome assessment used by service providers in the United Kingdom, Australia, and New Zealand (Wing et al. 1996). It includes symptoms (problems with hallucinations, delusions, and depressed mood), behaviors (aggression, deliberate self-harm, alcohol and substance use), activity limitations (problems with ADL, occupation, and activities), and even problems with living conditions among its 12 items, with four subscales. The status of this measure as a unidimensional scale is open to doubt; internal consistency is modest, and factor analytical studies have identified up to five dimensions (Pirkis et al. 2005). Responsiveness to change has not been demonstrated convincingly (Pirkis et al. 2005); the measure is, perhaps, better viewed as providing a health-status profile across relevant domains.

The best established and most widely used generic health status measure, the Medical Outcomes Study 36-item Short-Form Health Survey (SF-36), includes assessment of symptoms and impairments (pain, depression, and anxiety), general health, physical activity limitations (lifting, bending, climbing, walking), role limitations, and participation restriction (interference with social activities) (McHorney et al. 1993, 1994; Ware and Sherbourne 1992). However, scores from these items are not combined into a single summary score. Careful psychometric analysis led to the identification of eight subscale domains (physical function, role-physical, bodily pain, general health perceptions, vitality, social function, role-emotional, and mental health). Subsequently, the originators of the scale proposed mental-component summary (MCS) and physical-component summary (PCS) scores derived from factor analysis with orthogonal rotation (Ware et al. 1994). Although there is no doubt that the SF-36 is capable of capturing the effects of mental disorder on functioning (Creed et al. 2002; Wells et al. 1989), its structure does not allow these effects to be compared with those of physical health conditions, on a single metric. Furthermore, the orthogonal rotation used to derive the MCS and PCS scores has been shown, empirically, to bias estimation of physical impairment in those with impaired mental health, and vice versa; a sample of primary-care patients treated for depression had better PCS scores than did the general population, despite impairment on physical functioning domains that loaded on the PCS, and improvements in these domains after treatment were not reflected in concomitant changes in the PCS (Simon et al. 1998).

In summary, the conceptual basis for most generic disability instruments is relatively weak. Many of these instruments have been derived empirically, with item selection from much larger item sets that are largely based on psychometric criteria. WHO classifications have only recently begun to have an overt influence on instrument development (Harwood and Ebrahim 1995). The "holy grail" of a simple measure with a universal metric—capable of assessing the severity of disability across different regions, cultures, and health conditions—has yet to be achieved. These considerations informed the development of a new self-report instrument, the WHO Disability Assessment Schedule II (WHODAS II; World Health Organization 2009), conducted in parallel with the revision of the ICIDH classification. Equal attention was given to the conceptual basis of the instrument (to be consistent with both ICIDH and ICF) as to its psychometric robustness. WHODAS II addresses five domains of activity limitation: understanding/communication, getting around (mobility), self-care, getting along with people (interpersonal interaction), and life activities. A sixth domain, participation in society, assesses broader social aspects of disability. A key aim is to identify the consequences of any type of health condition that has an impact on everyday functioning, treating all disorders at parity in determination of level of functioning (Chopra et al. 2004). Psychometric testing of WHODAS II (www.who.int/icidh/whodas) has been rigorous. An early draft (89 items) was tested in field trials in 21 sites and 19 countries, partly to ensure cross-cultural applicability. On the basis of psychometric analyses and further field-testing in early 1999, the measure was shortened to 36 items, and a 12-item screening questionnaire was developed (Rehm et al. 2000).

The psychometric properties of WHODAS II have been explored in different clinical populations, including those with inflammatory arthritis (Baron et al. 2008), back pain (Chwastiak and Von Korff 2003), ankylosing spondylitis (van Tubergen et al. 2003), systemic sclerosis (Hudson et al. 2008), acquired hearing loss (Chisolm et al. 2005), psychosis (Chopra et al. 2004; McKibbin et al. 2004), and depression (Chwastiak and Von Korff 2003) as well as among mental health service users (Chávez et al. 2005) and persons undergoing rehabilitation for a variety of chronic disorders (Pösl et al. 2007). The WHODAS II performed well in all of these contexts, with high internal consistency, moderate to good test-retest reliability, and good concurrent validity against indicators of disease severity and disease-specific and other generic disability assessments. The WHO Web site reports a clear unidimensional structure for WHODAS II, with very high loadings of all six domain scores on a global disability latent variable (www.who.int/icidh/whodas). The shorter 12-item "screener" version of WHODAS II appears to have been little used to date (Andrews et al. 2010; Norton et al. 2004). This is surprising, because it takes only 5 minutes to administer and covers all six domains of the full 36-item WHODAS II (Üstün et al. 2009). In WHO pilot studies, the correlation between the score from the screener and the score from WHODAS II was 0.95, meaning that the screener explained more than 90% of the total variation of the full 36-item WHODAS II (Üstün et al. 2009). Confirmatory factor analysis indicated a unidimensional scale with good classical scaling properties. However, the screener was not found to be compatible with criteria of item response theory (IRT), reducing its cross-cultural applicability (Üstün et al. 2009). Accordingly, 5 of the 12 items (in the understanding and communicating, self-care, and participation domains) were subsequently replaced with others in the same domains from the 36-item version to improve IRT characteristics.

The principal purpose of the new analyses presented in this chapter is to assess the extent to which the WHODAS II functions as a truly generic disability measure, capable of quantifying the disabling consequences of different health conditions along a single metric. We address this question, with a view to epidemiological and health service research applications, by

1. Examining the scaling properties of the WHODAS II 12-item screener in survey populations of older people with depression, dementia, and physical impairment (the 10/66 Dementia Research Group's surveys in seven low- or middle-income countries); and
2. Comparing and contrasting the responsiveness characteristics of the full WHODAS II with those of other generic assessments in clinical samples of older people undergoing hip/knee arthroplasty or community treatment for depression.

Measuring Disability Across Health Conditions in Population Surveys

Background

The 36-item WHODAS II has been used previously in two population-based studies: the World Mental Health surveys of adults across 16 countries (Von Korff et al. 2008) and the Kwangju community survey of physical and psychiatric morbidity among older adults in South Korea (Kim et al. 2005). Findings from these surveys again supported internal consistency (Von Korff et al. 2008) and concurrent validity; in the World Mental Health surveys, WHODAS II scores were consistently correlated with the Sheehan Disability Scale (Von Korff et al. 2008). In Korea, physical health, depression, and cognitive function explained 40% of variance in WHODAS II scores; effects of sociodemographic variables were no longer apparent after controlling for these health outcomes. In the World Mental Health survey, confirmatory factor analysis provided only relatively weak support for unidimensionality in the four countries in which this was carried out (Von Korff et al. 2008). However, the domain subscale scores all loaded greater than 0.40 on a global disability latent variable, and to this extent the utility of a global disability score was supported. Previously, the 12-item WHODAS II screener had not been reported to have been used in population-based research.

Others have remarked on the skewed and zero-inflated character of the WHODAS II distribution and on the large distributional differences between survey populations from different countries (Buist-Bouwman et al. 2008; Von Korff et al. 2008). Standardizing WHODAS II distributions by dichotomizing at the ninetieth percentile for each population has been proposed (Von Korff et al. 2008). However, this has the disadvantage of both loss of measurement precision and loss of ability to model and explore country differences.

Method

Cross-sectional surveys were conducted in 11 geographically defined catchment area sites in seven low- or middle-income countries (India, China, Cuba, Dominican Republic, Venezuela, Mexico, and Peru). Door-to-door canvassing was conducted to enumerate all residents who were ages 65 years and older. All residents who consented to participate received the full 2- to 3-hour assessment, which comprised participant and informant interviews, physical examination, and phlebotomy. Interviews were carried out in participants' homes. The target sample size for each country was 2,000–3,000 (see Table 10–1). China, India, Peru, and Mexico split recruitment between urban and rural sites; other countries included urban sites only. Local ethical committees and the King's College London ethical committee approved all studies.

Measures

The full 10/66 population-based study protocols have been published already in an open access journal (Prince et al. 2007a). Only those measures relevant to the current analyses are described here. Age was formally determined during interview from stated age, official documentation, and informant report, and, if discrepant, age according to an event calendar. We also recorded sex, marital status, and educational level (none, some but less than primary, completed primary, completed secondary, and tertiary). The 10/66 population-based study interview generates information regarding dementia diagnosis, mental disorders, physical health, anthropometry, demographics, an extensive dementia and chronic diseases risk-factor questionnaire, disability, health-service utilization, care arrangements, and caregiver strain (Prince et al. 2007a). Assessments relevant to the outcomes in this analysis were

- A structured clinical mental-state interview, the Geriatric Mental State, which applies a computer algorithm, AGECAT (Copeland et al. 1986), and identifies organicity (probable dementia), depression, anxiety, and psychosis

TABLE 10–1. Sample, by country and health status

Health status	Cuba	Dominican Republic	Peru	Venezuela	Mexico	China	India	Total
"Well"	2,144 (72.8%)	1,220 (60.7%)	1,411 (73.0%)	1,297 (65.8%)	1,408 (70.3%)	1,749 (80.9%)	1,515 (75.6%)	10,744 (71.5%)
Depression only	96 (3.3%)	89 (4.4%)	48 (2.5%)	25 (1.3%)	37 (1.8%)	2 (0.1%)	123 (6.1%)	420 (2.8%)
Dementia only	212 (7.2%)	107 (5.3%)	101 (5.2%)	75 (3.8%)	104 (5.2%)	78 (3.6%)	117 (5.8%)	794 (5.3%)
Physical impairment only	329 (11.2%)	302 (15.0%)	252 (13.0%)	408 (20.7%)	312 (15.6%)	242 (11.2%)	158 (7.9%)	2,003 (13.3%)
Comorbidity	163 (5.5%)	293 (14.6%)	121 (6.3%)	166 (8.4%)	142 (7.1%)	91 (4.2%)	91 (4.5%)	1,067 (7.1%)
Dependency	261 (10.0%)	237 (11.8%)	161 (8.3%)	209 (10.6%)	196 (9.8%)	237 (11.0%)	114 (5.8%)	1,415 (9.7%)
Mean WHODAS II score	13.4 (20.0)	16.5 (20.2)	12.3 (19.1)	10.8 (19.1)	10.5 (18.2)	8.0 (17.8)	19.4 (19.1)	13.0 (19.2)
Median WHODAS II score	5.6 (0–19.4)	8.3 (0–27.7)	5.6 (0–16.7)	2.8 (0–16.7)	2.8 (0–13.9)	0 (0–8.3)	13.9 (2.8–30.6)	5.6 (0–19.4)
Proportion (%) of nonzero scores	62.2	68.6	61.5	58.6	50.2	32.8	80.1	59.1
Mean score for those with nonzero scores	21.5 (21.7)	24.0 (20.5)	20.0 (20.9)	18.4 (17.8)	21.0 (21.0)	24.5 (23.6)	24.2 (18.4)	22.0 (20.6)
Total	2,944	2,011	1,933	1,971	2,003	2,162	2,004	15,028

Note. WHODAS II=World Health Organization Disability Assessment Schedule II.

- A cognitive test battery comprising the Community Screening Instrument for Dementia (CSI'D') COGSCORE (Hall et al. 1993)—incorporating the Consortium to Establish a Registry for Alzheimer's Disease (CERAD) animal-naming verbal fluency task—and the modified CERAD 10-word list learning task, with delayed recall (Ganguli et al. 1996)
- An informant interview, the CSI'D' RELSCORE (Hall et al. 1993), for evidence of cognitive and functional decline
- A participant health and risk-factor interview, covering self-reported diagnoses, impairments, and disability

Diagnoses

Information from these assessments was used to identify and describe health states as follows:

- Dementia, according to either the 10/66 dementia diagnosis algorithm (Prince et al. 2003) or the DSM-IV-TR dementia criterion (American Psychiatric Association 2000)
- Depression, as ICD-10 (World Health Organization 1992) depressive episode (mild, moderate, or severe), ascertained using the Geriatric Mental State (Copeland et al. 1986)
- Physical impairments, as self-reported arthritis or rheumatism; eyesight problems; hearing difficulty or deafness; persistent cough; breathlessness, difficulty breathing, or asthma; high blood pressure; heart trouble or angina; stomach or intestine problems; faints or blackouts; paralysis, weakness, or loss of one leg or arm; and skin disorders, such as pressure sores, leg ulcers, or severe burns (George and Fillenbaum 1985) [Each impairment was rated as present if it interfered with activities "a little" or "a lot."]

These three diagnostic groupings were used to define a summary variable coded as "well" (none of the above); depression only; dementia only; physical impairment only; and comorbidity (two or more of the above).

Disability

Global disability was assessed with the 12-item WHODAS II screener (Rehm et al. 2000), administered by an interviewer to an older participant. This brief version of the WHODAS II comprises two questions from each of the six domains covered in the full 36-item version plus two further questions to estimate the number of disability days experienced in the last month. The global disability score was calculated using the SPSS algorithm provided by the WHO; this score ranges from zero (no disability) to 100 (maximum disability). Disability days were dichotomized at 15 or more days in the past month, as an independent criterion of severe disability. The interviewer administered open-ended questions to a key informant, to ascertain dependency: Who shares the home with the participant? What kind of help does the participant need inside and outside of the home? Who in the family is available to care for the participant? What help do you provide? Do you help to organize care for the participant? Is there anyone else in the family who is more involved in helping than you? What do they do? What about friends and neighbors? What do they do? The interviewer then coded whether the participant required no care, care some of the time, or care much of the time. Dependency (needing care at least some of the time) was used as a second independent criterion of severe disability.

Analyses

We report here the distribution of health conditions and WHODAS II disability scores (mean, median, proportion of nonzero scores, and mean for those scoring above zero) by country and the distribution of WHODAS II scores (box plots) by health condition. We also report the frequency responses for each WHODAS II item, by health condition. We carried out separate Mokken scale analyses within each health-condition group (depression only, dementia only, physical impairment only, and comorbidity) and for the sample as a whole, as nonparametric IRT tests for hierarchical scaling properties. These are present when items can be ordered by degree of difficulty, such that any individual who endorses a particular item also will endorse all the items ranked lower in difficulty. Scalability was measured by the Loevinger coefficient for each item (H_i) and for the whole scale (H); weak scalability was indicated by values between 0.3 and 0.4; moderate, from 0.4 to 0.5; and strong, above 0.5. We also checked for violations of monotonicity and violation of non-intersection (double monotonicity) between pairs of items. We tested for measurement invariance by estimating, for item difficulties, the between-health-condition Spearman-rank correlations and the overall intra-class correlation. The concurrent validity of the WHODAS II was assessed using receiver operating characteristic (ROC) curve analysis against two independent concurrent criteria: 15 or more disability days in the past month and dependency (needing care at least some of the time). For each health condition group, we report the area under the ROC curve with 95% confidence intervals, and the optimum cutpoint on the WHODAS II global disability score, maximizing the sum of sensitivity and specificity.

Results

In all, 15,028 participants were interviewed across the seven countries, with sample sizes varying between 1,933 and 2,162—other than in Cuba, where 2,944 were interviewed (Table 10–1). Overall,

420 participants (2.8%) had depression only, 794 (5.3%) had dementia only, 2,003 (13.3%) had physical impairment only, and 1,067 (7.1%) had some degree of comorbidity between these mental, cognitive, and physical disorders. There was much less variation in prevalence of these health conditions and of dependency—as rated by the interviewer—than there was in mean and median WHODAS II scores, which were particularly high in India and low in China, compared with other centers. This was mainly accounted for by the proportion of participants scoring 0%–67.2% in China and 19.9% in India—with little variation in mean WHODAS II scores once zero scores were excluded. Compared with participants with none of the health conditions (mean WHODAS II score=7.5, median=0), WHODAS II scores were elevated in all four health-condition groups (see Figure 10–1): highest in those with comorbidity (mean=42.1, median=36.1), then dementia (median=30.7, median=22.2), depression (mean=22.1, median=19.4), and physical impairment (mean=18.4, median=11.1).

Mokken-scale analysis indicated that the WHODAS II was a strong Mokken scale; Loevinger's H was 0.63 for the whole scale and exceeded 0.50 for each item (Table 10–2). There were no violations of monotonicity. Violations of non-intersection both were very few in number (three for standing; two for dealing with people you don't know; and one each for joining in community activities, concentrating, walking a kilometer, getting dressed, and maintaining a friendship) with respect to the number of active pairs (n=7,040) and were all close to the minimum specified threshold of 0.03. For the health condition subgroups, the WHODAS II was a moderate Mokken scale for participants with depression only and a strong Mokken scale for those with dementia or physical impairment only and those with comorbidity. For each health-condition category, the four items ranked with the highest item difficulty (difficulty reported only with high levels of trait disability) for the threshold between no difficulty and some difficulty were 1) getting dressed, 2) dealing with people you don't know, 3) maintaining a friendship, and 4) washing the whole body (Table 10–3). Walking a kilometer, standing for long periods, and household responsibilities were consistently ranked as low-item difficulty items (difficulty reported even with low levels of trait disability). The relatively close relationship between item difficulties across health conditions is illustrated graphically in Figure 10–2. Spearman rank correlation coefficients between health conditions exceeded 0.90, other than for those between dementia and depression (0.65), dementia and physical impairment (0.75), and dementia and comorbidity (0.75). The overall intraclass correlation coefficient was 0.87 (0.73–0.96). Closer inspection revealed a modest degree of differential item functioning for participants with dementia, with respect to two items: item difficulties were 1) ranked lower for patients with dementia, compared with other groups, for learning a

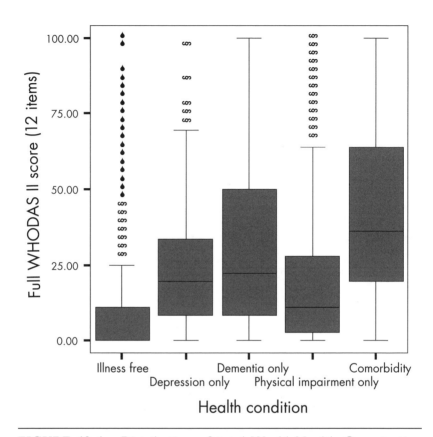

FIGURE 10–1.   Distribution of total World Health Organization Disability Assessment Schedule II (WHODAS II) score, by health condition.

new task (indicating endorsement of this item at lower levels of trait disability for dementia only), and 2) ranked higher for being emotionally affected (indicating endorsement of this item only at higher levels of trait disability for dementia only).

For each health-condition group, the WHODAS II discriminated effectively between participants with and without dependency needs and those with more or fewer than 15 disability days in the last month (Table 10–4). The optimum cutpoint for identification of severe disability, according to these criteria, was almost identical for participants with pure depression, dementia, and physical impairment but was somewhat higher for those with comorbidity.

TABLE 10–2. Mokken analysis Loevinger's H values (coefficients of scalability)

HEALTH CONDITION WHODAS II ITEM	DEPRESSION (n=420)	DEMENTIA (n=794)	PHYSICAL IMPAIRMENT (n=2,003)	COMORBIDITY (n=1,067)	ALL
1. Standing	0.48	0.52	0.58	0.55	0.61
2. Household responsibilities	0.54	0.69	0.62	0.63	0.68
3. Learning a new task	0.46	0.64	0.51	0.60	0.59
4. Joining in community activities	0.46	0.69	0.59	0.61	0.66
5. How much emotionally affected	0.46	0.50	0.51	0.45	0.57
6. Concentrating	0.38	0.63	0.45	0.55	0.58
7. Walking a kilometer	0.51	0.59	0.59	0.60	0.64
8. Washing whole body	0.44	0.67	0.56	0.63	0.65
9. Getting dressed	0.51	0.68	0.58	0.65	0.68
10. Dealing with people you don't know	0.48	0.61	0.47	0.57	0.58
11. Maintaining a friendship	0.49	0.64	0.50	0.60	0.62
12. Carrying out work and everyday activities	0.52	0.71	0.60	0.65	0.68
Whole scale	**0.48**	**0.63**	**0.56**	**0.59**	**0.63**

Note. WHODAS II=World Health Organization Disability Assessment Schedule II.

TABLE 10–3. Distribution of responses to individual WHODAS II items by health condition, with item difficulties from Mokken analysis

WHODAS II ITEM		"WELL" (n=10,744)	DEPRESSION ONLY (n=420)	DEMENTIA ONLY (n=794)	PHYSICAL IMPAIRMENT ONLY (n=2,003)	COMORBIDITY (n=1,067)	ALL
Standing for long periods (30 minutes)	0	68.8%	39.7%	46.8%	48.3%	27.2%	61.2%
	1	14.8%	23.0%	16.8%	13.5%	10.1%	14.6%
	2	10.8%	23.0%	15.5%	18.9%	21.5%	13.2%
	3	3.5%	6.9%	8.3%	10.4%	17.3%	5.7%
	4	2.1%	7.4%	12.5%	8.9%	23.9%	5.2%
Item difficulty (rank)			0.40 (10)	0.47 (8)	0.48 (11)	0.27 (10)	0.61 (12)
Household responsibilities	0	79.2%	46.7%	43.7%	57.3%	29.0%	70.0%
	1	11.6%	24.6%	16.1%	16.4%	14.3%	13.0%
	2	6.3%	17.5%	13.1%	15.6%	21.6%	9.3%
	3	2.0%	7.2%	9.0%	5.6%	11.9%	3.7%
	4	0.9%	4.1%	18.1%	5.2%	23.2%	4.0%
Item difficulty (rank)			0.47 (9)	0.44 (10)	0.57 (9)	0.29 (9)	0.70 (9)
Learning a new task	0	80.6%	54.1%	36.4%	65.6%	31.3%	72.1%
	1	11.1%	24.4%	15.7%	15.4%	16.1%	12.7%
	2	4.7%	12.9%	15.7%	11.4%	15.7%	7.2%
	3	2.2%	3.6%	11.0%	3.5%	11.5%	3.5%
	4	1.3%	5.0%	21.3%	4.2%	25.4%	4.5%
Item difficulty (rank)			0.54 (7)	0.36 (12)	0.66 (7)	0.31 (8)	0.72 (8)

TABLE 10–3. Distribution of responses to individual WHODAS II items by health condition, with item difficulties from Mokken analysis (*continued*)

WHODAS II ITEM		"WELL" (n=10,744)	DEPRESSION ONLY (n=420)	DEMENTIA ONLY (n=794)	PHYSICAL IMPAIRMENT ONLY (n=2,003)	COMORBIDITY (n=1,067)	ALL
Joining in community activities	0	83.9%	54.7%	45.4%	64.0%	34.4%	74.9%
	1	9.5%	20.6%	14.8%	12.8%	12.4%	10.7%
	2	4.0%	13.9%	11.6%	12.5%	15.2%	6.6%
	3	1.3%	5.0%	9.3%	4.7%	11.0%	3.0%
	4	1.3%	5.8%	18.9%	6.1%	27.1%	4.8%
Item difficulty (rank)			0.55 (6)	0.46 (9)	0.64 (8)	0.34 (7)	0.75 (7)
How much emotionally affected	0	77.6%	32.3%	52.4%	51.3%	24.1%	67.8%
	1	13.2%	26.8%	21.2%	18.3%	16.9%	14.9%
	2	7.1%	23.2%	13.3%	20.2%	31.1%	11.3%
	3	1.6%	12.0%	6.6%	7.1%	16.0%	3.9%
	4	0.5%	5.7%	6.5%	3.2%	11.9%	2.1%
Item difficulty (rank)			0.32 (12)	0.53 (5)	0.51 (10)	0.24 (11)	0.68 (10)
Concentrating	0	90.3%	52.4%	52.7%	77.0%	42.0%	82.1%
	1	6.7%	28.5%	16.5%	13.6%	16.4%	9.4%
	2	2.3%	14.1%	11.0%	5.9%	18.3%	4.7%
	3	0.5%	3.6%	7.5%	2.1%	8.9%	1.7%
	4	0.2%	1.4%	12.2%	1.5%	14.4%	2.1%
Item difficulty (rank)			0.52 (8)	0.52 (6)	0.77 (5)	0.42 (5)	0.82 (5)

TABLE 10–3. Distribution of responses to individual WHODAS II items by health condition, with item difficulties from Mokken analysis (*continued*)

WHODAS II ITEM	"WELL" (n=10,744)	DEPRESSION ONLY (n=420)	DEMENTIA ONLY (n=794)	PHYSICAL IMPAIRMENT ONLY (n=2,003)	COMORBIDITY (n=1,067)	ALL
Walking a kilometer						
0	72.5%	36.1%	38.6%	47.2%	22.0%	62.8%
1	11.7%	23.9%	16.9%	12.4%	10.8%	12.3%
2	8.6%	18.9%	14.3%	16.2%	16.6%	10.7%
3	4.1%	7.7%	9.3%	11.9%	13.3%	6.2%
4	3.2%	13.4%	20.9%	12.3%	37.4%	8.0%
Item difficulty (rank)		0.36 (11)	0.39 (11)	0.47 (12)	0.22 (12)	0.63 (11)
Washing whole body						
0	93.8%	78.5%	62.7%	83.0%	52.3%	87.4%
1	3.8%	11.5%	10.4%	7.0%	10.7%	5.3%
2	1.3%	4.3%	7.4%	4.7%	10.9%	2.8%
3	0.6%	3.8%	5.5%	1.5%	7.8%	1.6%
4	0.5%	1.9%	14.0%	3.8%	18.4%	2.9%
Item difficulty (rank)		0.78 (4)	0.63 (4)	0.83 (4)	0.52 (4)	0.87 (4)

TABLE 10–3. Distribution of responses to individual WHODAS II items by health condition, with item difficulties from Mokken analysis *(continued)*

WHODAS II ITEM		"WELL" (n=10,744)	DEPRESSION ONLY (n=420)	DEMENTIA ONLY (n=794)	PHYSICAL IMPAIRMENT ONLY (n=2,003)	COMORBIDITY (n=1,067)	ALL
Getting dressed	0	96.5%	86.8%	71.8%	88.0%	58.8%	91.2%
	1	2.3%	6.9%	8.7%	5.3%	11.3%	3.8%
	2	0.7%	3.1%	4.7%	3.0%	10.9%	2.0%
	3	0.2%	2.2%	4.4%	1.2%	5.0%	1.0%
	4	0.2%	1.0%	10.4%	2.6%	14.0%	2.1%
Item difficulty (rank)			0.87 (2)	0.72 (1)	0.88 (2)	0.59 (3)	0.91 (1)
Dealing with people you don't know	0	94.8%	87.8%	68.0%	86.2%	63.6%	89.9%
	1	3.8%	6.7%	13.7%	8.4%	12.7%	5.6%
	2	1.1%	3.1%	7.0%	3.7%	9.8%	2.4%
	3	0.1%	1.7%	2.9%	0.9%	5.0%	0.8%
	4	0.2%	0.7%	8.5%	0.9%	8.9%	1.3%
Item difficulty (rank)			0.88 (1)	0.68 (3)	0.86 (3)	0.64 (1)	0.90 (2)

TABLE 10–3.   Distribution of responses to individual WHODAS II items by health condition, with item difficulties from Mokken analysis (*continued*)

WHODAS II ITEM		"WELL" (n=10,744)	DEPRESSION ONLY (n=420)	DEMENTIA ONLY (n=794)	PHYSICAL IMPAIRMENT ONLY (n=2,003)	COMORBIDITY (n=1,067)	ALL
Maintaining a friendship	0	95.2%	85.6%	68.4%	88.7%	62.5%	90.4%
	1	3.5%	6.9%	11.3%	6.6%	11.4%	5.0%
	2	0.8%	4.8%	6.1%	3.3%	11.4%	2.3%
	3	0.1%	1.4%	4.3%	0.7%	4.7%	0.8%
	4	0.2%	1.2%	9.9%	0.8%	9.9%	1.5%
Item difficulty (rank)			0.85 (3)	0.69 (2)	0.89 (1)	0.63 (2)	0.90 (2)
Carrying out work, everyday activities	0	85.5%	57.3%	49.5%	66.0%	34.9%	76.6%
	1	8.8%	18.7%	15.9%	13.3%	15.1%	10.5%
	2	3.9%	14.6%	11.7%	12.7%	18.7%	6.9%
	3	1.1%	5.3%	7.0%	4.5%	10.8%	2.7%
	4	0.7%	4.1%	15.8%	3.5%	20.4%	3.3%
Item difficulty (rank)			0.57 (5)	0.50 (7)	0.66 (6)	0.35 (6)	0.77 (6)

Note.   0=no difficulty; 1=mild difficulty; 2=moderate difficulty; 3=severe difficulty; 4=extreme difficulty/cannot do. WHODAS II=World Health Organization Disability Assessment Schedule II.

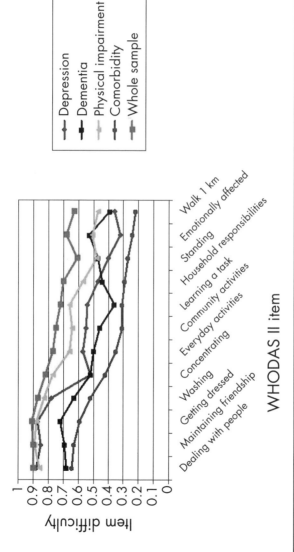

FIGURE 10–2. Item difficulties (Mokken-scale analysis), by health status.

WHODAS II=World Health Organization Disability Assessment Schedule II.

TABLE 10–4. Receiver operating characteristic analysis of discriminating ability of WHODAS II against two independent criteria of severe disability (dependency and 15 or more disability days), by health status

HEALTH STATUS	CRITERION = DEPENDENCY (SOME NEEDS FOR CARE)				CRITERION = 15 OR MORE DISABILITY DAYS			
	AUROC	OPTIMUM CUTPOINT	SENSITIVITY	SPECIFICITY	AUROC	OPTIMUM CUTPOINT	SENSITIVITY	SPECIFICITY
Depression	0.80 (0.72–0.87)	26.4	0.71	0.75	0.78 (0.72–0.83)	26.4	0.64	0.74
Dementia	0.79 (0.75–0.82)	26.3	0.75	0.72	0.85 (0.83–0.88)	26.4	0.78	0.73
Physical impairment	0.84 (0.81–0.87)	26.4	0.77	0.75	0.83 (0.81–0.86)	23.6	0.66	0.79
Comorbidity	0.86 (0.83–0.88)	43.1	0.80	0.79	0.82 (0.80–0.85)	37.5	0.79	0.72
Whole sample	**0.88 (0.87–0.89)**	**23.6**	**0.85**	**0.77**	**0.86 (0.85–0.87)**	**15.3**	**0.74**	**0.77**

Note. AUROC=area under receiver operating characteristic curve; WHODAS II=World Health Organization Disability Assessment Schedule II.

Discussion

Scales compatible with criteria of IRT provide a robust basis for measurement and valid comparisons between subgroups. Item characteristics are an essential property of the item and should be invariant with respect to the group to which they are administered and the test within which they are contained. By contrast, scales that are consistent with classical test theory but incompatible with IRT are group and test dependent and need to be redefined for each new sample and setting (Hambleton et al. 1991). Rehm et al. (2000), in their analysis (using WHO pilot data) of an earlier version of the 12-item WHODAS II screener, found the screener was not compatible with IRT principles. In our analysis of data from older respondents from seven low- and middle-income countries, we found strong evidence from Mokken-scale analysis to support the unidimensionality and IRT compatibility of the revised version of the 12-item screener, currently recommended by the WHO.

Furthermore, our findings also support group invariance for the WHODAS II with respect to assessment of disability across physical, mental, and cognitive disorders in older people. The WHODAS II was a moderate-to-strong Mokken scale in all of these subgroups. Absolute values of item difficulties varied between subgroups, because these confound differences between positions on the latent-disability variable of the four health condition subgroups, and differences between health conditions, with respect to the item's location on the latent variable (Gillespie et al. 1988). However, the rank ordering of item difficulties was highly correlated between health conditions. Differential item functioning was mainly apparent in the group with dementia only, in which, compared with other groups, learning a new task had a lower item difficulty (understandable in the context of isolated cognitive impairment in early dementia) and being emotionally affected had a higher item difficulty (again, to be expected given the difficulties of accessing mood through self-report in persons with dementia). We also examined the relationship between scores on the WHODAS II and two external criteria of severe disability—dependency and 15 or more disability days—using ROC analysis across the different health conditions. Optimal cutpoints were almost identical for the pure dementia, depression, and physical-impairment subgroups and somewhat higher for the comorbidity subgroup. This raises the possibility that use of multidomain generic measures, such as the WHODAS II, may have the effect of overestimating externally rated disability in persons with comorbidity, relative to those with single conditions.

Overall, the pattern of findings from these psychometric analyses is consistent with the WHO's aim of constructing a measure capable of identifying the consequences of any type of health condition, treating all disorders at parity. This has been achieved largely through selection of items that are not condition specific and capable of being endorsed by participants with mental, cognitive, and substance use disorders as well as physical health conditions. The focus on activity limitation and participation restriction, rather than impairment, has certainly been helpful in this regard. For the full 36-item WHODAS II, used in the European Study of the Epidemiology of Mental Disorders part of the World Mental Health Survey, this property has been convincingly demonstrated—persons with mental and physical disorders showed impairment in all WHODAS II domains with respect to those lacking these disorders (Buist-Bouwman et al. 2006). Mental disorders were as disabling as physical disorders on total WHODAS II score, self-care, getting along, and participation. On life activities and communicating/understanding, respondents with a mental disorder functioned slightly worse than individuals with a physical disorder, whereas respondents with physical disorders had more difficulty getting around. Our demonstration of robust IRT scaling properties, and group invariance, for the 12-item WHODAS II screener is a new finding and a considerable bonus, with respect to facilitating research into the relative impact and burden of health conditions across cultures. The cross-cultural robustness of the WHODAS II remains to be established formally. Cross-cultural measurement invariance between Mediterranean and non-Mediterranean countries has been demonstrated for the full 36-item WHODAS II using confirmatory factor analysis (CFA) (Hall et al. 1993). However, because of the filter questions used in the World Mental Health version of the WHODAS II, IRT analyses were not applied to these data sets. The 10/66 Dementia Research Group surveys are not limited in this way, and we will be addressing the issue of cross-cultural measurement invariance, using CFA and Mokken analysis, in a future paper.

Measuring Change in Disability Across Health Conditions in Health Service Research

Background

Two types of responsiveness to changes in disability have been described. *Internal* responsiveness is the ability to measure change over time or before and after an intervention of known clinical effectiveness. *External* responsiveness "reflects the extent to which changes in a measure…relate to corresponding changes in a reference measure of health status," a sort of "gold standard" (Husted et al. 2000). The internal responsiveness of the WHODAS II has been assessed with respect to clinical interventions for depression (Chwastiak and Von Korff 2003), anxiety disorders (Perini et al. 2006), low-back pain (Chwastiak and Von Korff 2003), and rehabilitation for a variety of chronic physical conditions (Pösl et al. 2007). Only one previous study has compared the responsiveness of the WHODAS II with that of other measures across physical and mental disorders (Chwastiak and Von Korff 2003). External responsiveness has been examined only with respect to symptom change for anxiety disorders (Perini et al. 2006).

We chose to study two index conditions, depression and arthritis, for their high levels of associated disability and effectiveness of available treatments and to evaluate outcome measures in both "physical" and "mental" conditions. To facilitate comparison, both treatment groups consisted of older adults.

Method

Our method of approach was to conduct a longitudinal naturalistic study of the responsiveness of different measures of health status, disability, and quality of life in the face of surgical and mental health interventions of established clinical effectiveness. Participants were assessed twice, within 2 weeks of beginning treatment and 4 months after the intervention had started.

Participants

Two clinical samples were identified. The first sample comprised patients who had been placed on a waiting list for primary hip or knee arthroplasty for osteoarthritis at a South London teaching hospital. These patients were recruited at their preoperative assessments 2 weeks before surgery. The second sample comprised patients with late-life depression referred to community-based Mental Health of the Elderly secondary-care teams, which offered a range of interventions to patients older than 65 years in a relatively deprived area of London. These patients were identified (by their key workers) as having depression for which a new episode of treatment was planned. Treatment consisted of antidepressant medication, with additional electroconvulsive therapy where indicated. Patients were included in this study if they scored more than 15 on the Hamilton Depression Rating Scale (Hamilton 1960) and met diagnostic criteria for one or more of the depressive disorders listed in ICD-10.

Assessments

Assessments included both clinician-rated impairment-specific measures and health-related quality-of-life instruments: *Clinician-*

rated impairment-specific measures were used for the arthroplasty and depression samples. Arthroplasty participants were rated preoperatively with one of two commonly used clinical measures—the Harris Hip Score (Harris 1969) or the Knee Society Clinical Rating Scale (Insall et al. 1989), as appropriate—which assessed pain, joint function, and mobility. Participants in the depression sample were rated at recruitment with the 17-item Hamilton Depression Rating Scale (Hamilton 1960), a semistructured psychiatrist-administered interview.

Health-related quality-of-life instruments used included

- *Disability:* WHODAS II (Murray and Lopez 1996). Each of the six domains—understanding/communication, getting around, self-care, getting along with others, life activities, and participation restriction—is scaled to produce a score ranging from 0 to 100, with higher scores reflecting greater disability. A weighted summed score of global disability is calculated, reflecting contributions of both activity limitation and participation restriction to overall disability.
- *Handicap:* The London Handicap Scale (Harwood and Ebrahim 1995). This scale was designed to measure the ICIDH construct of handicap: "disadvantages experienced by the individual as a result of impairments and disabilities"; thus, handicaps reflect interaction with, and adaptation to, an individual's surroundings. The six 6-point scales assess disadvantage in "survival roles" of mobility, physical independence, orientation, occupation, social integration, and economic self-sufficiency and provide a weighted summary measure of handicap.
- *Health status:* SF-36 (Ware and Sherbourne 1992). The SF-36 has assumed preeminence in the field of health status measurement; a wealth of work supports its psychometric robustness. It has eight domain scales of physical functioning: physical function, physical role difficulties, emotional role difficulties, social function, mental health, vitality, bodily pain, and health perceptions. Subscale scores range from 0 to 100, with higher scores indicating better functioning. SF-36 begins with a single summary global health question.
- *Quality of life:* WHO Quality of Life BREF (WHOQOL-BREF, World Health Organization 1998a). The WHOQOL-BREF is a 26-item self-completed short form comprising four summary quality of life scales—physical, psychological, social, and environmental—and a single summary global quality-of-life question. The group that developed WHOQOL defined quality of life as

> individuals' perception of their position in life in the context of the culture and value systems in which they live and in relation to their goals, expectations, standards and concerns. It is a

broad-ranging concept affected in a complex way by the person's physical health, psychological state, level of independence, social relationships and their relationship to salient features of their environment. (World Health Organization 1998b)

A 100-item instrument based on this concept, the WHOQOL, has been developed and extensively field tested in general populations (World Health Organization 1998b).

Analysis

Demographic and clinical characteristics of the samples were described. Responsiveness to change of the WHODAS II was measured using four indices for each health-related quality-of-life measure for each clinical group. Measures of internal responsiveness were effect size and standardized response mean. The *effect size,* the most commonly used index of response, is the difference in mean score before and after treatment divided by the standard deviation of the baseline measure. Effect sizes of 0.8 or greater are deemed to reflect large changes, 0.5–0.8 moderate changes, and 0.2–0.5 small changes (Kazis et al. 1989). The *standardized response mean* is the mean change in score divided by the standard deviation of the change in scores. It standardizes the change in a measure relative to between-patient variability in change scores. The two indices of external responsiveness were the correlation of changes in WHODAS II scores with changes in two global outcomes, self-rated on five-point Likert scales: the global health rating from the SF-36 and the global quality-of-life rating from the WHOQOL-BREF.

Results

Of 72 prearthroplasty patients, 65 (90%) were reinterviewed 4 months later. Of the 49 patients with depression, 40 (82%) were reinterviewed 4 months later; 2 had died, and 7 refused follow-up. The depressed patients were older than the arthroplasty patients (mean age=78 years, range=65–95, vs. mean age=70 years, range=52–86) and were less likely to be married (15% vs. 47%). There were no baseline differences on any health-related quality-of-life measure between patients lost to follow-up and those who completed the study. At baseline, arthroplasty patients and depressed patients had similar overall levels of disability and handicap, as measured by the WHODAS II and London Handicap Scale (Tables 10–5 and 10–6). However, compared with the arthroplasty patients, the depressed patients were more disabled in the understanding/communicating, self-care, and getting along with others domains of the WHODAS II; had a worse quality of life in all areas except physical; and were less impaired in the physical function and bodily pain subscales of the SF-36. They were much more impaired than arthroplasty patients in the emotional role, vitality, and mental health subscales of the SF-36. Overall, differences between the two patient groups in baseline domain/subscale patterns of disability were more striking for the SF-36 than for either the WHODAS II or the WHOQOL.

For the arthroplasty group, 55% underwent knee arthroplasty, and the others underwent hip arthroplasty. Demographic and baseline health-related quality-of-life scores did not differ between the two types of operation, except for WHODAS II self-care and SF-36 physical-role functioning, for which those undergoing hip replacement were more limited. The two groups were combined for subsequent analyses. For the depression group, treatment consisted of antidepressant medication in all cases, and additional electroconvulsive therapy in four cases; those who had the additional electroconvulsive therapy were not substantially different from the others on the quality-of-life assessments at baseline.

Internal responsiveness was assessed with two unit-free indices of magnitude of change in the measures, effect size and standardized response mean. Postarthroplasty, the knee- and hip-impairment scores showed large changes (>0.8) on both indices of response (see Table 10–5). The WHODAS II showed large changes on the global-disability score and the getting-around domain and moderate changes (>0.5) on the life-activities and understanding/communication domains. Of the SF-36 subscales, bodily pain showed a large, and social functioning a moderate, change. For the WHOQOL-BREF, only the physical quality-of-life domain was moderately responsive. Four months after commencement of treatment for late-life depression, the Hamilton Depression Rating Scale was highly responsive (Table 10–6). The WHODAS II showed just under moderate responsiveness in all domains, except getting around and getting along with others. The SF-36 mental health, vitality, and emotional-role functioning subscales were highly, or moderately, responsive, depending on the index of change used. WHOQOL-BREF physical and psychological quality-of-life subscales also were moderately responsive.

External responsiveness was assessed through correlation of changes in test measures with changes in the global health rating from the SF-36 and the global quality-of-life rating from the WHO-QOL-BREF (Tables 10–5 and 10–6). Among patients with arthritis, changes in global health ratings were significantly (>0.31) correlated with changes in the WHODAS II global disability score and getting around and participation domains; changes in the SF-36 bodily pain and health perceptions subscales; and changes in the WHO-QOL-BREF physical and social quality-of-life domains. Global quality-of-life changes were significantly correlated with changes in all domains of the WHOQOL-BREF and with changes in the SF-36 emotional-role functioning and mental health subscales. For patients with depression, changes in global health were significantly (>0.34) correlated with SF-36 mental health, emotional-role, and health perception subscales only. The WHOQOL-BREF physical, psychological, and environmental quality-of-life domains were correlated with overall quality-of-life change, as was the Hamilton Depression Rating Scale score; SF-36 emotional-role, mental health, and vitality subscales; and the London Handicap Scale.

Discussion

The purpose of this study was to evaluate the responsiveness of the WHODAS II relative to that of other established assessments of disability, health status, and quality of life. We did not aim to evaluate individual interventions or compare their relative effectiveness. Internal responsiveness to change is a vital component of the external validity of an outcome measure for health services research. Condition-specific measures indicated large changes in impairments targeted by interventions. Measures applicable across health conditions invariably showed lower responsiveness. However, half of the WHOQOL-BREF domains were insensitive to these major health interventions, although physical quality of life improved in both groups and psychological quality of life improved in those patients with depression. Likewise, in each clinical group, several SF-36 subscales were moderately responsive or unchanging, and those that did show marked responses were predictable from the condition being treated—mental health, vitality, and emotional role for depression and bodily pain; physical and social function for arthroplasty. WHODAS II demonstrated moderate (>0.4), but still useful, responsiveness across a broader range of domains and in the overall disability score for both depression and arthroplasty groups.

Our findings are broadly comparable with those of the few other studies that have compared, directly, the responsiveness of the WHODAS II with that of the SF-36 or SF-12. For patients with depression, the effect size for the WHODAS II global disability score (0.47) was a little smaller than that reported in two previous studies for depression treatment in primary care (0.65) (Chwastiak and Von Korff 2003) and "rehabilitation" for depression (0.69) (Pösl et al. 2007). In our study, as in others that have looked at responsiveness to depression interventions (Chwastiak and Von Korff 2003; Pösl et al. 2007), understanding/communicating, self-care, life activities, and participation were the most responsive WHODAS domains. For the SF-36, in our study, as with others (Chwastiak and Von Korff 2003; Pösl et al. 2007), responsiveness was limited to the mental health, vitality, and role emotional domains. The responsiveness of the WHODAS II also has been assessed in patients with social phobia and panic/agoraphobia who were undergoing group cognitive-behavioral therapy

TABLE 10–5. Responsiveness to change of the WHODAS II, WHOQOL-BREF, SF-36, and London Handicap scales, compared 4 months after lower limb arthroplasty

Scale	Baseline mean (SD)	Change score (95% CI)	Effect size	SRM	Health change correlation	QOL change correlation
Harris Hip Score (0–100)	44.4 (10.8)	38.1 (32.2, 44.0)	3.53	2.54	0.16	-0.01
Knee Society Clinical Rating (0–200)	92.2 (27.2)	32.8 (21.6, 44.1)	1.21	1.03	0.25	0.22
WHODAS II (0–100)						
Disability total	25.5 (10.8)	9.0 (6.2, 11.8)	0.83	0.90	0.45	-0.06
Understanding	5.7 (7.7)	3.8 (2.0, 5.6)	0.49	0.54	0.11	-0.01
Getting around	59.3 (18.9)	22.7 (17.0, 28.4)	1.20	1.06	0.38	-0.13
Self-care	16.5 (13.9)	4.7 (0.5, 8.9)	0.34	0.30	0.13	0.14
Getting on with others	10.0 (12.2)	-1.5 (-5.2, 2.2)	-0.12	-0.10	0.13	-0.03
Life activities	33.4 (24.6)	14.8 (7.9, 21.8)	0.60	0.54	0.22	-0.21
Participation	29.2 (21.9)	8.4 (3.0, 13.9)	0.39	0.40	0.46	-0.15
WHOQOL-BREF (0–20)						
Physical	10.6 (2.5)	1.3 (0.7, 1.9)	0.52	0.54	0.36	0.37
Psychological	13.9 (2.2)	-0.5 (-1.2, 0.3)	-0.21	-0.16	0.19	0.43
Social	15.1 (2.7)	0.3 (-0.7, 1.2)	0.09	0.07	0.32	0.47
Environment	13.4 (1.9)	-0.2 (-0.8, 0.4)	-0.09	-0.08	0.15	0.41

TABLE 10–5. Responsiveness to change of the WHODAS II, WHOQOL-BREF, SF-36, and London Handicap scales, compared 4 months after lower limb arthroplasty *(continued)*

Scale	Baseline Mean (SD)	Change Score (95% CI)	Effect Size	SRM	Health Change Correlation	QOL Change Correlation
SF-36						
Physical function	30.8 (21.6)	9.9 (2.8, 17.0)	0.46	0.38	0.31	0.23
Role—physical	20.8 (32.9)	5.9 (−6.5, 18.4)	0.18	0.12	0.22	0.12
Role—emotional	54.2 (43.1)	5.4 (−8.1, 18.8)	0.13	0.11	0.14	0.39
Social function	51.4 (26.1)	16.9 (7.9, 26.0)	0.64	0.49	0.19	0.06
Vitality	42.7 (21.1)	4.9 (−0.1, 10.0)	0.23	0.25	0.21	0.28
Mental health	68.7 (20.4)	0.7 (−5.0, 6.3)	0.03	0.03	0.06	0.41
Bodily pain	32.4 (23.2)	19.7 (12.3, 27.1)	0.85	0.70	0.38	0.26
Health perceptions	53.1 (21.2)	3.9 (−1.6, 9.3)	0.18	0.20	0.61	0.27
London Handicap Scale (0–100)	68.3 (10.6)	4.6 (1.8, 7.3)	0.43	0.41	−0.09	0.07

Note. External responsiveness was assessed through correlation of changes in test measures with changes in global health rating from the SF-36 and global-quality-of-life rating from the WHOQOL-BREF. Correlations of health-related QOL subscale changes with changes in Likert ratings for health and quality of life; correlations >0.31 were significant at P<0.05, and correlations >0.43 were significant at P<0.001.

CI=confidence interval; QOL=quality of life; SF-36=Short Form–36; SRM=standardized response mean; WHODAS II=World Health Organization Disability Assessment Schedule II; WHOQOL-BREF=World Health Organization Quality of Life–BREF.

TABLE 10–6. Responsiveness to change of the WHODAS II, WHOQOL-BREF, SF-36 and London Handicap scales, compared 4 months after starting treatment for late-life depression

SCALE	BASELINE MEAN (SD)	CHANGE SCORE (95% CI)	EFFECT SIZE	SRM	HEALTH CHANGE CORRELATION	QOL CHANGE CORRELATION
Hamilton Depression Rating Scale (0–47)	22.3 (5.26)	11.5 (8.8, 14.2)	2.19	1.35	0.31	0.43
WHODAS II (0–100)						
Global disability	29.2 (13.8)	6.5 (1.5, 11.4)	0.47	0.46	0.13	0.41
Understanding	26.4 (18.7)	7.6 (1.3, 13.8)	0.41	0.39	0.06	0.24
Getting around	40.7 (29.7)	4.1 (−2.2, 10.4)	0.14	0.21	0.18	0.27
Self-care	23.8 (18.2)	9.0 (2.8, 15.2)	0.49	0.47	0.00	0.14
Getting on with others	16.2 (13.0)	1.9 (−3.6, 7.3)	0.14	0.11	−0.03	0.07
Life activities	31.0 (29.6)	12.0 (2.7, 21.3)	0.41	0.41	0.22	0.25
Participation	35.3 (13.8)	7.5 (0.7, 14.3)	0.43	0.38	0.00	0.22
WHOQOL-BREF						
Physical	11.2 (2.9)	1.9 (0.9, 2.9)	0.66	0.63	0.32	0.60
Psychological	9.1 (2.9)	2.2 (1.2, 3.3)	0.77	0.70	0.34	0.64
Social	13.7 (3.3)	0.4 (−1.1, 1.8)	0.11	0.08	0.19	0.23
Environment	12.6 (2.2)	0.7 (−0.1, 1.6)	0.33	0.28	0.12	0.40
SF-36						
Physical function	43.2 (26.0)	3.1 (6.6, 34.7)	0.12	0.12	0.00	0.23
Role—physical	25.7 (36.9)	12.9 (−5.6, 31.3)	0.35	0.23	0.21	0.23
Role—emotional	12.0 (23.7)	33.3 (15.9, 50.8)	1.41	0.64	0.35	0.41

TABLE 10–6. Responsiveness to change of the WHODAS II, WHOQOL-BREF, SF-36 and London Handicap scales, compared 4 months after starting treatment for late-life depression *(continued)*

SCALE	BASELINE MEAN (SD)	CHANGE SCORE (95% CI)	EFFECT SIZE	SRM	HEALTH CHANGE CORRELATION	QOL CHANGE CORRELATION
SF-36 *(continued)*						
Social function	45.3 (25.7)	9.4 (–4.8, 23.6)	0.36	0.21	0.07	0.31
Mental health	29.7 (21.4)	21.8 (12.2, 31.5)	1.02	0.73	0.47	0.56
Vitality	23.5 (20.9)	18.2 (9.0, 27.4)	0.87	0.64	0.07	0.47
Bodily pain	66.1 (36.0)	6.6 (–4.9, 18.0)	0.18	0.19	–0.05	–0.13
Health perceptions	42.8 (20.8)	5.4 (–1.9, 12.7)	0.27	0.25	0.62	0.21
London Handicap Scale (0–100)	61.6 (15.9)	3.5 (–1.3, 8.2)	0.22	0.23	0.04	0.51

Note. External responsiveness was assessed through correlation of changes in test measures with changes in global health rating from the SF-36 and global QOL rating from the WHOQOL-BREF. Correlations of health-related QOL subscale changes with changes in Likert ratings for health and quality of life; correlations >0.34 were significant at $P<0.05$, correlations >0.43 were significant at $P<0.001$.

CI=confidence interval; QOL=quality of life; SF-36=Short Form–36; SRM=standardized response mean; WHODAS II=World Health Organization Disability Assessment Schedule II; WHOQOL-BREF=World Health Organization Quality of Life–BREF.

(Perini et al. 2006). The WHODAS II effect sizes for agoraphobia (0.57) and social phobia (0.69) were smaller than those for the SF-12 MCS for panic/agoraphobia (0.90) and for social phobia (0.95). However, external responsiveness against impairment-specific symptom scales was greater for the WHODAS than for the SF-12 MCS for social phobia and comparable for panic/agoraphobia (Perini et al. 2006). For our arthroplasty group, the effect size for the WHODAS II global disability score (0.83) was larger than that previously reported for primary-care interventions for back pain (0.60) (Chwastiak and Von Korff 2003), which probably reflects the relative effectiveness of these interventions. In both studies, getting around, life activities, participation, self-care, and communication/understanding were the most responsive domains. In both studies, responsiveness for the SF-36 was limited to large effects on bodily pain and moderate effects on social function and physical function. The one other study that assessed responsiveness for physical health conditions reported small but statistically significant effect sizes across most WHODAS II domains for musculoskeletal and cardiovascular diseases and breast cancer (Pösl et al. 2007); a fundamental weakness of this study was that the content of the "rehabilitation" interventions was not described, and their effectiveness apparently had not been established. In all of these studies, there appears to be a trade-off between the responsiveness of a scale or subscale and its scope. The more impairment focused a scale, the more responsive it is to an intervention targeting that impairment. However, the pattern of change in WHODAS II scores across activity limitation and participation domains suggests that mental and physical interventions have broad effects on disability beyond those detected by the more impairment-focused SF-36 subscales. Scales that focus on symptoms or impairments may not capture the full benefits of these interventions; however, some degree of responsiveness may have to be sacrificed to achieve this goal.

For our test of external responsiveness, we chose to correlate changes in health-related quality-of-life measures with changes in self-rated global outcomes, hence judging responsiveness with respect to patient-observed improvement (Burvill et al. 1990). In the group that underwent arthroplasty, the WHODAS II performed well when change in health was used as the external comparator but poorly when the criterion was change in quality of life. Conversely, for patients treated for depression, the WHODAS II generally performed better when change in quality of life was the external criterion. In both groups, for the SF-36, the health perceptions subscale was more responsive with respect to patient-rated changes in health, whereas emotional role, mental health, and vitality subscales were more responsive with respect to changes in quality of life. For both clinical groups, changes in the WHOQOL-BREF domain scores were strongly correlated with changes in self-rated global quality of life, indicating good longitudinal internal consistency. Clearly, the choice of gold standard is critical in assessment of external responsiveness; both the nature of the construct used as an external comparator (health status, satisfaction, or quality of life) and the perspective from which it is rated may result in different responsiveness characteristics for the same measure.

One limitation of our study was the relatively short interval between intervention and follow-up assessment. Previous studies have shown clinical responses in these populations in this time frame (Drewett et al. 1992; Heiligenstein et al. 1995). Although wider effects on disability and quality of life may take longer to appear, this should not have impeded assessment of relative responsiveness of the different measures. The WHODAS II seems to be a useful instrument for capturing broad effects of health service interventions on disability as a generic, broadly defined construct. It was less responsive than more narrowly focused impairment-specific outcome measures. For both patient groups, it was more responsive than the London Handicap Scale and seems more capable of detecting changes in less predictable domains than either the SF-36 or WHOQOL-BREF.

Conclusion

The WHO ICF classification describes the effects of health conditions in limiting activities and behaviors and restricting the participation of individuals in society. These processes can be seen as representing a final common pathway through which different disorders—acute and chronic, mental or physical, alone or in combination—can exert their effects and result in disadvantages. The WHODAS II disability assessment scale, developed to be consistent with the ICF classification, has been shown to have robust psychometric properties across a wide variety of diagnoses and disorders. It seems to be capable of capturing the disabling consequences of mental, cognitive, and physical health conditions and is equally responsive to effective interventions for depression, anxiety, and musculoskeletal disorders.

Through analyses presented in this chapter, we have demonstrated that the 12-item WHODAS II screener, by dint of its hierarchical measurement properties, can be used to make meaningful comparisons of the extent of disability across diverse health conditions. This desirable property yet has to be demonstrated for the full 36-item WHODAS II.

The SF-36 has assumed preeminence in the field of health status measurement; a wealth of work supports its psychometric robustness. However, throughout the development of the SF-36 and its component summary scores, there has been an explicit assumption that physical health and mental health are, to an important extent, separate entities and that consequences of impairment in one entity are distinct from those in the other, therefore, separate metrics should be used to quantify the entities. The initial premise is highly questionable; there is now a considerable research literature attesting to the protean links between physical and mental disorders (Prince et al. 2007b). Mental disorders are prominent among risk factors and sequelae of communicable and noncommunicable diseases, accidents, and injuries; the extensive comorbidity with mental disorders has important implications for treatment outcome of many physical health conditions (Prince et al. 2007b). The decision to use separate metrics for consequences of physical and mental disorders imposes significant limitations on the utility of SF-36 and SF-12 for population and health services research. Both measures have been used successfully in national mental health surveys (Bijl and Ravelli 2000; Das-Munshi et al. 2007; Grant et al. 2005; Sanderson and Andrews 2002) to assess relative burdens of different mental disorders (Bijl and Ravelli 2000; Grant et al. 2005; Sanderson and Andrews 2002) and the contributions of these burdens to impaired physical functioning in people with diabetes (Das-Munshi et al. 2007). Unlike the WHODAS II, the SF-36 cannot be used to assess the relative burden arising from physical and mental disorders. This is an important issue for mental health; analysis of GBD data, using the common disability-adjusted life-year metric, reveals that, at country level, the proportion of health care budgets spent on mental health is much smaller than the proportion of disease burden attributable to mental health conditions for countries at all levels of economic development (Saxena et al. 2007). Likewise, although the SF-36 captures the benefits of mental health interventions on mental health outcomes, it cannot be used to compare the effectiveness and cost-effectiveness of physical and mental health interventions.

The use of a broadly based, conceptually driven instrument, such as the WHODAS II, should aid future research into relative disease burden. The disability-adjusted life-year has been criticized from a variety of perspectives. It imposes a somewhat medicalized model of disability, anchored as it is to expert opinion of disability levels associated with diagnostic groups (Mont 2007b). Disability weights may be improved through the inclusion of lay opinion (Mont 2007b; Williams 1999) or by measuring disability directly in health surveys, using a simple generic measure such as the WHODAS II (Sanderson and Andrews 2001; Williams 1999). More radically, Williams (1999) has challenged the basic premise of the GBD enterprise, from a health-economic perspective. What is required, in his view, to inform policymaking and prioritization is not an understanding of the relative burden of different diseases but rather an understanding of the relative effectiveness of interventions:

> We do not need to know the GBD, but the marginal impact of a health technology upon it. Priority setting is to be driven by a comparison of incremental gains with incremental costs....Health technology assessment is a more urgent, more focused, and more useful field of endeavor for priority setting purposes than calculating the GBD. (Williams 1999)

Cost-effectiveness analyses for mental health interventions in low- and middle-income countries suggest ratios on the order of US $500–$5,000 per averted disability-adjusted life-year; this is unfavorable when compared with vaccination programs or tuberculosis control but is equivalent to interventions for other chronic disorders: for example, antiretroviral treatments for HIV/AIDS, secondary prevention of hypertension, or glycemic control for diabetes (Patel et al. 2003). Such work is in its infancy. Evidence-based advocacy for mental health requires that future trials of effectiveness of mental health interventions include generic outcomes that facilitate direct comparisons with interventions more routinely provided in general health care settings, particularly in low- and middle-income settings, where the mental health treatment gap is most pronounced. Modeling, conducted as part of the recent *The Lancet* Series on Global Mental Health, indicated that comprehensive community-based mental health services could be provided for an incremental per capita cost of only US $2 in low-income countries and US $4–$6 in middle-income countries (Lancet Global Mental Health Group et al. 2007). This presents policymakers with the bill without yet a clear understanding of the benefits associated with such a fundamental health service reform.

References

American Psychiatric Association: Diagnostic and Statistical Manual of Mental Disorders, 4th Edition, Text Revision. Washington, DC, American Psychiatric Association, 2000

Andrews G, Kemp A, Sunderland M, et al: Normative data for the 12-item WHO Disability Assessment Schedule 2.0. PLoS ONE 4(12):e8343, 2009

Baron M, Schieir O, Hudson M, et al: The clinimetric properties of the World Health Organization Disability Assessment Schedule II in early inflammatory arthritis. Arthritis Rheum 59:382–390, 2008

Bijl RV, Ravelli A: Current and residual functional disability associated with psychopathology: findings from the Netherlands Mental Health Survey and Incidence Study (NEMESIS). Psychol Med 30:657–668, 2000

Buist-Bouwman MA, De Graaf R, Vollebergh WA, et al: Functional disability of mental disorders and comparison with physical disorders: a study among the general population of six European countries. Acta Psychiatr Scand 113:492–500, 2006

Buist-Bouwman MA, Ormel J, de Graaf R, et al: Psychometric properties of the World Health Organization Disability Assessment Schedule used in the European Study of the Epidemiology of Mental Disorders. Int J Methods Psychiatr Res 17:185–197, 2008

Burvill PW, Mowry B, Hall WD: Quantification of physical illness in psychiatric research in the elderly. Int J Geriatr Psychiatry 5:161–170, 1990

Chávez LM, Canino G, Negrón G, et al: Psychometric properties of the Spanish version of two mental health outcome measures: World Health Organization Disability Assessment Schedule II and Lehman's Quality of Life Interview. Ment Health Serv Res 7:145–159, 2005

Chisolm TH, Abrams HB, McArdle R, et al: The WHO-DAS II: psychometric properties in the measurement of functional health status in adults with acquired hearing loss. Trends Amplif 9:111–126, 2005

Chopra PK, Couper JW, Herrman H: The assessment of patients with long-term psychotic disorders: application of the WHO Disability Assessment Schedule II. Aust N Z J Psychiatry 38:753–759, 2004

Chwastiak LA, Von Korff M: Disability in depression and back pain: evaluation of the World Health Organization Disability Assessment Schedule (WHO DAS II) in a primary care setting. J Clin Epidemiol 56:507–514, 2003

Copeland JR, Dewey ME, Griffiths-Jones HM: A computerised psychiatric diagnostic system and case nomenclature for elderly subjects: GMS and AGECAT. Psychol Med 16:89–99, 1986

Creed F, Morgan R, Fiddler M, et al: Depression and anxiety impair health-related quality of life and are associated with increased costs in general medical inpatients. Psychosomatics 43:302–309, 2002

Das-Munshi J, Stewart R, Ismail K, et al: Diabetes, common mental disorders, and disability: findings from the UK National Psychiatric Morbidity Survey. Psychosom Med 69:543–550, 2007

Drewett RF, Minns RJ, Sibly TF: Measuring outcome of total knee replacement using quality of life indices. Ann R Coll Surg Engl 74:286–289, 1992

Fuster V, Voûte J: MDGs: chronic diseases are not on the agenda. Lancet 366:1512–1514, 2005

Ganguli M, Chandra V, Gilbey J, et al: Cognitive test performance in a community-based nondemented elderly sample in rural India: the Indo-US Cross National Dementia Epidemiology Study. Int Psychogeriatr 8:507–524, 1996

George LK, Fillenbaum GG: OARS methodology: a decade of experience in geriatric assessment. J Am Geriatr Soc 33:607–615, 1985

Gillespie M, Tenvergert EM, Kingma J: Using Mokken methods to develop robust cross-national scales: American and West German attitudes toward abortion. Soc Indic Res 20:181–203, 1988

Grant BF, Hasin DS, Stinson FS, et al: Prevalence, correlates, co-morbidity, and comparative disability of DSM-IV generalized anxiety disorder in the USA: results from the National Epidemiological Survey on Alcohol and Related Conditions. Psychol Med 35:1747–1759, 2005

Hall KS, Hendrie HH, Brittain HM, et al: The development of a dementia screening interview in two distinct languages. Int J Methods Psychiatr Res 3:1–28, 1993

Hambleton RK, Rogers HJ, Swaminathan H: Fundamentals of Item Response Theory. Thousand Oaks, CA, Sage, 1991

Hamilton M: A rating scale for depression. J Neurol Neurosurg Psychiatry 23:56–62, 1960

Harris WH: Traumatic arthritis of the hip after dislocation and acetabular fractures: treatment by mold arthroplasty: an end-result study using a new method of result evaluation. J Bone Joint Surg Am 1:737–755, 1969

Harwood R, Ebrahim S: Manual of the London Handicap Scale. Nottingham, UK, University of Nottingham, 1995

Harwood R, Prince M, Mann A, et al: The prevalence of diagnoses, impairments, disabilities and handicaps in a population of elderly people living in a defined geographic area: the Gospel Oak Project. Age Ageing 27:707–714, 1998

Heiligenstein JH, Ware JE Jr, Beusterien KM, et al: Acute effects of fluoxetine versus placebo on functional health and well-being in late-life depression. Int Psychogeriatr 7(suppl):125–137, 1995

Hudson M, Steele R, Taillefer S, et al: Quality of life in systemic sclerosis: psychometric properties of the World Health Organization Disability Assessment Schedule II. Arthritis Rheum 59:270–278, 2008

Husted JA, Cook RJ, Farewell VT, et al: Methods for assessing responsiveness: a critical review and recommendations. J Clin Epidemiol 53:459–468, 2000

Insall JN, Dorr LD, Scott RD, et al: Rationale of the Knee Society clinical rating system. Clin Orthop Relat Res (248):13–14, 1989

Kazis LE, Anderson JJ, Meenan RF: Effect sizes for interpreting changes in health status. Med Care 27:S178–S189, 1989

Kim JM, Stewart R, Glozier N, et al: Physical health, depression and cognitive function as correlates of disability in an older Korean population. Int J Geriatr Psychiatry 20:160–167, 2005

Lancet Global Mental Health Group, Chisholm D, Flisher AJ, et al: Scale up services for mental disorders: a call for action. Lancet 370:1241–1252, 2007

Lindesay J: The Guy's/Age Concern survey: physical health and psychiatric disorder in an urban elderly community. Int J Geriatr Psychiatry 5:171–178, 1990

McHorney CA, Ware JE Jr, Raczek AE: The MOS 36-Item Short-Form Health Survey (SF-36), II: psychometric and clinical tests of validity in measuring physical and mental health constructs. Med Care 31:247–263, 1993

McHorney CA, Ware JE Jr, Lu JF, et al: The MOS 36-item Short-Form Health Survey (SF-36), III: tests of data quality, scaling assumptions, and reliability across diverse patient groups. Med Care 32:40–66, 1994

McKibbin C, Patterson TL, Jeste DV: Assessing disability in older patients with schizophrenia: results from the WHODAS-II. J Nerv Ment Dis 192:405–413, 2004

Mont D: Measuring Disability Prevalence. Social Protection Discussion Paper No. 0706. Washington, DC, World Bank, 2007a. Available at: http://siteresources.worldbank.org/SOCIALPROTECTION/Resources/SP-Discussion-papers/Disability-DP/0706.pdf. Accessed July 22, 2009.

Mont D: Measuring health and disability. Lancet 369:1658–1663, 2007b

Murray CJL, Lopez AD (eds): The Global Burden of Disease: A Comprehensive Assessment of Mortality and Disability From Diseases, Injuries and Risk Factors in 1990 and Projected to 2020. Cambridge, MA, Harvard University Press, 1996

Norton J, de Roquefeuil G, Benjamins A, et al: Psychiatric morbidity, disability and service use amongst primary care attenders in France. Eur Psychiatry 19:164–167, 2004

Organisation for Economic Co-operation and Development: Transforming Disability Into Ability: Policies to Promote Work and Income Security for Disabled People. Paris, Organisation for Economic Co-operation and Development, 2003

Patel V, Chisholm D, Rabe-Hesketh S, et al: Efficacy and cost-effectiveness of drug and psychological treatments for common mental disorders in general health care in Goa, India: a randomised, controlled trial. Lancet 361:33–39, 2003

Perini SJ, Slade T, Andrews G: Generic effectiveness measures: sensitivity to symptom change in anxiety disorders. J Affect Disord 90:123–130, 2006

Pirkis JE, Burgess PM, Kirk PK, et al: A review of the psychometric properties of the Health of the Nation Outcome Scales (HoNOS) family of measures. Health Qual Life Outcomes 3:76, 2005

Pösl M, Cieza A, Stucki G: Psychometric properties of the WHODASII in rehabilitation patients. Qual Life Res 16:1521–1531, 2007

Prince MJ: The classification and measurement of disablement and its applications for clinical gerontology. Rev Clin Gerontol 8:227–240, 1998

Prince M, Acosta D, Chiu H, et al: Dementia diagnosis in developing countries: a cross-cultural validation study. Lancet 361:909–917, 2003

Prince M, Ferri CP, Acosta D, et al: The protocols for the 10/66 Dementia Research Group population-based research programme. BMC Public Health 7:165, 2007a

Prince M, Patel V, Saxena S, et al: No health without mental health. Lancet 370:859–877, 2007b

Rehm J, Üstün TB, Saxena S: On the development and psychometric testing of the WHO screening instrument to assess disablement in the general population. Int J Methods Psychiatr Res 8:110–122, 2000

Sanderson K, Andrews G: Mental disorders and burden of disease: how was disability estimated and is it valid? Aust N Z J Psychiatry 35:668–676, 2001

Sanderson K, Andrews G: Prevalence and severity of mental health-related disability and relationship to diagnosis. Psychiatr Serv 53:80–86, 2002

Saxena S, Thornicroft G, Knapp M, et al: Resources for mental health: scarcity, inequity, and inefficiency. Lancet 370:878–889, 2007

Simon GE, Revicki DA, Grothaus L, et al: SF-36 summary scores: are physical and mental health truly distinct? Med Care 36:567–572, 1998

Üstün TB, Kostanjsek N, Chatterji S, et al. (eds): Measuring Health and Disability: Manual for WHO Disability Assessment Schedule (WHODAS 2.0). Geneva, Switzerland, World Health Organization, 2009

van Tubergen A, Landewe R, Heuft-Dorenbosch L, et al: Assessment of disability with the World Health Organisation Disability Assessment Schedule II in patients with ankylosing spondylitis. Ann Rheum Dis 62:140–145, 2003

Von Korff M, Crane PK, Alonso J, et al: Modified WHODAS-II provides valid measure of global disability but filter items increased skewness. J Clin Epidemiol 61:1132–1143, 2008

Ware JE Jr, Sherbourne CD: The MOS 36-item short-form health survey (SF-36), I: conceptual framework and item selection. Med Care 30:473–483, 1992

Ware J, Kosinski M, Keller SD: SF-36 Physical and Mental Component Summary Scales: A User's Manual. Boston, MA, The Health Institute, New England Medical Center, 1994

Wells KB, Stewart A, Hays RD, et al: The functioning and well-being of depressed patients: results from the Medical Outcomes Study (see comments). JAMA 262:914–919, 1989

Williams A: Calculating the global burden of disease: time for a strategic reappraisal? Health Econ 8:1–8, 1999

Wing JK, Curtis RH, Beevor AK: HoNOS: Health of the Nation Outcome Scales. Report on Research July 1993–December 1995. London, Royal College of Psychiatrists, 1996

World Health Organization: International Classification of Impairments Disabilities and Handicaps: A Manual of Classification Relating to the Consequences of Disease. Albany, NY, World Health Organization, 1980

World Health Organization: International Statistical Classification of Diseases and Related Health Problems, 10th Revision. Geneva, World Health Organization, 1992

World Health Organization: The World Health Organization Quality of Life assessment (WHOQOL): position paper from the World Health Organization. Soc Sci Med 41:1403–1409, 1995

World Health Organization: Development of the World Health Organization WHOQOL-BREF quality of life assessment. The WHOQOL Group. Psychol Med 28:551–558, 1998a

World Health Organization: The World Health Organization Quality of Life Assessment (WHOQOL): development and general psychometric properties. Soc Sci Med 46:1569–1585, 1998b

World Health Organization: International Classification of Functioning, Disability and Health (ICF). Geneva, World Health Organization, 2001

World Health Organization: WHO Statistical Information System: Working Paper Describing Data Sources, Methods and Results for Projections of Mortality and Burden of Disease for 2005, 2015 and 2030. Geneva, World Health Organization, 2006

World Health Organization: World Health Organization Disability Assessment Schedule II (WHODAS II). Geneva, Switzerland, World Health Organization, 2009. Available at: http://www.who.int/icidh/whodas. Accessed July 29, 2009.

PART IV

IDENTIFYING IMPORTANT
CULTURE- AND GENDER-RELATED
EXPRESSIONS OF DISORDERS

CHAPTER 11

Assessing Mental Disorders and Service Use Across Countries

The WHO World Mental Health Survey Initiative

Philip S. Wang, M.D., Dr.P.H.
Sergio Aguilar-Gaxiola, M.D., Ph.D.
Jordi Alonso, M.D., Ph.D.
Sing Lee, M.B., B.S., F.R.C.Psych.
Michael Schoenbaum, Ph.D.
T. Bedirhan Üstün, M.D.
Ronald C. Kessler, Ph.D.
Ronny Bruffaerts, Ph.D.
Guilherme Borges, M.Sc., Dr.Sc.
Giovanni de Girolamo, M.D.
Oye Gureje, M.D., Ph.D., D.Sc.
Josep Maria Haro, M.D., M.P.H., Ph.D.

Portions of this chapter, including tables, have appeared previously in Ronald C. Kessler and T. Bedirhan Üstün (eds): *The WHO World Mental Health Surveys Global Perspective on the Epidemiology of Mental Disorders.* New York, Cambridge University Press, © World Health Organization, 2008. Used with permission. The views and opinions expressed are those of the authors and should not be construed to represent the views of any sponsoring organization, agencies, or the U.S. Government.

Stanislav Kostyuchenko, M.D.
Viviane Kovess Masféty, M.Sc., M.D., Ph.D.
Daphna Levinson, Ph.D.
Herbert Matschinger, Ph.D.
Zeina Mneimneh, M.P.H., M.Sc.
Mark Oakley Browne, Ph.D.
Johan Ormel, Ph.D.
José Posada-Villa, M.D.
Soraya Seedat, M.B.Ch.B., F.C.Psych., Ph.D.
Hisateru Tachimori, Ph.D.
Adley Tsang, B.So.Sci.

Although assessments of mental disorders and service use within countries have been possible for more than half a century, comparisons across countries have been more challenging, due largely to the inconsistent manner in which methods have been applied (Hagnell 1966; Langner and Michael 1963; Leighton 1959). This situation changed with the development of the Diagnostic Interview Schedule (DIS) in the 1980s (Bland et al. 1988). Because the DIS was the first psychiatric diagnostic interview that could be administered by lay interviewers, it became possible to conduct parallel psychiatric epidemiological surveys in different countries (Bland et al. 1988; Hwu et al. 1989; Lépine et al. 1989; Robins and Regier 1991). Results from these early cross-national surveys laid the groundwork for the World Health Organization (WHO) World Mental Health (WMH) Survey Initiative (http://www.hcp.med.harvard.edu/wmh/) (Weissman et al. 1994, 1996a, 1996b, 1997).

Other diagnostic schedules, such as the Composite International Diagnostic Interview (CIDI), have been developed subsequently. Still, innovations in the DIS and these early cross-national surveys continue to be used in psychiatric epidemiological efforts throughout the globe (Andrade et al. 1996, 2002; Bijl et al. 1998; Caraveo et al. 1998; Kessler et al. 1994; Kýlýç 1998; Vega et al. 1998; Wittchen 1998), and indeed, some of the key initial findings have been replicated in subsequent efforts, such as the WMH survey.

For example, across surveys/countries, about one-third of respondents are typically found to have met criteria for a mental disorder at some point in their lifetimes (World Health Organization International Consortium of Psychiatric Epidemiology 2000), but the majority of those meeting such criteria for mental disorders reported never receiving any specific treatment (Alegria et al. 2000;

Bijl et al. 2003). Important questions have been raised regarding such findings (Regier et al. 1998, 2000). Could many of these episodes of mental disorders have been mild or self-limited? If so, would it be prudent to treat them, even in economically advantaged societies, let alone in low-resource settings?

Answering these questions has been difficult because earlier cross-national surveys mainly estimated the prevalence of disorders but not their severity or consequences. Some investigators have created post hoc measures of the severity of mental disorders. In secondary analyses of earlier DIS and CIDI surveys that used such measures, as many as half of mental disorders have been estimated to be mild; however, even though use of treatments was typically correlated with disorder severity, even one- to two-thirds of the most disabled cases did not receive any treatment (Bijl et al. 2003; Narrow et al. 2002).

The current WMH initiative builds on, and markedly expands, earlier cross-national psychiatric epidemiological efforts. Whereas previous cross-national surveys have been conducted mainly in industrialized Western countries, the WMH survey includes countries across all geographic regions and across the spectrum of economic development. This breadth considerably increases the fraction of the world's population for which WMH findings can provide information. Additional WMH survey innovations, intended to increase the accuracy of cross-national comparisons, include a high degree of consistency and coordination across country surveys. To overcome limits in earlier cross-national efforts, the WMH survey instruments contain rigorous assessments of disorder severity as well as of associated disability. Finally, the WMH survey instruments include standardized questions about mental health services received, including their intensity and adequacy.

In the remainder of this chapter, we first raise some important methodological issues that should be considered when interpreting findings from the WMH initiative. Next, we briefly cover some WMH survey results that have emerged to date. We close with some suggestions for future directions, based on WMH survey findings, for researchers, clinicians, and policymakers charged with meeting the mental health needs of their countries' citizenry.

Methodological Issues

Assessing Mental Disorders, Severity, and Disability Across Countries

There are several important methodological considerations to bear in mind when making assessments of mental disorders and service use across countries (Haro et al. 2008; Kessler et al. 2008). First, it is not clear to what extent nosologic systems to classify mental disorders, which were developed mainly in Western and developed nations, reflect the disorders present in other countries. For example, the *Diagnostic and Statistical Manual of Mental Disorders* (DSM) and *International Classification of Diseases* (ICD) classification systems might not capture relevant local forms of psychopathology or their symptom expression. Because of this, there may be locally relevant syndromes in some countries that are not CIDI diagnoses, whereas some disorders assessed by diagnostic instruments, such as the CIDI, may not exist in all countries. With regard to the latter, it has been reassuring, in the WMH initiative, that culturally competent teams, including local mental health clinicians within each collaborating country, have not identified instances in which the disorders assessed by the CIDI do not exist. However, more intriguing are possibilities that some disorders assessed by the CIDI are expressed differently across countries. One such possibility that is the subject of investigation is whether social anxiety disorder is sometimes expressed differently in Asian countries, where great value is placed on not offending others (Choy et al. 2008). Additional questions that have been researched include whether variants of some disorders, which may not be fully captured by the CIDI, exist within specific cultures (Tseng 2006).

Another important methodological consideration for cross-national comparisons is whether the accuracy and thresholds of diagnoses made, using instruments such as the CIDI, differ between countries (Chang et al. 2008). The country-specific concepts and wording used to describe psychopathological constructs could substantially affect the reliability and validity of diagnoses. Furthermore, in countries in which free speech may have been curtailed, or in which there has been no experience with anonymous public-opinion surveying, participants may be hesitant to endorse symptoms of mental disorders. The accuracy of diagnoses also could depend, critically, on the rigor with which surveys are translated and monitored for quality and data are cleaned and coded, as well as other important aspects of survey implementation. That good concordance has been observed, in WMH survey clinical reappraisal studies, between CIDI diagnoses and diagnoses made in blind clinical re-interviews, provides some reassurance regarding the diagnostic accuracy of WMH survey results in some countries. However, it is important to keep in mind that these clinical reappraisal studies were limited largely to developed Western countries. In fact, the observation that countries with the lowest prevalence rates also had the highest proportions of treated respondents who were classified as subthreshold cases provides some indications that mental disorders may have been underestimated in these countries. To more definitively address these issues and make potential future revisions to the WMH survey methodology, clinical reappraisal studies examining cross-national differences in the accuracy of CIDI diagnoses have been undertaken in countries from all global regions and levels of economic development.

As mentioned earlier, assessing both the prevalence and the severity of mental disorders has been an important challenge in cross-national surveys. In part so that policymakers can know how many untreated cases are in need of mental health services, the WMH CIDI includes standard measures of the severity of specific mental disorders. All WMH surveys also contain measures of disability, including global functioning measures such as the WHO Disability Assessment Schedule (WHODAS; World Health Organization 1998) as well as disorder-specific measures of disability such as the Sheehan Disability Scale (Leon et al. 1997).

Assessing Treatment and Treatment Adequacy Across Countries

Important methodological considerations for cross-national assessment of mental health service use include recognizing the tremendous variation in what constitutes mental health treatment both within and across countries. Sources of this variation include the broad range of physicians from whom patients can receive mental health treatments, including general medical providers, such as internists and family practitioners; mental health specialists, such as psychiatrists and behavioral neurologists; and other specialty physicians, such as obstetricians-gynecologists. The specific treatment modalities employed by these physicians, such as pharmacotherapies and talk therapies, also can differ depending on physicians' specialization and training. Considerable additional variation comes from the wide spectrum of other professionals offering mental health services, which includes mental health specialists, such as psychologists, marriage, and family counselors; psychiatric social workers; human services personnel, such as human services caseworkers; religious and spiritual advisers; and complementary alternative medicine providers, such as traditional healers, acupuncturists, and self-help group moderators. To capture this range of possible treatment sources systematically and allow for cross-national comparisons, the WMH survey has employed an extensive and standardized module on mental health services and pharmacotherapy.

An additional goal of the WMH survey has been to assess the timeliness, intensity, and adequacy of treatments. By shedding light on the patterns and correlates of failing to receive any treatment, receiving treatment only after long delays, or receiving treatment that fails to meet the recommendations in evidence-based practice guidelines, researchers and policymakers see how to better develop and target interventions to address unmet needs for effective treatment.

Results From the World Mental Health Survey Initiative

Lifetime Mental Disorders

Results emerging from the WMH Survey Initiative regarding the occurrence of mental disorders over respondents' lifetimes indicate that such experiences are quite common across countries. The fraction of respondents with at least one lifetime disorder exceeded one-third in five WMH survey countries (Colombia, France, New Zealand, Ukraine, United States), one-fourth in six additional countries (Belgium, Germany, Lebanon, Mexico, the Netherlands, South Africa), and one-sixth in another four countries (Israel, Italy, Japan, Spain), as can be seen in Table 11–1. Lower lifetime prevalences were observed in the two remaining countries, China (Beijing/Shanghai) and Nigeria, although some evidence suggests that methodological biases may have lowered these prevalence estimates (Gureje et al. 2006; Shen et al. 2006).

The WMH survey lifetime prevalence concerning the four specific classes of diagnoses studied indicated that all four classes are significant public health concerns across the globe. In 10 countries surveyed, the most prevalent class was anxiety disorders; mood disorders were the most prevalent in all the remaining WMH survey countries except for one. Among those countries that had surveys containing relatively complete assessments of impulse-control disorders, this class of diagnoses was generally the least prevalent; in most of the remainder, substance use disorders were generally the least prevalent. However, it is important to point out that estimates of rates of substance use disorders may have been lowered because surveys in Western European countries did not assess illegal drug abuse or dependence; estimates of the lifetime prevalence of substance use disorders also may have been lowered because the presence of abuse was required in order for substance dependence to be assessed (Hasin and Grant 2004).

In most WMH survey countries, many respondents experienced more than one lifetime mental disorder. Thus, for example, the sum of the prevalence estimates for the four separate disorder classes was between 30% and 50% higher than the prevalence estimates of having any lifetime disorder, across countries surveyed.

WMH data on the lifetime occurrence of mental disorders also revealed surprising consistency across countries in the typical ages at onset for disorders. Standardized age-at-onset distributions indicated that impulse-control disorders generally have the earliest median ages at onset, ranging from 7 to 9 years of age for attention-deficit/hyperactivity disorder, 7 to 15 for oppositional defiant disorder, 9 to 14 for conduct disorder, and 13 to 21 for intermittent explosive disorder. For anxiety disorders, ages at onset appeared to be distributed in a more bimodal fashion, with phobias and separation anxiety disorder having very early ages (median, 7–14 years) and generalized anxiety disorder, panic disorder, and posttraumatic stress disorder having later ages (median, 24–50 years). For mood disorders, ages at onset typically ranged between the late 20s and early 40s (median age, 29–43 years). The ages at onset for substance use disorders varied considerably more across WMH countries; however, one consistent pattern that was observed across surveys was that relatively few ages at onset occurred prior to the mid-teens, but they did increase rapidly thereafter in adolescence and early adulthood.

A final result concerning lifetime mental disorders in the WMH survey, which confirms earlier cross-national research, is the fairly consistent finding that lifetime risk appears to be greatest in more recent cohorts (World Health Organization International Consortium of Psychiatric Epidemiology 2000). Results from survival analyses conducted on WMH data have shown that the relative risks for anxiety, mood, and substance use disorders are generally higher in more recent cohorts compared with older ones; such cohort effects were not observed for impulse-control disorders, however (results not shown but available on request).

Failure and Delay in Help Seeking After First Onset of Mental Disorders

Table 11–2 presents the proportions of lifetime cases of anxiety disorders in which the respondents made treatment contact in the year of disorder onset. These proportions ranged from 0.8% in Nigeria to 36.4% in Israel. The proportion of lifetime cases of anxiety disorders in which the respondents made treatment contact by age 50 years ranged from 15.2% in Nigeria to 95.0% in Germany. Among those cases of lifetime mental disorders in which the respondents eventually did make treatment contact, median delays were generally longer in developing, than developed, countries and ranged from 3.0 years in Israel to 30.0 years in Mexico.

Specifically, for lifetime cases of mood disorders, the proportion of respondents making initial treatment contact in the year of onset ranged from 6.0% in Nigeria and China to 52.1% in the Netherlands (Table 11–3). By age 50 years, the proportion of cases of lifetime mood disorders in which the respondents made treatment contact ranged from 7.9% in China to 98.6% in France. Median delays among cases

TABLE 11–1. Lifetime prevalence and projected lifetime risk, as of age 75 years, of DSM-IV-TR/CIDI disorders

	ANY ANXIETY DISORDER					ANY MOOD DISORDER				
	PREVIOUS			PROJECTED LIFETIME RISK		PREVIOUS			PROJECTED LIFETIME RISK	
	%	n^a	SE	%	SE	%	n^a	SE	%	SE
WHO Regional Office for the Americas										
Colombia	25.3	948	1.4	30.9	2.5	14.6	666	0.7	27.2	2.0
Mexico	14.3	684	0.9	17.8	1.6	9.2	598	0.5	20.4	1.7
United States	31.0	2,692	1.0	36.0	1.4	21.4	2,024	0.6	31.4	0.9
WHO Regional Office for Africa										
Nigeria	6.5	169	0.9	7.1	0.9	3.3	236	0.3	8.9	1.2
South Africa	15.8	695	0.8	30.1	4.4	9.8	439	0.7	20.0	2.4
WHO Regional Office for the Eastern Mediterranean										
Lebanon	16.7	282	1.6	20.2	1.8	2.6	352	0.9	20.1	1.2
WHO Regional Office for Europe										
Belgium	13.1	219	1.9	15.7	2.5	14.1	367	1.0	22.8	1.7
France	22.3	445	1.4	26.0	1.6	21.0	648	1.1	30.5	1.4
Germany	14.6	314	1.5	16.9	1.7	9.9	372	0.6	16.2	1.3
Israel	5.2	252	0.3	10.1	0.9	10.7	524	0.5	21.2	1.6
Italy	11.0	328	0.9	13.7	1.2	9.9	452	0.5	17.3	1.2
Netherlands	15.9	320	1.1	21.4	1.8	17.9	476	1.0	28.9	1.9
Spain	9.9	375	1.1	13.3	1.4	10.6	672	0.5	20.8	1.2
Ukraine	10.9	371	0.8	17.3	2.0	15.8	814	0.8	25.9	1.5
WHO Regional Office for the Western Pacific										
People's Republic of China	4.8	159	0.7	6.0	0.8	3.6	185	0.4	7.3	0.9
Japan	6.9	155	0.6	9.2	1.2	7.6	183	0.5	14.1	1.7
New Zealand	24.6	3,171	0.7	30.3	1.5	20.4	2,755	0.5	29.8	0.7

Note. CIDI=Composite International Diagnostic Interview; WHO=World Health Organization.
[a]The numbers reported here are the numbers of respondents with the disorders indicated in the column heading. In the case of anxiety and substance use disorders, the denominators are the numbers of respondents in the Part 2 sample. In the case of mood disorders, the denominators are the numbers of respondents in the Part 1 sample. In the case of impulse-control disorders and any disorders, the denominators are the number of respondents age 44 years in the Part 2 sample.
[b]Projected lifetime risk to age 65 years, due to the sample including only respondents up to age 65.
[c]Cell size was too small to be included in analysis.
[d]Impulse-control disorders not assessed.

ANY IMPULSE-CONTROL DISORDER					ANY SUBSTANCE USE DISORDER					ANY DISORDER				
PREVIOUS			PROJECTED LIFETIME RISK		PREVIOUS			PROJECTED LIFETIME RISK		PREVIOUS			PROJECTED LIFETIME RISK	
%	n^a	SE	%	SE	%	n^a	SE	%	SE	%	n^a	SE	%	SE
9.6	273	0.8	10.3	0.9	9.6	345	0.6	12.8	1.0	39.1	1,432	1.3	55.2[b]	6.0
5.7	152	0.6	5.7	0.6	7.8	378	0.5	11.9	1.0	26.1	1,148	1.4	36.4[b]	2.1
25.0	1,051	1.1	25.6	1.1	14.6	1,144	0.6	17.4	0.6	47.4	3,929	1.1	55.3	1.2
0.3	9	0.1	—[c]	–	3.7	119	0.4	6.4	1.0	12.0	440	1.0	19.5	1.9
—[d]	–	–	–	–	13.3	505	0.9	17.5	1.2	30.3	1,290	1.1	47.5	3.7
4.4	53	0.9	4.6	1.0	2.2	27	0.8	–	—[c]	25.8	491	1.9	32.9	2.1
5.2	31	1.4	5.2	1.4	8.3	195	0.9	10.5	1.1	29.1	519	2.3	37.1	3.0
7.6	71	1.3	7.6	1.3	7.1	202	0.5	8.8	0.6	37.9	847	1.7	47.2	1.6
3.1	31	0.8	3.1	0.8	6.5	228	0.6	8.7	0.9	25.2	573	1.9	33.0	2.5
—[d]	–	–	–	–	5.3	261	0.3	6.3	0.4	17.6	860	0.6	29.7	1.5
1.7	27	0.4	—[c]	–	1.3	56	0.2	1.6	0.3	18.1	612	1.1	26.0	1.9
4.7	37	1.1	4.8	1.1	8.9	210	0.9	11.4	1.2	31.7	633	2.0	42.9	2.5
2.3	40	0.8	2.3	0.8	3.6	180	0.4	4.6	0.5	19.4	842	1.4	29.0	1.8
8.7	91	1.1	9.7	1.3	15.0	293	1.3	18.8	1.7	36.1	1,074	1.5	48.9	2.5
4.3	37	0.9	4.9	0.9	4.9	128	0.7	6.1	0.8	13.2	419	1.3	18.0	1.5
2.8	11	1.0	—[c]	–	4.8	69	0.5	6.2	0.7	18.0	343	1.1	24.4	1.8
—[d]	–	–	–	–	12.4	1,767	0.4	14.6	0.5	39.3	4,815	0.9	48.6	1.5

TABLE 11–2.   Proportional treatment contact in the year of onset of any anxiety disorder and median duration of delay among cases in which the respondents subsequently made treatment contact

	MAKING TREATMENT CONTACT IN YEAR OF ONSET, % (SE)	MAKING TREATMENT CONTACT BY AGE 50 YEARS, % (SE)	MEDIAN DURATION OF DELAY IN YEARS, % (SE)
WHO Regional Office for the Americas			
Colombia	2.9 (0.6)	41.6 (3.9)	26.0 (1.5)
Mexico	3.6 (1.1)	53.2 (18.2)	30.0 (5.1)
United States	11.3 (0.7)	87.0 (2.4)	23.0 (0.6)
WHO Regional Office for Africa			
Nigeria	0.8 (0.5)	15.2 (2.6)	16.0 (4.2)
WHO Regional Office for the Eastern Mediterranean			
Lebanon	3.2 (1.1)	37.3 (11.5)	28.0 (3.9)
WHO Regional Office for Europe			
Belgium	19.8 (2.8)	84.5 (4.9)	16.0 (3.5)
France	16.1 (1.8)	93.3 (1.9)	18.0 (1.8)
Germany	13.7 (1.8)	95.0 (2.3)	23.0 (2.3)
Israel	36.4 (0.9)	90.7 (1.3)	3.0 (0.1)
Italy	17.1 (2.1)	87.3 (8.5)	28.0 (2.2)
Netherlands	28.0 (3.7)	91.1 (2.8)	10.0 (1.6)
Spain	23.2 (2.0)	86.6 (5.2)	17.0 (3.2)
WHO Regional Office for the Western Pacific			
People's Republic of China	4.2 (2.0)	44.7 (7.2)	21.0 (3.1)
Japan	11.2 (2.4)	63.1 (6.2)	20.0 (2.4)
New Zealand	12.5 (0.8)	84.2 (2.5)	21.0 (0.8)

Note.   WHO=World Health Organization.

of mood disorders in which the respondents eventually made treatment contact ranged from 1 year in five countries (i.e., Belgium, the Netherlands, Spain, China, and Japan) to 14 years in Mexico.

For lifetime cases of substance use disorders, the proportion of respondents who made treatment contact in the year of disorder onset ranged from 0.9% in Mexico to 18.6% in Spain (see Table 11–4). The proportion of lifetime cases of substance use disorders in which the respondents made treatment by age 50 years ranged from 19.8% in Nigeria to 86.1% in Germany. Median delays for lifetime cases of substance use disorders in which respondents eventually

TABLE 11–3. Proportional treatment contact in the year of onset of any mood disorder and median duration of delay among cases in which the respondents subsequently made treatment contact

	MAKING TREATMENT CONTACT IN YEAR OF ONSET, % (SE)	MAKING TREATMENT CONTACT BY AGE 50 YEARS, % (SE)	MEDIAN DURATION OF DELAY IN YEARS, % (SE)
WHO Regional Office for the Americas			
Colombia	18.7 (2.7)	66.6 (3.7)	9.0 (1.6)
Mexico	16.0 (2.2)	69.9 (8.5)	14.0 (3.1)
United States	35.4 (1.2)	94.8 (2.5)	4.0 (0.2)
WHO Regional Office for Africa			
Nigeria	6.0 (1.7)	33.3 (7.2)	6.0 (3.3)
WHO Regional Office for the Eastern Mediterranean			
Lebanon	12.3 (2.0)	49.2 (5.2)	6.0 (2.1)
WHO Regional Office for Europe			
Belgium[a]	47.8 (2.7)	93.7 (2.5)	1.0 (0.3)
France[a]	42.7 (2.1)	98.6 (1.4)	3.0 (0.3)
Germany[a]	40.4 (3.8)	89.1 (5.0)	2.0 (0.4)
Israel[a]	31.9 (0.8)	92.7 (0.5)	6.0 (0.3)
Italy[a]	28.8 (3.0)	63.5 (5.9)	2.0 (0.5)
Netherlands[a]	52.1 (2.9)	96.9 (1.7)	1.0 (0.3)
Spain[a]	48.5 (2.3)	96.4 (3.1)	1.0 (0.3)
WHO Regional Office for the Western Pacific			
People's Republic of China	6.0 (2.2)	7.9 (2.6)	1.0 (2.0)
Japan	29.6 (4.0)	56.8 (7.3)	1.0 (0.7)
New Zealand	41.4 (1.3)	97.5 (1.0)	3.0 (0.2)

Note. WHO=World Health Organization.
[a]Used major depressive episode instead of any mood disorder.

made treatment contact ranged from 6.0 years in Spain to 18.0 years in Belgium.

For lifetime anxiety disorders, female sex was significantly associated with higher likelihood of making initial treatment contact in four countries (France, Germany, New Zealand, and the United States; results not shown but available on request). There were significant, generally monotonic, relationships between being in younger cohorts and higher probabilities of treatment contact in all but two countries

TABLE 11–4. Proportional treatment contact in the year of onset of any substance use disorder and median duration of delay among cases in which the respondents subsequently made treatment contact

	MAKING TREATMENT CONTACT IN YEAR OF ONSET, % (SE)	MAKING TREATMENT CONTACT BY AGE 50 YEARS, % (SE)	MEDIAN DURATION OF DELAY IN YEARS, % (SE)
WHO Regional Office for the Americas			
Colombia	3.6 (0.8)	23.1 (7.1)	11.0 (5.0)
Mexico	0.9 (0.5)	22.1 (4.8)	10.0 (3.3)
United States[a]	10.0 (0.8)	75.5 (3.8)	13.0 (1.2)
WHO Regional Office for Africa			
Nigeria[a]	2.8 (1.7)	19.8 (7.2)	8.0 (1.8)
WHO Regional Office for the Eastern Mediterranean			
Lebanon[a]	_[b]	_[b]	_[b]
WHO Regional Office for Europe			
Belgium	12.8 (4.8)	61.2 (17.7)	18.0 (5.8)
France	15.7 (5.4)	66.5 (14.1)	13.0 (3.7)
Germany	13.2 (5.7)	86.1 (8.6)	9.0 (3.9)
Israel	2.0 (0.5)	48.0 (2.4)	12.0 (0.5)
Italy[a]	_[b]	_[b]	_[b]
Netherlands	15.5 (5.4)	66.6 (7.9)	9.0 (3.1)
Spain	18.6 (7.6)	40.1 (14.1)	6.0 (4.9)
WHO Regional Office for the Western Pacific			
People's Republic of China[a]	2.8 (1.8)	25.7 (9.0)	17.0 (3.7)
Japan[a]	9.2 (5.1)	31.0 (7.8)	8.0 (4.6)
New Zealand	6.3 (0.8)	84.8 (15.4)	17.0 (1.3)

Note.   WHO=World Health Organization.
[a]Assessed in the Part 2 sample.
[b]Disorder was omitted as a result of insufficient cases ($n<30$).

(Lebanon and Mexico). In all but one country (Israel), for lifetime cases of anxiety disorders with earlier ages at onset, the respondents were significantly less likely to make treatment contact.

Being female was significantly associated with higher likelihoods of lifetime treatment contact for mood disorders in three countries (Mexico, New Zealand, and the United States). Probabilities of life-time treatment contacts for mood disorders were significantly higher among younger cohorts in all but five countries (China, Germany, Italy, Japan, and Mexico). For cases of mood disorders with earlier ages at onset, the respondents were significantly less likely to make treatment contacts in all but two countries (China and Nigeria).

For substance use disorders, females were significantly more likely to make initial treatment contact in one country (New Zealand). The probabilities of initial treatment contact were significantly higher among younger cohorts in all but 5 of the 13 countries in which this relationship was examined (China, France, Germany, the Netherlands, and Nigeria). For cases of substance use disorders with earlier ages at onset, the respondents were significantly less likely to make initial treatment contacts in all but 5 of the 13 countries in which this was examined (China, France, Japan, Mexico, and Nigeria).

Prevalence and Severity of 12-Month Mental Disorders

Among respondents, the prevalence of any mental disorder in the year prior to being surveyed ranged between 6.0% in Nigeria and 27.0% in the United States (Table 11–5). The most common class of 12-month disorders was anxiety disorders in all but three countries, with prevalence ranging between 3.0% and 19.0%. (Most common in Israel, as well as Ukraine, were mood disorders, whereas impulse-control disorders were most common in China.) The next most common class was mood disorders in all but three countries. (South Africa had a higher prevalence of substance disorders, and China and the United States had higher prevalences of impulse-control disorder, ranging between 1.1% and 9.7%.) The 12-month prevalences of substance disorders (0.2%–6.4%) and impulse-control disorders (0.1%–10.5%) were generally lower across most countries.

The proportions of cases that could be categorized as serious ranged from 12.8% to 36.8%; 12.5%–47.6% of cases could be classified as moderate and 28.0%–74.7% as mild (Table 11–6). Positive associations were observed between the overall prevalence of any 12-month disorder and both the proportion of cases classified as serious (Pearson $r=0.46$; $P<0.001$) and the proportion of cases classified as either serious or moderate (Pearson $r=0.77$; $P<0.001$).

Use of Services in the 12 Months Prior to Survey

Among respondents, the prevalence of use of any mental health services during the prior 12 months ranged widely from 1.6% in Nigeria

TABLE 11–5. Twelve-month prevalence of CIDI/DSM-IV disorders

	Anxiety, % (SE)	Mood, % (SE)	Impulse Control,[a] % (SE)	Substance, % (SE)	Any, % (SE)
WHO Regional Office for the Americas					
Colombia	14.4 (1.0)	7.0 (0.5)	4.4 (0.4)	2.8 (0.4)	21.0 (1.0)
Mexico	8.4 (0.6)	4.7 (0.3)	1.6 (0.3)[b]	2.3 (0.3)	13.4 (0.9)
United States	19.0 (0.7)	9.7 (0.4)	10.5 (0.7)	3.8 (0.4)	27.0 (0.9)
WHO Regional Office for Africa					
Nigeria	4.2 (0.5)	1.1 (0.1)	0.1 (0.0)[c,d]	0.9 (0.2)	6.0 (0.6)
South Africa	8.2 (0.6)[e,f]	4.9 (0.4)[g]	1.9 (0.3)[c,d,h]	5.8 (0.5)	16.7 (1.0)
WHO Regional Office for the Eastern Mediterranean					
Lebanon	12.2 (1.2)	6.8 (0.7)	2.6 (0.7)[d]	1.3 (0.8)	17.9 (1.7)
WHO Regional Office for Europe					
Belgium	8.4 (1.4)	5.4 (0.5)[g]	1.7 (1.0)[b]	1.8 (0.4)[i]	13.2 (1.5)
France	13.7 (1.1)	6.5 (0.6)[g]	2.4 (0.6)[b]	1.3 (0.3)[i]	18.9 (1.4)
Germany	8.3 (1.1)	3.3 (0.3)[g]	0.6 (0.3)[b]	1.2 (0.2)[i]	11.0 (1.3)
Israel	3.6 (0.3)[e,f]	6.4 (0.4)	—(—)[b,c,d,h]	1.3 (0.2)	10.0 (0.5)
Italy	6.5 (0.6)	3.4 (0.3)[g]	0.4 (0.2)[b]	0.2 (0.1)[i]	8.8 (0.7)
Netherlands	8.9 (1.0)	5.1 (0.5)[g]	1.9 (0.7)[b]	1.9 (0.3)[i]	13.6 (1.0)
Spain	6.6 (0.9)	4.4 (0.3)[g]	0.5 (0.2)[b]	0.7 (0.2)[i]	9.7 (0.8)
Ukraine	6.8 (0.7)[e,f]	9.0 (0.6)[g]	5.7 (1.0)[c,d]	6.4 (0.8)	21.4 (1.3)

TABLE 11–5. Twelve-month prevalence of CIDI/DSM-IV disorders *(continued)*

	ANXIETY, % (SE)	MOOD, % (SE)	IMPULSE CONTROL,[a] % (SE)	SUBSTANCE, % (SE)	ANY, % (SE)
WHO Regional Office for the Western Pacific					
People's Republic of China	3.0 (0.5)	1.9 (0.3)	3.1 (0.7)[c,d]	1.6 (0.4)	7.1 (0.9)
Japan	4.2 (0.6)[e]	2.5 (0.4)	0.2 (0.1)[c,d,h]	1.2 (0.4)	7.4 (0.9)
New Zealand	15.0 (0.5)[e]	8.0 (0.4)	(—)[b,c,d,h]	3.5 (0.2)	20.7 (0.6)

Note. Anxiety disorders include agoraphobia, adult separation anxiety disorder, generalized anxiety disorder, panic disorder, posttraumatic stress disorder, social phobia, and specific phobia. Mood disorders include bipolar disorders, dysthymia, and major depressive disorder. Impulse-control disorders include intermittent explosive disorder and reported persistence, in the past 12 months, of symptoms of three child or adolescent disorders (attention-deficit/hyperactivity disorder, conduct disorder, and oppositional defiant disorder). Substance disorders include alcohol or drug abuse, with or without dependence. In the case of substance dependence, respondents who met full criteria at some time in their life and who continue to have any symptoms are considered to have 12-month dependence, even if they currently do not meet full criteria for the disorder. Organic exclusions were made as specified in DSM-IV-TR (American Psychiatric Association 2000).

CIDI=Composite International Diagnostic Interview; WHO=World Health Organization.

[a]Impulse-control disorders restricted to 39 years and younger (China, Ukraine, Nigeria) or to age 44 years and younger (all other countries).
[b]Intermittent explosive disorder was not assessed.
[c]Attention-deficit/hyperactivity disorder was not assessed.
[d]Oppositional defiant disorder was not assessed.
[e]Adult separation anxiety disorder was not assessed.
[f]Specific phobia was not assessed.
[g]Bipolar disorders were not assessed.
[h]Conduct disorder was not assessed.
[i]Only alcohol abuse with or without dependence was assessed. No assessment was made of other drug abuse with or without dependence.

TABLE 11–6. Prevalence of 12-month CIDI/DSM-IV disorders by severity across countries

	SERIOUS, % (SE)	MODERATE, % (SE)	MILD, % (SE)
WHO Regional Office for the Americas			
Colombia	23.1 (2.1)	41.0 (2.6)	35.9 (2.1)
Mexico	25.7 (2.4)	33.9 (2.2)	40.5 (2.6)
United States	25.2 (1.4)	39.2 (1.2)	35.7 (1.4)
WHO Regional Office for Africa			
Nigeria	12.8 (3.8)	12.5 (2.6)	74.7 (4.2)
South Africa	25.7 (1.8)	31.5 (2.2)	42.8 (2.2)
WHO Regional Office for the Eastern Mediterranean			
Lebanon	22.4 (3.1)	42.6 (4.7)	35.0 (5.5)
WHO Regional Office for Europe			
Belgium	31.8 (4.2)	37.8 (3.3)	30.4 (4.8)
France	18.5 (2.5)	42.7 (3.0)	38.8 (3.6)
Germany	21.3 (2.5)	42.6 (4.6)	36.1 (4.3)
Israel	36.8 (2.4)	35.2 (2.3)	28.0 (2.1)
Italy	15.9 (2.7)	47.6 (3.8)	36.5 (3.9)
Netherlands	30.7 (3.4)	31.0 (3.7)	38.3 (4.6)
Spain	19.3 (2.4)	42.3 (4.0)	38.4 (4.7)
Ukraine	22.9 (1.8)	39.4 (2.9)	37.7 (3.5)
WHO Regional Office for the Western Pacific			
People's Republic of China	13.8 (3.7)	32.2 (4.9)	54.0 (4.6)
Japan	13.2 (3.1)	45.5 (5.3)	41.3 (4.6)
New Zealand	25.3 (1.0)	40.8 (1.4)	33.9 (1.2)

Note.   CIDI=Composite International Diagnostic Interview; WHO=World Health Organization.

to 17.9% in the United States, with generally lower proportions recorded in developing, versus developed, countries (Table 11–7) as well as in countries spending less on overall health care (Table 11–8). Greater proportions used the general medical sector than mental health specialty sectors in most countries; however, in three countries (Mexico, Colombia, and Israel) this situation was reversed. Generally smaller proportions of respondents used the human services and complementary and alternative medical sectors.

Significant, generally monotonic, relationships were observed between the severity of 12-month disorders and the likelihood of 12-month service use in all countries except China (Table 11–9). The proportion of cases in which respondents used services during the prior 12 months was generally lower in developing, than in developed, countries across all severity categories. Nevertheless, in absolute terms, only from 11.0% of respondents with serious cases in China to 62.1% of respondents with serious cases in Belgium received any treatments in these 12 months. For moderate and mild cases, the proportions of respondents using 12-month services were typically even lower. The proportion of respondents who did not meet criteria for 12-month mental disorders but used services during the 12 months ranged from 1.0% in Nigeria to 13.4% in South Africa.

Other WMH survey findings, which suggest that treatment resources may not be being distributed as allocated, include those from analyses of the relationship between disorder severity and use of the mental health specialty sector (results not shown but available on request). Significant relationships between severity and 12-month service use existed in only six WMH countries, and even in those countries, meaningful proportions of respondents in mild and noncases received treatments from mental health specialty sectors.

Among respondents who initiated treatments, the proportion who subsequently received any follow-up care ranged between 70.2% in Germany and 94.5% in Italy (Table 11–10). In general, smaller proportions of respondents received any follow-up care in low- and middle-income countries than in high-income countries. Although there were statistically significant relationships between the severity of mental disorders and the proportion of respondents receiving any follow-up care in seven countries, all countries had meaningful proportions of both severe cases in which respondents did not receive any follow-up care and apparent noncases in which respondents did receive care.

Among respondents using services, the proportions receiving treatments that met a definition for being potentially minimally adequate ranged between 10.4% in Nigeria and 42.3% in France (Table 11–11). Again, lower-income countries generally had smaller proportions than higher-income countries (a notable exception to this pattern was the United States, in which the proportion was 18.1%). There were statistically significant relationships between the severity of disorders and the proportion of respondents who received minimally adequate treatment in only five countries; again, all countries had meaningful percentages of both severe cases in which respondents failed to receive minimally adequate treatment and apparent noncases in which respondents did.

Conclusion

When one is interpreting the results from the WMH survey, it is important to keep some potential limitations in mind. Information

TABLE 11–7. Twelve-month service use by sectors in the WMH surveys

| | AMONG RESPONDENTS[a] | | | | | | | | | | | | | | |
| | ANY TREATMENT | | | MENTAL HEALTH SPECIALTY | | | GENERAL MEDICAL | | | HUMAN SERVICES | | | CAM | | |
COUNTRY	n	%	SE	n	%	SE	n	%	SE	n	%	SE	n	%	SE
WHO Regional Office for the Americas															
Colombia	217	5.5	0.6	126	3.0	0.4	82	2.3	0.4	19	0.5	0.2	10	0.2	0.1
Mexico	240	5.1	0.5	121	2.8	0.3	92	1.7	0.3	15	0.3	0.1	45	1.0	0.2
United States	1,477	17.9	0.7	738	8.8	0.5	773	9.3	0.4	266	3.4	0.3	247	2.8	0.2
WHO Regional Office for Africa															
Nigeria	57	1.6	0.3	5	0.1	0.1	42	1.1	0.2	14	0.5	0.2	1	0.0	0.0
South Africa	675	15.4	1.0	108	2.5	0.4	440	10.2	0.8	169	3.7	0.4	161	3.7	0.3
WHO Regional Office for the Eastern Mediterranean															
Lebanon	77	4.4	0.6	18	1.0	0.3	53	2.9	0.5	11	0.8	0.3	0	0.0	0.0
WHO Regional Office for Europe															
Belgium	187	10.9	1.4	96	5.2	0.7	147	8.2	1.3	6	0.4	0.2	12	0.7	0.3
France	272	11.3	1.0	111	4.4	0.5	214	8.8	0.9	10	0.4	0.2	9	0.5	0.3
Germany	183	8.1	0.8	100	3.9	0.6	102	4.2	0.6	16	1.0	0.4	15	0.6	0.2
Israel	421	8.8	0.4	215	4.4	0.3	169	3.6	0.3	71	1.6	0.2	42	0.8	0.1
Italy	141	4.3	0.4	55	2.0	0.3	107	3.0	0.3	15	0.4	0.1	4	0.1	0.0
Netherlands	202	10.9	1.2	105	5.5	1.0	141	7.7	1.1	14	0.6	0.2	27	1.5	0.4
Spain	375	6.8	0.5	200	3.6	0.4	249	4.4	0.4	11	0.1	0.1	20	0.2	0.1
Ukraine	212	7.2	0.8	39	1.2	0.3	135	4.0	0.7	47	1.7	0.4	29	1.0	0.3
WHO Regional Office for the Western Pacific															
People's Republic of China	74	3.4	0.6	19	0.6	0.2	41	2.3	0.5	6	0.3	0.1	18	0.7	0.3
Japan	92	5.6	0.9	43	2.4	0.5	47	2.8	0.5	8	0.8	0.5	13	0.6	0.2
New Zealand	1,592	13.8	0.5	585	5.2	0.3	1,122	9.2	0.4	203	1.6	0.2	265	2.6	0.3
χ^2_{16}	764.6* (< 0.001)			679.6* (< 0.001)			732.2* (< 0.001)			262.9* (< 0.001)			388.0* (<0.001)		

Note.   CAM=complementary and alternative medicine; WHO=World Health Organization; WMH=World Mental Health.
*Significant at the .05 level, two-sided test.
[a]Percentages among respondents are based on entire Part 2 samples.
[b]Percentages are based on respondents using any 12-month services.

| AMONG RESPONDENTS USING SERVICES[b] | | | | | | | | | | | |
| MENTAL HEALTH SPECIALTY | | | GENERAL MEDICAL | | | HUMAN SERVICES | | | CAM | | |
n	%	SE	n	%	SE	n	%	SE	n	%	SE
126	53.4	4.8	82	41.7	5.1	19	9.2	2.8	10	3.7	1.4
121	53.6	4.2	92	33.1	4.0	15	6.2	2.0	45	20.0	3.4
738	48.8	1.7	773	51.8	1.3	266	18.8	1.1	247	15.6	1.0
5	8.3	3.7	42	66.6	10.1	14	30.9	10.2	1	1.1	1.1
108	16.3	2.2	440	66.4	2.5	169	24.0	1.9	161	23.8	2.1
18	22.3	5.7	53	66.6	7.4	11	17.5	6.1	0	0.0	0.0
96	47.9	4.4	147	75.5	3.8	6	3.7	1.8	12	6.5	2.9
111	39.4	3.6	214	78.4	3.3	10	3.4	1.2	9	4.3	2.1
100	48.5	4.8	102	51.7	5.1	16	12.2	4.5	15	7.4	2.5
215	50.5	2.6	169	40.4	2.6	71	18.0	2.0	42	9.6	1.5
55	47.1	5.1	107	70.9	4.8	15	9.1	2.4	4	1.5	0.7
105	51.0	6.0	141	71.2	6.1	14	5.4	1.6	27	13.5	3.8
200	52.2	3.6	249	64.9	3.4	11	2.1	0.8	20	3.5	1.0
39	17.2	3.8	135	55.4	7.1	47	24.1	5.1	29	14.4	4.0
19	18.0	5.9	41	68.5	6.8	6	7.4	3.8	18	21.2	7.3
43	42.5	5.5	47	50.2	8.2	8	15.0	6.7	13	11.1	4.7
585	37.6	1.8	1,122	66.5	1.8	203	11.5	1.1	265	19.0	1.7
232.4* (< 0.001)			207.3* (< 0.001)			201.8* (< 0.001)			223.1* (< 0.001)		

about mental health service use and lifetime mental disorders was assessed through respondent recall, which may be inaccurate and/or decrease in accuracy as the recall period gets longer (Jenkins et al. 1997; Shiffman et al. 2008; Stone and Broderick 2007). For this reason, the WMH has generally focused on gathering information that may be less vulnerable to biased recall (e.g., less frequent or more vividly remembered events, such as past suicide attempts or psychiatric hospitalizations) over longer periods. In addition, more detailed questions about past experiences generally have been reserved for recall over more proximal time periods, whereas the least detail was asked about lifetime experiences.

Nearly all of the surveys are cross-sectional, and the WMH survey is not useful generally for identifying temporal trends. For this reason, some WMH survey countries, such as the United States, have added trend surveys (i.e., new samples to monitor changes in the study population), panel surveys (i.e., repeat surveys on the same respondents to study within-person changes), or mixed panel trend surveys. However, even in countries where only cross-sectional surveys have been conducted, other features may make it possible to draw some inferences about temporal patterns from retrospective reports. For example, special wording sequences and probes to prime respondents' memories have made it possible to conduct the analyses of lifetime prevalence, age at disorder onset, and delays in initial treatment seeking presented here.

Finally, it is important to consider whether apparent differences between countries in the occurrence of mental disorders or service use may be due to any of the potential limitations discussed in the "Methodological Issues" section (Chang et al. 2008; Cooke et al. 2004; Simon et al. 2002). As mentioned, investigations of these possibilities are currently under way (Haro et al. 2008; Kessler et al. 2008). However, until results from these follow-up studies become available, it may be prudent to focus mainly on important similarities that have emerged to date and to be cautious when trying to make substantive interpretations for any cross-national differences observed.

Like findings from earlier cross-national surveys, WMH survey findings on the prevalence of mental disorders in the prior year indicate that the experience of recent episodes of mental illness is highly prevalent and associated with substantial impairments in role functioning (Kessler and Frank 1997; Ormel et al. 1994; Weissman et al. 1994, 1996a, 1996b, 1997; Wells et al. 1989). As discussed, the likelihood that potential biases make these estimates of the occurrence and seriousness of mental disorders conservative only underscores the need for urgent public attention (Allgulander 1989; Eaton et al. 1992; Kessler and Merikangas 2004; Kessler et al. 1994).

Unfortunately, the data on current mental health services received in the past year by people with mental illness demonstrate very considerable levels of unmet need for treatment worldwide. Even among those with the most serious disorders in developed countries, approximately half received no mental health care in the prior year, and the situation is even more dire in developing countries. Again, the likelihood that most biases would make these estimates of unmet need for treatment conservative only underscores the problem. Furthermore, among people with mental illness who do receive

TABLE 11–8. Healthcare spending and level of economic development of each WMH country

COUNTRY	NATIONAL HEALTH CARE BUDGET AS PERCENTAGE OF TOTAL GDP[a]	MENTAL HEALTH CARE BUDGET AS PERCENTAGE OF NATIONAL HEALTH CARE BUDGET[b]	LEVEL OF ECONOMIC DEVELOPMENT
Nigeria	3.4	–[c]	Low
People's Republic of China—Beijing	5.5	2.4	Low–middle
People's Republic of China—Shanghai	5.5	2.4	Low–middle
Colombia	5.5	0.1	Low–middle
South Africa	8.6	–[c]	Low–middle
Ukraine	4.3	–[c]	Low–middle
Lebanon	12.2	–[c]	High–middle
Mexico	6.1	1.0	High–middle
Belgium	8.9	6.0	High
France	9.6	8.0	High
Germany	10.8	–[c]	High
Israel	8.7	6.2	High
Italy	8.4	–[c]	High
Japan	8.0	5.0	High
Netherlands	8.9	7.0	High
New Zealand	8.3	11.0	High
Spain	7.5	–[c]	High
United States	13.9	6.0	High

Note. GDP=gross domestic product; WMH=World Mental Health. [a]World Health Organization Project Atlas: Resources for Mental Health and Neurological Disorders. Available at: http://www.who.int/globalatlas/dataQuery/default.asp. [b]World Health Organization Mental Health Atlas. Available at: http://www.who.int/mental_health/evidence/mhatlas05/en/index.html. [c]Figures not available.

TABLE 11–9. Percentages using 12-month services by severity of mental disorders in the WMH surveys

COUNTRY	SEVERE			MODERATE			MILD			NONE			TEST OF DIFFERENCE IN PROBABILITY OF TREATMENT BY SEVERITY	
	n	%[a]	SE	n	%[a]	SE	n	%[a]	SE	n	%[a]	SE	χ^2_3	P
WHO Regional Office for the Americas														
Colombia	54	27.8	4.8	47	10.3	2.0	30	7.8	1.6	86	3.4	0.6	96.1*	< 0.001
Mexico	52	25.8	4.3	53	17.9	2.9	33	11.9	2.3	102	3.2	0.4	132.9*	< 0.001
United States	385	59.7	2.4	394	39.9	1.3	219	26.2	1.7	479	9.7	0.6	668.5*	< 0.001
WHO Regional Office for Africa														
Nigeria	8	21.3	11.9	6	13.8	7.4	14	10.0	3.0	29	1.0	0.3	27.7*	< 0.001
South Africa	45	26.2	3.6	66	26.6	3.9	67	23.1	3.2	497	13.4	0.9	41.0*	< 0.001
WHO Regional Office for the Eastern Mediterranean														
Lebanon	22	20.1	5.2	19	11.6	3.1	7	4.0	1.6	29	3.0	0.7	34.9*	< 0.001
WHO Regional Office for Europe														
Belgium	46	62.1	9.2	30	38.4	8.3	13	12.7	4.6	98	6.8	1.1	227.1*	< 0.001
France	56	48.0	6.4	70	29.4	4.0	43	22.4	3.4	103	7.0	1.1	82.6*	< 0.001
Germany	30	40.6	8.9	39	23.9	4.7	27	20.5	5.2	87	5.9	0.9	54.5*	< 0.001
Israel	81	53.9	4.0	54	32.6	3.7	19	14.4	3.2	267	6.0	0.4	368.1*	< 0.001
Italy	29	51.6	6.5	38	25.9	4.2	21	17.8	4.5	53	2.2	0.4	192.7*	< 0.001
Netherlands	57	49.2	6.6	36	31.3	7.2	15	16.1	6.0	94	7.7	1.3	66.8*	< 0.001
Spain	79	58.7	4.9	93	37.4	5.0	35	17.3	4.3	168	3.9	0.5	446.1*	< 0.001
Ukraine	49	25.7	3.2	68	21.2	3.6	19	7.6	2.6	76	4.4	0.8	81.2*	< 0.001

TABLE 11–9. Percentages using 12-month services by severity of mental disorders in the WMH surveys *(continued)*

COUNTRY	SEVERE			MODERATE			MILD			NONE			TEST OF DIFFERENCE IN PROBABILITY OF TREATMENT BY SEVERITY	
	n	%ᵃ	SE	n	%ᵃ	SE	n	%ᵃ	SE	n	%ᵃ	SE	χ^2_3	P
WHO Regional Office for the Western Pacific														
People's Republic of China	5	11.0	5.4	11	23.5	10.9	3	1.7	1.2	55	2.9	0.6	16.1*	0.001
Japanᵇ	10	24.2	5.0	16	24.2	5.0	9	12.8	4.4	57	4.5	0.9	44.5*ᵇ	<0.001
New Zealand	458	56.6	2.2	421	39.8	1.9	184	22.2	1.9	529	7.3	0.5	644.8*	<0.001
χ^2_{16}ᶜ	186.9* (<0.001)			145.6* (<0.001)			104.1* (<0.001)			330.0* (<0.001)				

Note. Percentages are based on entire Part 2 samples.

WHO=World Health Organization; WMH=World Mental Health.

*Significant at the .05 level, two-sided test.

ᵃPercentages are based on respondents using any services, within each level of severity.

ᵇSevere and moderate cases were combined into one category for Japan, and the percentage using services was displayed in both columns.

The χ^2 test was two degrees of freedom for this country.

ᶜχ^2_{16} is from a model predicting any 12-month service use among respondents, within each level of severity.

TABLE 11–10. Percentages receiving follow-up treatment[a] among respondents using services in the WMH surveys

Country	Any Severity n	%[b]	SE	Severe n	%[c]	SE	Moderate n	%[c]	SE	Mild n	%[c]	SE	None n	%[c]	SE	Test of difference in probability of follow-up treatment by severity χ²[2d]	P
WHO Regional Office for the Americas
Colombia	158	72.0	4.3	49	92.6	3.5	31	73.1	7.9	20	61.7	11.3	58	63.6	7.9	12.3*	0.006
Mexico	180	74.5	4.4	40	85.5	4.2	41	76.6	6.7	25	84.3	6.9	74	67.8	7.7	6.0	0.11
United States	1,313	86.8	1.4	362	93.2	1.7	354	88.4	2.0	187	83.0	2.9	410	83.3	2.6	17.2*	0.001
WHO Regional Office for Africa
Nigeria	47	76.3	8.7	6	—[e]	—[e]	6	—[e]	—[e]	13	74.6	9.2	22	74.6	9.2	0.4	0.51
South Africa	601	89.1	1.7	42	93.9	3.9	63	95.7	3.0	58	87.4	3.7	438	88.0	2.2	3.0	0.39
WHO Regional Office for the Eastern Mediterranean
Lebanon	62	78.9	6.9	17	84.1	4.4	15	84.1	4.4	7	75.7	10.2	23	75.7	10.2	0.8	0.37
WHO Regional Office for Europe
Belgium	165	84.3	3.9	42	84.4	9.5	27	84.3	10.4	12	—[e]	—[e]	84	83.1	5.1	3.1	0.38
France	235	86.0	3.9	49	87.5	4.7	65	97.3	1.6	35	89.7	4.4	86	80.0	6.9	7.8	0.05
Germany	152	70.2	5.1	28	89.2	8.5	37	97.1	0.7	23	—[e]	—[e]	64	61.1	7.4	66.4*	< 0.001
Israel	364	86.1	1.8	73	90.7	3.2	48	89.2	4.2	17	—[e]	—[e]	226	83.6	2.4	3.3	0.34
Italy	129	94.5	1.5	28	—[e]	—[e]	34	93.1	3.7	19	—[e]	—[e]	48	94.4	2.4	1.3	0.73
Netherlands	183	85.9	4.3	53	96.4	2.1	35	98.9	1.2	15	—[e]	—[e]	80	78.5	7.2	10.0*	0.007
Spain	341	88.8	2.6	73	95.3	1.9	86	92.6	3.0	33	90.8	6.2	149	84.7	4.7	5.8	0.12
Ukraine	167	79.1	3.8	44	92.3	3.6	51	82.3	4.5	14	—[e]	—[e]	58	71.8	7.0	12.5*	0.006

TABLE 11–10. Percentages receiving follow-up treatment[a] among respondents using services in the WMH surveys (continued)

Country	Any Severity			Severe			Moderate			Mild			None			Test of Difference in Probability of Follow-up Treatment by Severity	
	n	%[b]	SE	n	%[c]	SE	n	%[c]	SE	n	%[c]	SE	n	%[c]	SE	χ^2_{2d}	P
WHO Regional Office for the Western Pacific																	
People's Republic of China	56	77.6	6.0	4	—[e]	—[e]	6	—[e]	—[e]	3	80.8	6.8	43	80.8	6.8	1.0	0.33
Japan	83	89.8	2.6	9	—[e]	—[e]	13	—[e]	—[e]	9	91.2	3.3	52	91.2	3.3	0.9	0.33
New Zealand	1,394	85.7	1.3	421	92.5	1.4	368	88.7	1.8	151	83.5	3.2	454	81.0	2.8	15.1*	0.002
χ^2_{16}[f]	67.1* (<0.001)			25.4 (0.06)			71.5* (<0.001)			21.3 (0.13)			47.9* (<0.001)				

Note. WHO=World Health Organization; WMH=World Mental Health.

*Significant at the 0.05 level, two-sided test.

[a]Follow-up treatment was defined as receiving two or more visits to any service sector or being in ongoing treatment at interview.

[b]Percentages are based on entire Part 2 samples.

[c]Percentages are those receiving follow-up treatment, among those in treatment, within each level of severity.

[d]One degree of freedom chi-square tests were performed for Nigeria, Lebanon, Japan, and People's Republic of China, where combined severe and moderate was compared against combined mild and none category. Three-degree-of-freedom tests were performed for all other countries.

[e]Percentages not reported if the number of cases with any treatment in a level of severity <30.

[f]χ^2_{16} is from a model predicting follow-up treatment among respondents, in each level of severity, that used any 12-month services.

TABLE 11–11. Percentages receiving minimally adequate treatment[a] among respondents using services in the WMH surveys

COUNTRY	ANY SEVERITY			SEVERE			MODERATE			MILD			NONE			TEST OF DIFFERENCE IN PROBABILITY OF MINIMALLY ADEQUATE TREATMENT, BY SEVERITY	
	n	%[b]	SE	n	%[c]	SE	n	%[c]	SE	n	%[c]	SE	n	%[c]	SE	χ²[d]	P
WHO Regional Office for the Americas																	
Colombia	33	14.7	3.4	11	23.1	8.5	7	21.7	10.5	3	6.3	4.6	12	10.1	3.5	4.7	0.20
Mexico	42	15.2	2.7	8	11.3	4.5	13	28.6	6.3	6	19.8	5.8	15	11.3	4.0	10.5*	0.014
United States	302	18.1	1.1	160	41.8	3.2	101	24.8	2.1	41	4.9	0.8	—	—	—	114.0*	<0.001
WHO Regional Office for Africa																	
Nigeria	1	10.4	9.8	0	—[e]	—[e]	0	—[e]	—[e]	0	12.4	11.8	1	12.4	11.8		
South Africa	0	—[f]	—[f]	0	—[f]	—[f]	0	—[f]	—[f]	0	—[f]	—[f]	0	—[f]	—[f]		
WHO Regional Office for the Eastern Mediterranean																	
Lebanon	18	24.5	7.1	5	24.0	6.2	3	24.0	6.2	3	24.8	10.7	7	24.8	10.7	0.0	0.95
WHO Regional Office for Europe																	
Belgium	78	33.6	5.2	23	42.5	8.5	12	35.5	12.6	5	—[e]	—[e]	38	29.4	6.2	1.7	0.63
France	113	42.3	5.4	29	57.9	8.5	28	36.5	6.6	15	41.5	9.7	41	40.2	8.3	3.4	0.34
Germany	91	42.0	6.1	21	67.3	10.7	21	53.3	8.4	14	—[e]	—[e]	35	35.4	8.8	6.1	0.11
Israel	148	35.1	2.5	28	34.4	5.4	21	40.3	6.8	6	—[e]	—[e]	93	34.3	3.1	0.7	0.87
Italy	45	33.0	5.1	12	—[e]	—[e]	11	35.7	9.4	6	—[e]	—[e]	16	29.9	7.4	3.5	0.32
Netherlands	98	34.4	5.0	37	65.7	9.2	19	34.1	10.2	10	—[e]	—[e]	32	21.9	5.2	23.2*	<0.001
Spain	152	37.3	3.3	41	47.5	7.5	37	43.6	5.6	20	44.8	9.9	54	30.1	4.4	8.5*	0.037
Ukraine	0	—[f]	—[f]	0	—[f]	—[f]	0	—[f]	—[f]	0	—[f]	—[f]	0	—[f]	—[f]		

TABLE 11–11. Percentages receiving minimally adequate treatment[a] among respondents using services in the WMH surveys *(continued)*

COUNTRY	ANY SEVERITY			SEVERE			MODERATE			MILD			NONE			TEST OF DIFFERENCE IN PROBABILITY OF MINIMALLY ADEQUATE TREATMENT, BY SEVERITY	
	n	%[b]	SE	n	%[c]	SE	n	%[c]	SE	n	%[c]	SE	n	%[c]	SE	χ^2_{2d}	P
WHO Regional Office for the Western Pacific																	
People's Republic of China	19	24.1	7.0	0	—[e]	—[e]	3	—[e]	—[e]	2	20.1	5.9	14	20.1	5.9	0.8	0.36
Japan	35	31.8	6.8	6	—[e]	—[e]	6	—[e]	—[e]	5	27.9	7.0	18	27.9	7.0	4.4*	0.037
New Zealand	0	—[f]	—[f]	0	—[f]	—[f]	0	—[f]	—[f]	0	—[f]	—[f]	0	—[f]	—[f]	—[f]	—[f]
χ^2_{13}[g]	117.0* (<0.001)			41.0* (<0.001)			31.2* (0.002)			25.9* (0.011)			96.7* (<0.001)				

Note. WHO=World Health Organization; WMH=World Mental Health. *Significant at the 0.05 level, two-sided test.
[a]Minimally adequate treatment was defined as receiving eight or more visits to any service sector, or four or more visits and at least one month of medication, or being in ongoing treatment at interview. [b]Percentages based on entire Part 2 samples. [c]Percentages are those receiving minimally adequate treatment among those in treatment, within each level of severity. [d]The test was not performed for Nigeria because there was only one (unweighted) case with adequate treatment. One degree of freedom chi-square tests were performed for Lebanon, Japan, and People's Republic of China, where combined severe and moderate was compared against combined mild and none category. Two-degree of freedom test was performed for the United States, where the mild and none categories were collapsed. Three-degree-of-freedom tests were performed for all other countries. [e]Percentages not reported if the number of cases with any treatment in a level of severity <30. [f]The questions on pharmacoepidemiology were not asked in Ukraine, South Africa, or New Zealand. [g]χ^2_{13} is from a model predicting minimally adequate treatment, among respondents in each level of severity that used any 12-month services.

treatment, fewer than half—that is, fewer than one-quarter overall—receive even minimally *effective* treatment. Little is known about the safety and efficacy of non–health care services from complementary and alternative medicine and human services sectors that is received by some patients (Niggemann and Gruber 2003). Approximately one-quarter of respondents starting treatments did not receive any follow-up care, and only a minority of treatments met minimal standards for adequacy (Agency for Health Care Policy and Research 1993; American Psychiatric Association 2006; Lehman and Steinwachs 1998; Wang et al. 2005).

In the face of these findings of widespread unmet needs for mental health treatment, it may be of additional concern that many respondents *not* meeting criteria for 12-month disorders *did* receive treatment. However, a recent analysis of WMH data from the United States found that many of these apparent noncases may actually have been using services appropriately; for example, for secondary prevention of lifetime disorders or for subthreshold syndromes associated with substantial role impairment (Druss et al. 2007).

The generally low level of investment by most countries in treating mental disorders, both in absolute terms and given their relative societal burdens, makes the prevailing high levels of unmet need worldwide not surprising (Lopez et al. 2006; Saxena et al. 2003). For example, developing countries often expend less than 1% of their already limited health care budgets on mental health services (Saxena et al. 2003). However, in addition to suggesting that more treatment resources are needed, the WMH surveys also identify some ways that countries could optimize their investments, no matter their size.

Notwithstanding their potential limitations, the WMH findings may be of benefit to nations seeking ways to make the most efficient use of their constrained health care resources (Saxena et al. 2003; World Health Organization 2001). For example, the lifetime data from the WMH survey on typical treatment-seeking processes after the first onset of mental disorders suggest the potential value of focusing on early intervention, before many negative sequelae from mental illnesses occur, such as persistence or severity of primary disorders and, possibly, occurrence of secondary disorders (Kohn et al. 2004). Interventions to reduce long periods of untreated mental illness could comprise public awareness, screening, aggressive outreach, and prompt initiation of, or referral for, treatment and could be applied in schools, at clinics, or in health care systems (Aseltine and DeMartino 2004; Beidel et al. 2000; Carleton et al. 1996; Connors 1994; Jacobs 1995; Morrissey-Kane and Prinz 1999; Multimodal Treatment Study of Children With ADHD Cooperative Group 1999; Regier et al. 1988; Velicer et al. 1995; Weaver 1995).

Similarly, the finding that so many serious cases are untreated suggests the need for programs targeting the most vulnerable patients. Optimizing a country's limited resources may also require employing the general medical sector as an access point, with the specialty sector serving to care for the most serious cases (Rosenheck et al. 1998). Clearly, no matter how resources are allocated, the WMH findings indicate that substantial improvement is needed in the continuity and quality of care being received. Interventions—for use at the local level—to improve treatment initiation, reduce dropout, and enhance adequacy have been developed and, in many cases, have proven to be effective and cost-effective (Wang et al. 2007). Policies, delivery system redesigns, and means of financing also are critical to ensure uptake of such interventions.

What does the future hold for the WMH Survey Initiative? One likely next step would be to expand to include both new participating countries and new scientific agendas. For example, national surveys have been added in Iraq and India, as well as a regional survey in Brazil. Other countries, such as China, are conducting surveys in other regions using enhanced methods based on the experience of their initial surveys. Analyses being conducted by WMH work groups have moved beyond basic description to shedding light on new areas, including the following:

- Studies of sociodemographic groups at increased risk for mental disorders, using a cross-national framework
- Identification of other substantive risk factors for mental disorders, such as childhood adversities and traumatic events
- Exploration of reasons for failing to receive treatment and prematurely dropping out
- Comprehensive accounting of societal burdens from mental illness, including educational attainment, marital outcomes, role functioning, and work productivity
- Documentation of the global experience of suicidality, including ideation, plans, gestures, and attempts
- Identification of patterns of comorbidity between mental disorders and general medical conditions
- Documentation of health preferences and utilities associated with mental and general medical conditions throughout the world
- Evaluation of key nosological issues that will inform the DSM-5 and ICD-11 revision process

These analyses have been described by investigators involved (Borges et al. 2006; Demyttenaere et al. 2007; Gureje et al 2008; Gyrd-Hansen 2005; Lee et al. 2009; Nock and Kessler 2006; Nock et al. 2008; Ormel et al. 2007; Scott et al. 2007, 2008; Torrance 2006). A more detailed description of this ongoing work can be found on the WMH Web site at www.hcp.med.harvard.edu. These findings, together with the basic descriptive epidemiology of mental disorders, will help inform the ongoing update of the Global Burden of Disease initiative (Murray et al. 2007).

Finally, future WMH efforts will focus on informing the design and targeting of interventions within countries. Through methodological developments in quasi-experimental methods and analytic techniques, it may be increasingly possible to make provisional causal inferences based on descriptive WMH epidemiological data (Brookhart et al. 2007; Lu 1999; Schneeweiss et al. 2007). To achieve this objective, individual-level WMH survey data could be linked with those of the WHO Project Atlas, as well as the WHO Assessment Instrument for Mental Health Systems, on existing policies, delivery systems, and financing of mental health care (Mezzich 2003; Saxena et al. 2003). Such linked data sets could become important tools for studying impacts of health care policies, delivery system designs, and levels or mechanisms of financing mental health services on use and quality of treatments. Through this approach, the WMH Survey Initiative could provide policymakers and other stakeholders worldwide with information to guide future decision making and ultimately improve the care outcomes of people with mental disorders.

Acknowledgments

These surveys are carried out in conjunction with the World Health Organization (WHO) World Mental Health (WMH) Survey Initiative. We thank the WMH staff for assistance with instrumentation, fieldwork, and data analysis. These activities were supported by the U.S. National Institute of Mental Health (NIMH; R01MH070884); the John D. and Catherine T. MacArthur Foundation; the Pfizer Foundation; the U.S. Public Health Service (R13-MH066849, R01-MH069864, R01 DA016558); the Fogarty International Center (FIRCA R03-TW006481); the Pan American Health Organization; the Eli Lilly and Company Foundation; Ortho-McNeil Pharmaceutical, Inc.; GlaxoSmithKline; Bristol-Myers Squibb; and Shire. A complete list of WMH publications can be found at http://www.hcp.med.harvard.edu/wmh/. The Chinese WMH Survey Initiative is supported by the Pfizer Foundation. The Colombian National Study of Mental Health is supported by the Ministry of Social Protection. The ESEMeD project is funded by the European Commission (Contracts QLG5-1999-01042; SANCO 2004123), the Piedmont Region (Italy); Fondo de Investigación Sanitaria, Instituto de Salud Carlos III, Spain (FIS 00/0028); Ministerio de Ciencia y Tecnología, Spain (SAF 2000–158-CE); Departament de Salut, Generalitat de Catalunya, Spain; Instituto de Salud Carlos III (CIBER CB06/02/0046, RETICS RD06/0011 REM-TAP); and other local agencies as well as by an unrestricted educational grant from GlaxoSmithKline. The Israel National Health Survey is funded by the Ministry of Health, with support from the Israel National Institute for Health Policy and Health Services Research and the National Insurance Institute of Israel. The WMH Japan Survey is supported by the Grant for Research on Psychiatric and Neurological Diseases and Mental Health (H13-SHOGAI-023, H14-TOKUBETSU-026, H16-KOKORO-013) from the Japan Ministry of Health, Labour, and Welfare. The Lebanese National Mental Health Survey is supported by the Lebanese Ministry of Public Health; the WHO (Lebanon); Fogarty International; Act for Lebanon; anonymous private donations to IDRAAC, Lebanon; and unrestricted grants from Janssen Cilag, Eli Lilly, GlaxoSmithKline, Roche, and Novartis. The Mexican National Comorbidity Survey is supported by The National Institute of Psychiatry Ramon de la Fuente (INPRFM-DIES 4280) and by the National Council on Science and Technology (CONACyT-G30544-H), with supplemental support from the Pan American Health Organization. Te Rau Hinengaro: The New Zealand Mental Health Survey is supported by the New Zealand Ministry of Health, Alcohol Advisory Council, and the Health Research Council. The Nigerian Survey of Mental Health and Wellbeing is supported by the WHO (Geneva), the WHO (Nigeria), and the Federal Ministry of Health, Abuja, Nigeria. The South Africa Stress and Health Study is supported by the U.S. NIMH (R01-MH059575) and National Institute on Drug Abuse (NIDA), with supplemental funding from the South African Department of Health and the University of Michigan. The Ukraine Comorbid Mental Disorders during Periods of Social Disruption study is funded by the U.S. NIMH (RO1-MH61905). The U.S. National Comorbidity Survey Replication (NCS-R) is supported by the NIMH (U01-MH60220), with supplemental support from the NIDA, the Substance Abuse and Mental Health Services Administration, the Robert Wood Johnson Foundation (Grant 044708), and the John W. Alden Trust.

References

Agency for Health Care Policy and Research: Depression Guideline Panel: Treatment of Major Depression, Vol 2, No 5 (AHCPR 93–0551). Rockville, MD, U.S. Department of Health and Human Services, Agency for Health Care Policy and Research, 1993

Alegria M, Bijl RV, Lin E, et al: Income differences in persons seeking outpatient treatment for mental disorders: a comparison of the United States with Ontario and the Netherlands. Arch Gen Psychiatry 57:383–391, 2000

Allgulander C: Psychoactive drug use in a general population sample, Sweden: correlates with perceived health, psychiatric diagnoses, and mortality in an automated record-linkage study. Am J Public Health 79:1006–1010, 1989

American Psychiatric Association: Diagnostic and Statistical Manual of Mental Disorders, 4th Edition, Text Revision. Washington, DC, American Psychiatric Association, 2000

American Psychiatric Association: American Psychiatric Association Practice Guidelines for the Treatment of Psychiatric Disorders: Compendium 2006. Washington, DC, American Psychiatric Association, 2006

Andrade L, de Lolio C, Gentil V, et al: Lifetime prevalence of mental disorders in a catchment area in Sao Paulo, Brazil. Paper presented at the VII Congress of the International Federation of Psychiatric Epidemiology, Santiago, Chile, August 1996

Andrade L, Walters EE, Gentil V, et al: Prevalence of ICD-10 mental disorders in a catchment area in the city of Sao Paulo, Brazil. Soc Psychiatry Psychiatr Epidemiol 37:316–325, 2002

Aseltine RH Jr, DeMartino R: An outcome evaluation of the SOS Suicide Prevention Program. Am J Public Health 94:446–451, 2004

Beidel DC, Turner SM, Morris TL: Behavioral treatment of childhood social phobia. J Consult Clin Psychol 68:1072–1080, 2000

Bijl RV, van Zessen G, Ravelli A, et al: the Netherlands Mental Health Survey and Incidence Study (NEMESIS): objectives and design. Soc Psychiatry Psychiatr Epidemiol 33:581–586, 1998

Bijl RV, de Graaf R, Hiripi E, et al: The prevalence of treated and untreated mental disorders in five countries. Health Aff (Millwood) 22:122–133, 2003

Bland RC, Orn H, Newman SC: Lifetime prevalence of psychiatric disorders in Edmonton. Acta Psychiatr Scand Suppl 338:24–32, 1988

Borges G, Angst J, Nock MK, et al: A risk index for 12-month suicide attempts in the National Comorbidity Survey Replication (NCS-R). Psychol Med 36:1747–1757, 2006

Brookhart MA, Rassen JA, Wang PS, et al: Evaluating the validity of an instrumental variable study of neuroleptics: can between-physician differences in prescribing patterns be used to estimate treatment effects? Med Care 45:S116–122, 2007

Caraveo J, Martinez J, Rivera B: A model for epidemiological studies on mental health and psychiatric morbidity. Salud Mental 21:48–57, 1998

Carleton RA, Bazzarre T, Drake J, et al: Report of the Expert Panel on Awareness and Behavior Change to the Board of Directors, American Heart Association. Circulation 93:1768–1772, 1996

Chang SM, Hahm BJ, Lee JY, et al: Cross-national difference in the prevalence of depression caused by the diagnostic threshold. J Affect Disord 106:159–167, 2008

Choy Y, Schneier FR, Heimberg RG, et al: Features of the offensive subtype of Taijin-Kyofu-Sho in US and Korean patients with DSM-IV social anxiety disorder. Depress Anxiety 25:230–240, 2008

Connors CK: The Connors Rating Scales: use in clinical assessment, treatment planning and research, in Use of Psychological Testing for Treatment Planning and Outcome Assessment. Edited by Maruish M. Hillsdale, NJ, Lawrence Erlbaum, 1994, pp 570–578

Cooke DJ, Hart SD, Michie C: Cross-national differences in the assessment of psychopathy: do they reflect variations in raters' perceptions of symptoms? Psychol Assess 16:335–339, 2004

Demyttenaere K, Bruffaerts R, Lee S, et al: Mental disorders among persons with chronic back or neck pain: results from the World Mental Health Surveys. Pain 129:332–342, 2007

Druss BG, Wang PS, Sampson NA, et al: Understanding mental health treatment in persons without mental diagnoses: results from the National Comorbidity Survey Replication. Arch Gen Psychiatry 64:1196–1203, 2007

Eaton WW, Anthony JC, Tepper S, et al: Psychopathology and attrition in the epidemiologic catchment area surveys. Am J Epidemiol 135:1051–1059, 1992

Gureje O, Lasebikan VO, Kola L, et al: Lifetime and 12-month prevalence of mental disorders in the Nigerian Survey of Mental Health and Well-Being. Br J Psychiatry 188:465–471, 2006

Gureje O, Von Korff M, Kola L, et al: The relation between multiple pains and mental disorders: results from the World Mental Health Surveys. Pain 135:82–91, 2008

Gyrd-Hansen D: Willingness to pay for a QALY: theoretical and methodological issues. Pharmacoeconomics 23:423–432, 2005

Hagnell O: A prospective study of the incidence of mental disorder: a study based on 24,000 person years of the incidence of mental disorders in a Swedish population together with an evaluation of the aetiological significance of medical, social, and personality factors. The Lundby Project Lund. Stockholm, Svenska Bokforlaget, 1966

Haro JM, Arbabzadeh-Bouchez S, Brugha TS, et al: Concordance of the Composite International Diagnostic Interview Version 3.0 (CIDI 3.0) with standardized clinical assessments in the WHO World Mental Health Surveys, in The WHO World Mental Health Surveys: Global Perspectives on the Epidemiology of Mental Disorders. Edited by Kessler RC, Üstün TB. New York, Cambridge University Press, 2008, pp 114–130

Hasin DS, Grant BF: The co-occurrence of DSM-IV alcohol abuse in DSM-IV alcohol dependence: results of the National Epidemiologic Survey on Alcohol and Related Conditions on heterogeneity that differ by population subgroup. Arch Gen Psychiatry 61:891–896, 2004

Hwu HG, Yeh EK, Chang LY: Prevalence of psychiatric disorders in Taiwan defined by the Chinese Diagnostic Interview Schedule. Acta Psychiatr Scand 79:136–147, 1989

Jacobs DG: National depression screening day: educating the public, reaching those in need of treatment, and broadening professional understanding. Harv Rev Psychiatry 3:156–159, 1995

Jenkins R, Bebbington P, Brugha T, et al: The National Psychiatric Morbidity surveys of Great Britain: strategy and methods. Psychol Med 27:765–774, 1997

Kessler RC, Frank RG: The impact of psychiatric disorders on work loss days. Psychol Med 27:861–873, 1997

Kessler RC, Merikangas KR: The National Comorbidity Survey Replication (NCS-R): background and aims. Int J Methods Psychiatr Res 13:60–68, 2004

Kessler RC, McGonagle KA, Zhao S, et al: Lifetime and 12-month prevalence of DSM-III-R psychiatric disorders in the United States: results from the National Comorbidity Survey. Arch Gen Psychiatry 51:8–19, 1994

Kessler RC, Aguilar-Gaxiola S, Alonso J, et al: Prevalence and severity of mental disorders in the WMH Surveys, in The WHO World Mental Health Surveys: Global Perspectives on the Epidemiology of Mental Disorders. Edited by Kessler RC, Üstün TB. New York, Cambridge University Press, 2008, pp 534–540

Kohn R, Saxena S, Levav I, et al: The treatment gap in mental health care. Bull World Health Organ 82:858–866, 2004

Kýlýç C: Mental Health Profile of Turkey: Main Report. Ankara, Turkey, Ministry of Health Publications, 1998

Langner TS, Michael ST: Life Stress and Mental Health: The Midtown Manhattan Study. New York, Free Press of Glencoe, 1963

Lee S, Tsang A, Ruscio AM, et al: Implications of modifying the duration requirement of generalized anxiety disorder in developed and developing countries. Psychol Med 39:1163–1170, 2009

Lehman AF, Steinwachs DM: Translating research into practice: the Schizophrenia Patient Outcomes Research Team (PORT) treatment recommendations. Schizophr Bull 24:1–10, 1998

Leighton AH: My Name Is Legion: Stirling County Study, Vol 1. New York, Basic Books, 1959

Leon AC, Olfson M, Portera L, et al: Assessing psychiatric impairment in primary care with the Sheehan Disability Scale. Int J Psychiatry Med 27:93–105, 1997

Lépine JP, Lellouch J, Lovell A, et al: Anxiety and depressive disorders in a French population: methodology and preliminary results. Psychiatr Psychobiol 4:267–274, 1989

Lopez AD, Mathers CD, Ezzati M, et al (eds): Global Burden of Disease and Risk Factors. New York, Oxford University Press/World Bank, 2006

Lu M: The productivity of mental health care: an instrumental variable approach. J Ment Health Policy Econ 2:59–71, 1999

Mezzich JE: From financial analysis to policy development in mental health care: the need for broader conceptual models and partnerships. J Ment Health Policy Econ 6:149–150, 2003

Morrissey-Kane E, Prinz RJ: Engagement in child and adolescent treatment: the role of parental cognitions and attributions. Clin Child Fam Psychol Rev 2:183–198, 1999

Multimodal Treatment Study of Children With ADHD Cooperative Group: A 14-month randomized clinical trial of treatment strategies for attention-deficit/hyperactivity disorder: Multimodal Treatment Study of Children with ADHD. Arch Gen Psychiatry 56:1073–1086, 1999

Murray CJ, Lopez AD, Black R, et al: Global burden of disease 2005: call for collaborators. Lancet 370:109–110, 2007

Narrow WE, Rae DS, Robins LN, et al: Revised prevalence estimates of mental disorders in the United States: using a clinical significance criterion to reconcile 2 surveys' estimates. Arch Gen Psychiatry 59:115–123, 2002

Niggemann B, Gruber C: Side-effects of complementary and alternative medicine. Allergy 58:707–716, 2003

Nock MK, Kessler RC: Prevalence of and risk factors for suicide attempts versus suicide gestures: analysis of the National Comorbidity Survey. J Abnorm Psychol 115:616–623, 2006

Nock MK, Borges G, Bromet EJ, et al: Cross-national prevalence and risk factors for suicidal ideation, plans, and attempts. Br J Psychiatry 192:98–105, 2008

Ormel J, Von Korff M, Ustun TB, et al: Common mental disorders and disability across cultures: results from the WHO Collaborative Study on Psychological Problems in General Health Care. JAMA 272:1741–1748, 1994

Ormel J, Von Korff M, Burger H, et al: Mental disorders among persons with heart disease: results from World Mental Health surveys. Gen Hosp Psychiatry 29:325–334, 2007

Regier DA, Hirschfeld RM, Goodwin FK, et al: The NIMH Depression Awareness, Recognition, and Treatment program: structure, aims, and scientific basis. Am J Psychiatry 145:1351–1357, 1988

Regier DA, Kaelber CT, Rae DS, et al: Limitations of diagnostic criteria and assessment instruments for mental disorders: implications for research and policy. Arch Gen Psychiatry 55:109–115, 1998

Regier DA, Narrow WE, Rupp A, et al: The epidemiology of mental disorder treatment need: community estimates of medical necessity, in Unmet Need in Psychiatry: Problems, Resources, Responses. Edited by Andrews G, Henderson S. Cambridge, UK, Cambridge University Press, 2000, pp 41–58

Robins LN, Regier DA (eds): Psychiatric Disorders in America: The Epidemiologic Catchment Area Study. New York, Free Press, 1991

Rosenheck R, Armstrong M, Callahan D, et al: Obligation to the least well off in setting mental health service priorities: a consensus statement. Psychiatr Serv 49:1273–1274, 1290, 1998

Saxena S, Sharan P, Saraceno B: Budget and financing of mental health services: baseline information on 89 countries from WHO's project atlas. J Ment Health Policy Econ 6:135–143, 2003

Schneeweiss S, Setoguchi S, Brookhart A, et al: Risk of death associated with the use of conventional versus atypical antipsychotic drugs among elderly patients. CMAJ 176:627–632, 2007

Scott KM, Von Korff M, Ormel J, et al: Mental disorders among adults with asthma: results from the World Mental Health Survey. Gen Hosp Psychiatry 29:123–133, 2007

Scott KM, Bruffaerts R, Simon GE, et al: Obesity and mental disorders in the general population: results from the world mental health surveys. Int J Obes (London) 32:192–200, 2008

Shen YC, Zhang MY, Huang YQ, et al: Twelve-month prevalence, severity, and unmet need for treatment of mental disorders in metropolitan China. Psychol Med 36:257–267, 2006

Shiffman S, Stone AA, Hufford MR: Ecological momentary assessment. Annu Rev Clin Psychol 4:1–32, 2008

Simon GE, Goldberg DP, Von Korff M, et al: Understanding cross-national differences in depression prevalence. Psychol Med 32:585–594, 2002

Stone AA, Broderick JE: Real-time data collection for pain: appraisal and current status. Pain Med 8(suppl):S85–S93, 2007

Torrance GW: Utility measurement in healthcare: the things I never got to. Pharmacoeconomics 24:1069–1078, 2006

Tseng WS: From peculiar psychiatric disorders through culture-bound syndromes to culture-related specific syndromes. Transcult Psychiatry 43:554–576, 2006

Vega WA, Kolody B, Aguilar-Gaxiola S, et al: Lifetime prevalence of DSM-III-R psychiatric disorders among urban and rural Mexican Americans in California. Arch Gen Psychiatry 55:771–778, 1998

Velicer WF, Hughes S., Fava JL, et al: An empirical typology of subjects within stage of change. Addict Behav 20:299–320, 1995

Wang PS, Lane M, Olfson M, et al: Twelve-month use of mental health services in the United States: results from the National Comorbidity Survey Replication. Arch Gen Psychiatry 62:629–640, 2005

Wang PS, Aguilar-Gaxiola S, Alonso J, et al: Use of mental health services for anxiety, mood, and substance disorders in 17 countries in the WHO world mental health surveys. Lancet 370:841–850, 2007

Weaver AJ: Has there been a failure to prepare and support parish-based clergy in their role as frontline community mental health workers: a review. J Pastoral Care 49:129–147, 1995

Weissman MM, Bland RC, Canino GJ, et al: The cross national epidemiology of obsessive compulsive disorder. The Cross National Collaborative Group. J Clin Psychiatry 55(suppl):5–10, 1994

Weissman MM, Bland RC, Canino GJ, et al: Cross-national epidemiology of major depression and bipolar disorder. JAMA 276:293–299, 1996a

Weissman MM, Bland RC, Canino GJ, et al: The cross-national epidemiology of social phobia: a preliminary report. Int Clin Psychopharmacol 11(suppl):9–14, 1996b

Weissman MM, Bland RC, Canino GJ, et al: The cross-national epidemiology of panic disorder. Arch Gen Psychiatry 54:305–309, 1997

Wells JE, Bushnell JA, Hornblow AR, et al: Christchurch Psychiatric Epidemiology Study, part I: methodology and lifetime prevalence for specific psychiatric disorders. Aust N Z J Psychiatry 23:315–326, 1989

Wittchen HU: Early developmental stages of psychopathology study (EDSP): objectives and design. Eur Addict Res 4:18–27, 1998

World Health Organization: The WHO Disability Assessment Schedule II (WHO-DAS II). Geneva, Switzerland, World Health Organization, 1998

World Health Organization: The World Health Report 2001. Mental Health: New Understanding, New Hope, 2001. Geneva, Switzerland, Available at: http://www.who.int/whr2001. Accessed August 15, 2009.

World Health Organization International Consortium of Psychiatric Epidemiology: Cross-national comparisons of the prevalences and correlates of mental disorders. WHO International Consortium in Psychiatric Epidemiology. Bull World Health Organ 78:413–426, 2000

CHAPTER 12

The Intersection of Race, Ethnicity, Immigration, and Cultural Influences on the Nature and Distribution of Mental Disorders

An Examination of Major Depression

James S. Jackson, Ph.D.
Jamie M. Abelson, M.S.W.
Patricia A. Berglund, M.B.A.
Briana Mezuk, Ph.D.
Myriam Torres, M.S.
Rong Zhang, Ph.D.

Across the world, changing demographic, economic, and political conditions are altering the age structure and increasing the racial and ethnic composition of many societies. For example, in the United States, it is projected that within 25 years, about 40% of adults and 48% of children will be from racial and ethnic minority groups (Angel and Hogan 2004). However, the ability to identify, prevent, and treat mental illness effectively in different racial/ethnic and cultural groups has failed to keep pace with this growth and change. Little is known about either the perceptions of mental illness among many of these cultural groups or how to effectively engage them in the treatment process (Alarcón et al. 2002). Most research to date has been limited in ability to examine national differences—particularly between Western and non-Western diagnostic approaches—in perceptions of mental illness or in approaches to treatment. Existing data are often cross-sectional in nature, hampering the capability to examine change across time. Until recently, only a few studies have examined the influence of ethnicity, race, and culture on mental health within specific societies (e.g., Karlsen and Nazroo 2002; Noh and Kaspar 2003).

Although priorities of governments—such as those outlined in Healthy People 2010 (www.healthypeople.gov)—target improved quality of life for people of all ages, with a special emphasis on the elimination of existing health disparities, much work needs to be done to reach these important goals. Increased ethnic and racial diversity has been accompanied by new challenges to existing models of mental health, mental illness, and provision of effective mental health services. Western societies are becoming more complex with the growth of immigrant populations who bring cultural beliefs and practices that often differ in critical ways from their host cultures. Culture influences the meanings people impart to their health and illness as well as their willingness and capacity to productively interact with mental health professionals. Simultaneously, the immigrant experience of settling in a new country presents challenges and stressors that make immigrants vulnerable to mental health crises, particularly during the period of initial arrival and adjustment to their new environments (Vega and Rumbaut 1991).

In the United States and other developed countries, where health care and mental health care are embedded in Western medical systems, mental illness retains a stigma that makes people reluctant to seek treatment. This problem is often compounded in non-Western nations, where these conditions can be interpreted as punishment for past behavior. This is unfortunate, because mental disorders—such as schizophrenia, bipolar disorder, panic disorder, and major depression—are found worldwide, creating significant health problems across several continents (e.g., Demyttenaere et al. 2004). We believe that researchers and health care professionals all share a common goal to identify and eliminate the unnecessary suffering caused by mental illness in all societies; however, as yet, we lack a full understanding of cultural differences in the interpretation of mental illness and of how those cultural differences affect prevention and treatment of the illness in different societies. Significant creativity and innovation will be required to eliminate disparities in mental health both cross-nationally and in the United States. Epidemiological research focusing on population-group differences in psychopathology and within-group differences among racial/ethnic minorities will be particularly important, given the precarious economic and social situations of many minority Americans. Despite impressive advances in knowledge concerning the national distributions of psychopathology and the prevalences of help-seeking behavior and mental health service use, our knowledge of serious mental disorders and mental health among, and within, minority subgroup populations remains meager.

Cross-Cultural Measurement of Mental Illness

We believe that both intranational and cross-national approaches are essential to fully understand the predictors, influences, and consequences of mental health and illness across ethnic and cultural groups (Jackson et al. 2004). Intranational research allows for examination of ethnic differences in the prevalence of, and attitudes toward, mental illness, within a specific nation. The cross-national approach allows us to see how ethnic and cultural groups express similar problems across different political and economic bodies. By explicitly considering both intranational and cross-national research as a unified goal, we can better understand the dynamics of ethnic variation on mental health differentials within nations and extend this enhanced understanding to our analysis of comparative cross-national research. For example, are the mental health problems of Caribbeans the same among those living in the Caribbean as among those who have immigrated to the United States? By developing research designs that explicitly address ethnic and cultural differentials, our ability to perform sophisticated comparative research and develop effective and appropriate treatments will be greatly enhanced.

The majority of mental health research has been conducted in Western nations (Kessler and Üstün 2008). To date, very little research has focused on the cultural dimensions of mental health and the extent to which these cultural factors could adversely affect a person's mental well-being. Mental disorders are usually measured by diagnostic criteria provided in DSM-IV (American Psychiatric Association 1994) or, in some regions of the world, ICD-10 (World Health Organization 1992), and a formal diagnosis is made by a clinician. Unfortunately, few studies have been developed to validate these measures within non-Western (and non-English-speaking) nations, especially among minority racial and ethnic populations within these nations. Without uniformly validated diagnostic tools, comparative research is impossible. We believe previous research has seriously underestimated the extent to which culture influences physical and psychological health. This is particularly the case for cross-national comparisons of mental health and mental disorders. A key factor is the lack of standardized measures and scales that allow for a comparative-research framework. What is still needed, in part, is the equivalent of a thermometer—that is, an instrument that reliably measures the same construct across groups, just as a thermometer reliably measures body temperature regardless of group differences (W. Eaton, personal communication, November 2007). More fundamentally, however, there is a lack of uniform agreement across nations, and across cultures, as to what constitutes mental illness. For example, it is not clear at what point symptoms significantly impair a person's functioning at home, school, work, and in the community, thus constituting mental illness. Without a better understanding of the how, what, and where of these differences across cultures, ethnicities, and nations, we will continue to face challenges in defining systematic diagnostic measures.

New diagnostic and culturally sensitive approaches in the measurement of mental disorders and health have emerged in recent years. These techniques will be especially useful in the analysis of diverse populations, but the techniques need to be systematically examined and incorporated into a unified literature. The growing numbers of validation studies for depression scales, within specific countries, are examples of work that is under way but has not yet been fully catalyzed (e.g., Kessler and Üstün 2008). An increase in our attention to immigrant groups, using studies such as the Collaborative Psychiatric Epidemiology Surveys (CPES; http://www.icpsr. umich.edu/CPES/index.html), is also timely because it allows for development of new methodological approaches to measuring ethnic differentials in mental health, using data specially designed to test these kinds of questions (e.g., Alegría et al. 2009; Colpe et al. 2004).

A growing number of professionals have recognized the need for culturally relevant mental health research, and we have seen a growth in both culturally competent care and culturally sensitive approaches to the measurement of mental disorders. To some extent, the problem to be addressed is straightforward: how can we eliminate mental health disparities, given the ever-increasing diversity of the population both within and across nations and the growing movements of peoples across national borders? Changes in racial and ethnic composition of almost all national populations, along with growing economic and political crises worldwide, are resulting in higher numbers of persons who may be at risk of mental health crises. Although our ability to diagnose and medically treat mental health problems continues to improve, our ability to translate these gains cross-nationally, and across different ethnic groups, continues to lag. This disparity is a result of not only inattention to the problem but also technical complexities of validating established Western measures of disease as culturally appropriate measures that retain the same scale and meaning.

Influence of Environmental Living Conditions

In the United States, it is clear that the relative social and economic deprivation of African Americans, and many other minority groups (e.g., Puerto Rican, Vietnamese), compared with whites and other ethnic minorities (e.g., Chinese, Japanese) influences the distribution of psychopathology among ethnic and racial minorities (Williams and Harris-Reid 1999). Race, ethnicity, and sociocultural factors are important both in forming the context of mental health and illness and as sources of influence on normal development and on the nature, expression, and course of mental disorder (Jackson et al. 2004). We propose that these contextual factors have been viewed largely as nuisance variation in most research and thus have been considered unimportant in understanding basic cognitive, social, and pathological processes. We must place greater attention on studying these factors in the course of human psychological development, including development of psychopathology. Our research is predicated on this fairly basic set of assumptions that provides the scholarly and intellectual foundation for the work discussed in this chapter.

Our prior research suggests that disparities between race and ethnic groups in resources and environmental stressors contribute to critical differences in diagnosis, access to treatment, assignment to certain types of treatments, dropping out of treatment (premature termination), and treatment outcome (e.g., Neighbors et al. 1989). More research is needed in the areas of epidemiology, documentation of utilization rates, and impact of culturally specific intervention on increasing use, decreasing premature termination, and outcomes of treatment. There is preliminary evidence that cultural knowledge of African American and other race/ethnic groups helps because it is a necessary, but insufficient, "first step" in conducting good cross-cultural clinical interventions. Yet knowledge of culture alone cannot replace the necessity of developing adequate service delivery systems, good therapeutic skills, and effective follow-ups.

Under- or nonutilization of services is a problem for ethnic minorities, especially when use is viewed in relation to the prevalence of psychiatric morbidity in the general population (U.S. Department of Health and Human Services 2001). What is less clear is whether or not minorities are underrepresented in mental health care services in comparison with nonminorities receiving care, or whether minorities are underrepresented in comparison with their proportions in the population. One explanation for minority underutilization of services is the stigma attached to seeking mental health services and the fact that ethnic minorities are more likely to use alternative informal support systems or indigenous practitioners. The fact that minorities use informal support systems is well documented, but the hypothesis that they are more prone than nonminorities to engage in this form of help seeking is subject to question, given the fact that all groups rely heavily on their social networks for aid during crises. The literature on the underutilization of mental health services by ethnic minorities lacks an epidemiological focus that could improve documentation of the social, economic, and cultural factors that may influence perceptions of need and help seeking for mental health services.

Some recent work addresses discrete mental disorders and pathways into treatment, diagnostic divergence, and treatment efficacy and outcomes among different racial/ethnic groups (e.g., Alegría et al. 2009). We believe there is a need for more research that assesses risk factors, individual and family strengths, individual psychopathology, and service use—all within a context that stresses a focus on multiple (individual, family, community, organizational) levels of research and analysis. One consistent theme in our research over the past 30 years has been a concern with the influences of racial and cultural factors on these processes and their explication and empirical examination (Jackson et al. 2004).

Mental Health Status

Despite recent improvements in education and income, the socioeconomic status of African Americans is still relatively low in comparison with that of whites and several other minority groups (Jackson 2000). Consequentially, poor blacks and other groups live in neighborhoods that have problems, such as high rates of crime, low-quality schools, high unemployment, high levels of teenage pregnancy, inadequate housing, and inferior healthcare, to a much greater degree than do non-Hispanic white poor groups. Based on these social indicators, social scientists and other health scientists long have argued that the stress associated with disadvantaged status and exposure to discrimination increases the vulnerability of African Americans and other ethnic/racial minorities to mental and physical disorders (e.g., Nazroo 2003). Despite the attention given to estimating the relative effects of poor socioeconomic status on morbidity, we still do not fully understand how race/ethnicity and socioeconomic status interact to produce observed patterns of distress (Dohrenwend et al. 1992).

Reliance on global constructs, such as psychological distress, provides only limited information on group differences in psychiatric morbidity. The five-site National Institute of Mental Health Epidemiologic Catchment Area (ECA) Study on prevalence rates of specific psychiatric disorders employed methods that addressed some of the ambiguity inherent in the symptom-checklist approach and concerns of the selection bias of clinical studies (Robins and Regier 1991). With the exceptions of schizophrenia and phobias, the ECA study found roughly comparable rates of mental disorders for blacks and whites (Robins and Regier 1991). For example, age-adjusted analyses by sex and ECA site did not show any consistent excess among African Americans in lifetime or 6-month prevalence of depression (Somervell et al. 1989). Even more striking, results from the 1990 National Comorbidity Survey (NCS) found that rates of disorders for African Americans were consistently *below* those of whites; these unexpected differences were particularly pronounced for depression and substance abuse disorders (Kessler et al. 1994). The only exceptions to this trend were in the rates of phobia—blacks had slightly, but significantly, higher rates of agoraphobia than did whites (Magee et al. 1996). These findings ran counter to what was expected, given the poor living conditions of African Americans in the ECA and NCS samples, relative to whites. In general, however, psychiatric epidemiological studies have shown that the mental health of African Americans is better than would be expected, based on the assumed effects of discrimination and disadvantaged status (Jackson et al. 2004; Williams and Harris-Reid 1999). These data patterns will remain confusing as long as epidemiological studies of American minorities continue to focus solely on the demographic correlates of mental disorder. Clarification will require more comprehensive empirical investigations of prevalence rate differences of mental disorder, in conjunction with data on differences in exposure and responses to stressors, in samples with enough minorities to allow meaningful comparisons.

Stress and Adaptation

In the National Survey of Black Americans, and 20 years later, in the ongoing National Survey of American Life, we have used a stress-and-adaptation approach to understanding the distribution of distress and disorders among African Americans and other minority groups (Jackson et al. 2004). The life-stress paradigm provides a useful framework for considering and understanding the role of stressors in the lives of black persons and other groups discriminated against. Outlined in terms of this framework, the ongoing research 1) examines the nature and distribution of stressors and stress among major minority groups and whites by social, economic, and sociodemographic factors; 2) examines the influences of these stressors on mental disorders, severity of disorders, and psychological distress and impairment; and 3) explores the roles of psychological and social resources (e.g., mastery, self-esteem, informal emotional and instrumental support, religious involvement) in buffering the effects of stress on mental health and help seeking.

It also should be noted that although there are important commonalities in various racial and ethnic experiences, there is also considerable ethnic variation *within* the major minority populations; for example, Caribbeans constitute the largest black subgroup in the United States (Kent 2007). However, prior studies of minority mental health have not addressed the mental health consequences of such across- and within-group race/ethnic variation (e.g., Hispanic and Asian group differences). For example, it has been suggested that challenges—such as job stress, frustrated ambitions, discrimination from whites and other blacks, immigration status, and demands from relatives still residing in the Caribbean—have negative influences on the mental health of Caribbean subgroups (Nazroo 2003). Similar arguments can be made for Asian and Hispanic populations.

Major Depressive Episode and Major Depressive Disorder

In order to illustrate the effects of race, ethnicity, culture, and immigration on diagnosis, we use data from the CPES (2001–2003). This is a comprehensive epidemiological data set of more than 20,000 community-dwelling adults that includes the distributions, correlates, and risk factors for mental disorders among the general U.S. population, with special emphasis on ethnic minority groups. The three studies that comprise the CPES are: 1) the NCS Replication (NCS-R), a nationally representative survey on the prevalence of clinically significant mental disorders; 2) the National Survey of American Life, a nationally representative survey of African American and Caribbean black populations in the United States and non-Hispanic white respondents living in the same communities as African Americans; and 3) the National Latino and Asian American Survey, the first study of its kind to measure psychiatric epidemiology and service utilization among Hispanics and Asian Americans with a nationally representative sampling frame. All three studies used an expanded version of the World Health Organization's World Mental Health Composite International Diagnostic Interview (Kessler and Üstün 2004), a fully structured instrument administered by trained lay interviewers. Disorder diagnoses were based on DSM-IV (American Psychiatric Association 1994) criteria.

Nine racial/ethnic groups were identified in the CPES: Vietnamese, Filipino, Chinese, Cuban, Puerto Rican, Mexican, Caribbean black, African American, and non-Hispanic white. An "other" category was provided for each group, which includes individuals who do not fit into the nine identified groups and are too few in number to form separate ethnic groups. The assessment of major depressive episode (MDE) did not include Criterion B ("the symptoms do not meet criteria for a Mixed Episode") or Criterion E ("the symptoms are not better accounted for by Bereavement"). The algorithm for major depressive disorder (MDD) did not operationalize Criterion B ("the major depressive episode is not better accounted for by schizoaffective disorder") or the Criterion C "mixed episode" exclusion. Furthermore, the National Latino and Asian American Survey did not assess mania; therefore, our analyses of MDD were limited to within- and across-group differences for Caribbean blacks, African Americans, and whites.

Table 12–1 shows prevalence rates of lifetime MDE by racial/ethnic group and by gender and nativity across race/ethnicity groups. Analyses testing the difference between rates (not shown in table) revealed that Puerto Ricans and whites had significantly *higher* rates of lifetime MDE compared with all other groups. Within the Hispanic groups, the rates of lifetime MDE for Puerto Ricans, Cubans, and Mexicans were all significantly different from each other, with Mexicans having the lowest rate. The rates for Caribbean blacks and African Americans were comparable and did not differ from those of Cubans and Mexicans. The *lowest* rates of lifetime MDE were found among the Asian ethnic groups, with Filipinos having the lowest rate. However, the rates for Chinese were comparable with those for Caribbean blacks and African Americans.

Significant gender differences were in the expected direction, with females having higher rates of lifetime MDE than males among all groups, except for Vietnamese, Filipinos, and Caribbean blacks (see Table 12–1). Asians born outside the United States continued to have the lowest rates of lifetime MDE. Interestingly, rates for Chinese born in the United States were almost three times higher than Chinese born outside the United States. Other noteworthy nativity differences were between Mexicans, Caribbean blacks, and whites: all had higher rates if born in the United States. This pattern changed by gender, with Cuban, Puerto Rican, and African American females

TABLE 12–1. Major depressive episode[a] prevalence rates by race/ethnicity, gender, and nativity—lifetime

Group	Total, % (SE)	Male, % (SE)	Female, % (SE)	U.S. BORN Total, % (SE)	U.S. BORN Male, % (SE)	U.S. BORN Female, % (SE)	NON-U.S. BORN Total, % (SE)	NON-U.S. BORN Male, % (SE)	NON-U.S. BORN Female, % (SE)
Vietnamese				**6.99 (6.62)**	**0.00 (0.00)**	**10.71 (9.88)**	8.49 (1.87)	11.71 (3.50)	5.77 (1.62)
Filipino	7.23 (1.36)	5.95 (1.68)	8.25 (1.75)	11.99 (2.97)	10.13 (4.78)	13.71 (4.39)	5.18 (1.35)	3.96 (1.40)	6.10 (1.63)
Chinese	10.11 (1.60)	7.19 (1.61)	12.62* (2.29)	21.47 (3.49)	9.17 (2.45)	33.17* (5.86)	7.68 (1.52)	6.83 (1.83)	8.38 (2.06)
Other Asian	9.66 (1.25)	8.27 (1.61)	11.08 (2.03)	10.21 (2.35)	8.01 (3.06)	12.40 (3.41)	11.04 (1.73)	10.10 (2.28)	11.96 (2.65)
Cuban	17.39 (0.83)	13.01 (1.51)	22.23* (1.49)	14.85 (3.87)	13.85 (5.20)	16.21 (6.67)	17.79 (0.95)	12.86 (1.74)	23.06* (1.63)
Puerto Rican	22.22 (1.77)	16.73 (2.16)	27.48* (3.16)	21.19 (2.64)	16.89 (3.73)	24.87* (3.54)	23.46 (2.80)	16.56 (4.77)	31.06* (4.34)
Mexican	14.50 (0.74)	11.04 (1.06)	18.31* (0.96)	19.20 (1.37)	14.49 (1.41)	24.13* (1.95)	11.72 (1.06)	8.68 (1.49)	15.23* (1.87)
Other Latino	15.72 (1.18)	12.23 (2.20)	19.09* (1.58)	18.78 (2.21)	15.17 (4.30)	22.52 (2.75)	15.43 (1.69)	11.59 (2.68)	18.77* (2.24)

TABLE 12–1.   Major depressive episode[a] prevalence rates by race/ethnicity, gender, and nativity—lifetime (continued)

Group	TOTAL, % (SE)	MALE, % (SE)	FEMALE, % (SE)	U.S. BORN Total, % (SE)	U.S. BORN MALE, % (SE)	U.S. BORN FEMALE, % (SE)	NON-U.S. BORN TOTAL, % (SE)	NON-U.S. BORN MALE, % (SE)	NON-U.S. BORN FEMALE, % (SE)
Caribbean black	14.26 (2.25)	14.85 (4.58)	13.70 (2.02)	24.14 (5.12)	26.37 (8.71)	22.22 (4.32)	9.12 (2.06)	9.17 (3.35)	9.07 (1.42)
African American	12.26 (0.53)	8.93 (0.77)	14.92* (0.63)	13.07 (0.59)	9.72 (0.84)	15.67* (0.68)	13.36 (3.40)	**2.31 (1.65)**	29.62* (8.48)
Non-Latino white	20.35 (0.49)	15.99 (0.87)	24.43* (0.54)	26.06 (0.64)	20.81 (1.02)	30.81* (0.69)	17.18 (2.79)	10.19 (2.92)	23.55* (4.46)
None of the above[b]	29.29 (2.88)	26.42 (4.70)	31.39 (5.00)	38.98 (3.89)	33.74 (5.78)	42.53 (6.86)	**20.05 (12.80)**	**30.35 (24.81)**	**13.02 (11.21)**
Total	18.60 (0.44)	14.62 (0.68)	2.28* (0.47)	23.92 (0.59)	19.03 (0.85)	28.27* (0.64)	12.77 (0.67)	9.73 (0.83)	15.74* (1.05)

Note.   For any two groups, divide the absolute value of the difference between the prevalence rates by the largest standard error for the two rates; if result is >2, the difference is likely to be significant at the 5% level; otherwise, there likely is no difference between the two groups. For bolded data, prevalence rate or number of cases was too low to be reliable.
[a]Prevalence rates were weighted; standard errors were corrected for complex sample design.
[b]Includes racial/ethnic groups not identifying with any of the above groups (e.g., Native Americans or Arabs, who identified only as such).
*Within-group gender difference is significant at 0.05 level.

born outside the United States having significantly higher rates of lifetime MDE than females born in the United States.

Prevalence rates for 12-month MDE are shown in Table 12–2. The 12-month MDE rates show patterns similar to lifetime MDE. Puerto Ricans had a significantly higher rate than all other racial/ethnic groups, including whites, who had the second-highest rate (tests of significance not shown on table). The rate for whites was comparable with those of all ethnic groups except Asians. Asian ethnic groups had the lowest rates of 12-month MDE, and the groups were not different from each other. Although Vietnamese and Filipino groups had significantly lower rates of 12-month MDE than all other ethnic groups, the Chinese rate did not differ statistically from Caribbean black and African American rates.

The patterns across racial/ethnic groups were similar to those for lifetime MDE when gender and nativity were considered, with a few exceptions. All significant gender differences were as expected, with females having higher 12-month rates of MDE than males. Interestingly, males had higher rates than females among Caribbean blacks and Vietnamese, but these differences were not significant. Differences in rates by nativity also were evident, with those born in the United States generally having higher rates of 12-month MDE than those not born in the United States.

The rates of lifetime and 12-month MDD for Caribbean blacks, African Americans, and whites are shown in Tables 12–3 and 12–4. Consistent with previous findings, overall, whites and white females had higher rates of both lifetime and 12-month MDD than did Caribbean blacks and African Americans, and significant gender differences were evident among all groups except Caribbean blacks. Most lifetime rates for those born in the United States were much higher than for those born outside the United States, with the exception that African American women born outside the United States had higher rates. Another interesting finding is that whites born outside the United States had a lifetime MDD rate that was twice as high as that of Caribbean blacks born outside the United States. This pattern was even more striking in these groups for females born outside the United States. The nativity patterns did not hold for 12-month MDD.

Conclusion

Findings related to major depression from analyses of the CPES data set suggest a need to consider the intersection of race, immigration, culture, and ethnicity when assessing mood disorders in diverse populations. Patterns of consistency and difference were found both across and within racial/ethnic groups and by gender and nativity. Filipino and Vietnamese Asian ethnic groups living in the United States reported lower rates of MDE and MDD than all other groups, including Chinese. Puerto Ricans, however, consistently had the highest rates of these disorders. Although this work does not inform us about absolute rates of depression, it does illustrate the heterogeneity in expression and self-reports of symptoms meeting DSM-IV MDE/MDD criteria. For example, it may be that Puerto Ricans are comfortable expressing their feelings and acknowledging those feelings in the interview situation used in the CPES studies, especially in comparison with individuals from Asian groups. Or perhaps those groups who were found to have lower prevalence rates express depression in forms other than those identified by DSM-IV criteria (e.g., irritability vs. sadness or loss of interest). More detailed study will be needed to disentangle these alternative explanations. These results do show, however, that there is great value in examining within-group variation among Asians, blacks, and Hispanics because important differences have emerged that have implications for treatment and intervention.

It is striking that the commonly held view that women experience more depression than men was found to be generally true for most racial/ethnic groups. It is critical to note, however, that gender differences were not found among Caribbean blacks and most Asian ethnic groups. Trends in the data suggest a risk for depression among Caribbean black and Vietnamese males. Attention to the intersection of gender and culture are critical next steps to advance this work. Findings related to nativity strongly support the view that depression is less likely to be found in members of racial and ethnic groups who were born outside the United States in comparison with those who were born in the United States. It is possible that Asians actually experience lower rates of depression than other racial/ethnic groups, and females are at greater risk for depression than males, but additional symptom-level analyses, possibly extending DSM-IV criteria, are needed to fully understand the nature of disorders in different racial/ethnic groups.

In conclusion, there are large disparities in physical morbidities and mortality that are not reflected in the same disparities in serious mental disorders. Specifically, variation in the prevalence of depression across, and within, racial/ethnic groups needs to be understood in the context of other health burdens. For example, although African Americans have lower rates of MDE and MDD relative to non-Hispanic whites, they have substantially higher rates of physical health conditions known to be associated with depressive symptomology, including cardiovascular disease, most cancers, and type 2 diabetes. Understanding this health paradox is critical in understanding the nature of mental disorders and the types of services needed. We have speculated about possible causes of these physical and mental health rela-

TABLE 12–2. Twelve-month major depressive episode[a] prevalence rates by race/ethnicity, gender, and nativity

Group	Total, % (SE)	Male, % (SE)	Female, % (SE)	U.S. Born			Non-U.S. Born		
				Total, % (SE)	Male, % (SE)	Female, % (SE)	Total, % (SE)	Male, % (SE)	Female, % (SE)
Vietnamese	4.18 (1.12)	6.49 (2.38)	2.25 (0.84)	**6.99 (6.62)**	**0.00 (0.00)**	**10.71 (9.88)**	4.09 (1.13)	6.65 (2.44)	1.94 (0.79)
Filipino	4.17 (1.08)	4.19 (1.40)	4.16 (1.52)	7.48 (2.04)	6.53 (3.41)	8.36 (4.15)	2.75 (1.12)	**3.07 (1.51)**	**2.51 (1.29)**
Chinese	4.62 (1.23)	3.13 (1.22)	5.91 (1.59)	8.75 (2.10)	**4.60 (2.04)**	12.71 (4.01)	3.75 (1.33)	2.83 (1.38)	4.51 (1.64)
Other Asian	4.89 (0.93)	4.55 (1.35)	5.23 (1.35)	4.06 (1.72)	**1.83 (1.74)**	6.28 (2.86)	6.00 (1.37)	6.67 (2.08)	5.27 (1.69)
Cuban	7.96 (0.75)	5.41 (0.97)	10.79* (1.34)	**5.36 (2.81)**	**7.36 (4.26)**	**2.64 (2.55)**	8.38 (0.70)	5.06 (0.89)	11.92* (1.34)
Puerto Rican	11.85 (1.45)	10.04 (2.16)	13.59 (2.53)	10.71 (1.93)	9.23 (2.56)	11.99 (2.81)	13.23 (2.07)	10.91 (3.97)	15.78 (3.34)
Mexican	8.01 (0.59)	6.58 (0.91)	9.58* (0.90)	10.37 (1.16)	8.81 (1.31)	12.00 (1.67)	6.7 (0.63)	5.03 (1.08)	8.82 (1.39)
Other Latino	7.48 (0.82)	4.66 (1.09)	10.18* (1.16)	8.03 (1.31)	4.14 (1.44)	12.06* (1.90)	8.03 (1.32)	5.93 (1.75)	9.86* (1.55)

TABLE 12–2. Twelve-month major depressive episode[a] prevalence rates by race/ethnicity, gender, and nativity *(continued)*

| | | | | U.S. BORN | | | NON-U.S. BORN | | |
Group	TOTAL, % (SE)	MALE, % (SE)	FEMALE, % (SE)	TOTAL, % (SE)	MALE, % (SE)	FEMALE, % (SE)	TOTAL, % (SE)	MALE, % (SE)	FEMALE, % (SE)
Caribbean black	7.83 (1.67)	10.42 (3.72)	5.38 (1.19)	13.35 (3.73)	21.05 (7.52)	6.76 (1.93)	4.83 (1.10)	5.12 (1.86)	4.54 (0.99)
African American	6.79 (0.41)	4.54 (0.56)	8.58* (0.49)	7.21 (0.44)	4.87 (0.61)	9.03* (0.52)	7.97 (2.86)	**1.03** **(1.03)**	18.18* (6.44)
Non-Latino white	8.34 (0.32)	6.34 (0.43)	10.21* (0.47)	10.72 (0.43)	8.26 (0.53)	12.94* (0.62)	6.83 (1.92)	**3.35** **(1.76)**	10.01 (3.32)
None of the above[b]	14.70 (2.49)	13.22 (3.21)	15.78 (4.18)	19.86 (3.84)	16.56 (3.75)	22.09 (5.48)	**12.31** **(11.71)**	**30.35** **(24.81)**	**0.00** **(0.00)**
Total	8.12 (0.26)	6.22 (0.35)	9.87* (0.38)	10.32 (0.36)	7.93 (0.43)	12.44* (0.52)	6.56 (0.47)	5.27 (0.63)	7.83* (0.74)

Note. For any two groups, divide the absolute value of the difference between the prevalence rates by the largest standard error for the two rates; if result is >2, the difference is likely to be significant at the 5% level; otherwise, there likely is no difference between the two groups. For bolded data, prevalence rate or number of cases was too low to be reliable.
[a]Prevalence rates were weighted; standard errors were corrected for complex sample design.
[b]Includes racial/ethnic groups not identifying with any of the above groups (e.g., Native Americans or Arabs, who identified only as such).
*Within-group gender difference is significant at 0.05 level.

TABLE 12–3. Prevalence rates for lifetime major depressive disorder[a] by race/ethnicity, gender, and nativity

GROUP	TOTAL, % (SE)	MALE, % (SE)	FEMALE, % (SE)	U.S. BORN TOTAL, % (SE)	MALE, % (SE)	FEMALE, % (SE)	NON-U.S. BORN TOTAL, % (SE)	MALE, % (SE)	FEMALE, % (SE)
Caribbean black	12.85 (2.33)	14.02 (4.58)	11.74 (1.99)	21.18 (5.46)	25.50 (8.86)	17.48 (4.40)	8.48 (2.04)	8.35 (3.30)	8.61 (1.39)
African American	10.39 (0.47)	7.38 (0.69)	12.79* (0.62)	11.08 (0.53)	8.15 (0.77)	13.35* (0.67)	12.65 (3.49)	**2.31 (1.65)**	27.86* (8.40)
Non-Latino white	17.93 (0.54)	13.87 (0.81)	21.73* (0.53)	22.90 (0.69)	17.94 (0.96)	27.38* (0.71)	16.78 (2.78)	10.19 (2.92)	22.80* (4.45)
Total[b]	16.95 (0.49)	13.12 (0.73)	20.45* (0.48)	21.17 (0.65)	16.64 (0.86)	25.17* (0.67)	14.78 (2.01)	8.88 (2.12)	20.52* (3.31)

Note.   For any two groups, divide the absolute value of the difference between the prevalence rates by the largest standard error for the two rates; if result is >2, the difference is likely to be significant at the 5% level; otherwise, there likely is no difference between the two groups. For bolded data, prevalence rate or number of cases was too low to be reliable.
[a]Prevalence rates were weighted; standard errors were corrected for complex sample design.
[b]Includes Caribbean black, African American, and non-Latino white combined prevalence rates.
*Within-group gender difference is significant at 0.05 level.

TABLE 12–4.   Prevalence rates of 12-month major depressive disorder[a] by race/ethnicity, gender, and nativity

Group	Total, % (SE)	Male, % (SE)	Female, % (SE)	U.S. Born			Non-U.S. Born		
				Total, % (SE)	Male, % (SE)	Female, % (SE)	Total, % (SE)	Male, % (SE)	Female, % (SE)
Caribbean black	7.31 (1.74)	10.04 (3.72)	4.71 (1.02)	12.61 (4.02)	20.74 (7.57)	5.66 (1.67)	4.83 (1.08)	4.71 (1.83)	4.09 (0.90)
African American	5.30 (0.37)	3.12 (0.43)	7.04* (0.46)	5.63 (0.42)	3.45 (0.50)	7.32* (0.51)	7.97 (2.86)	**1.03** (**1.03**)	18.18* (6.44)
Non-Latino white	6.97 (0.29)	5.03 (0.39)	8.78* (0.39)	8.91 (0.39)	6.50 (0.49)	11.08* (0.53)	6.83 (1.92)	**3.35** (**1.76**)	10.01 (3.32)
Total[b]	6.76 (0.26)	4.85 (0.35)	8.51* (0.35)	8.44 (0.35)	6.13 (0.43)	10.48* (0.47)	6.48 (1.39)	3.34 (1.27)	9.54* (2.49)

Note.   For any two groups, divide the absolute value of the difference between the prevalence rates by the largest standard error for the two rates; if result is >2, the difference is likely to be significant at the 5% level; otherwise, there likely is no difference between the two groups. For bolded data, prevalence rate or number of cases was too low to be reliable.
[a]Prevalence rates were weighted; standard errors were corrected for complex sample design.
[b]Includes Caribbean black, African American, and non-Latino white combined prevalence rates.
*Within-group gender difference is significant at 0.05 level.

tionships, but more work is needed (Jackson and Knight 2006; Jackson et al. 2010). There is a need for new directions in research on mental health, including mental health services—especially studies substantively focused on racial, ethnic, and cultural variations—that use the most sophisticated analytic techniques currently available (Alarcón et al. 2002). This will require greater attention to how race, immigration, culture, and ethnicity (within the context of living arrangements and social and economic statuses) combine to influence diagnoses of serious mental disorders, service needs, intervention approaches, and treatments for an ever-growing population of ethnically, racially, and culturally diverse children and adults.

References

Alarcón RD, Bell CC, Kirmayer LJ, et al: Beyond the funhouse mirrors: research agenda on culture and psychiatric diagnosis, in A Research Agenda for DSM-V. Edited by Kupfer DJ, First MB, Regier DA. Washington, DC, American Psychiatric Association, 2002, pp 219–281

Alegría M, Woo M, Takeuchi D, et al: Ethnic and racial group–specific considerations, in Disparities in Psychiatric Care: Clinical and Cross-Cultural Perspectives. Edited by Ruiz P, Primm A. Baltimore, MD, Lippincott Williams & Wilkins, 2009, pp 306–318

American Psychiatric Association: Diagnostic and Statistical Manual of Mental Disorders, 4th Edition. Washington, DC, American Psychiatric Association, 1994

Angel JL, Hogan DP: Population aging and diversity in a new era, in Closing the Gap: Improving the Health of Minority Elders in the New Millennium. Edited by Whitfield KE. Washington, DC, Gerontological Society of America, 2004, pp 1–12

Colpe L, Merikangas K, Cuthbert B, et al: Guest editorial. Int J Methods Psychiatr Res 13:193–195, 2004

Demyttenaere K, Bruffaerts R, Posada-Villa J, et al: Prevalence, severity, and unmet need for treatment of mental disorders in the World Health Organization World Mental Health Surveys. JAMA 291:2581–2590, 2004

Dohrenwend BP, Levav I, Shrout PE, et al: Socioeconomic status and psychiatric disorders: the causation-selection issue. Science 255:946–952, 1992

Jackson JS (ed): New Directions: African Americans in a Diversifying Nation. Washington, DC, National Policy Association, Program for Research on Black Americans, University of Michigan, 2000

Jackson JS, Knight KM: Race and self-regulatory health behaviors: the role of the stress response and the HPA axis in physical and mental health disparities, in Social Structures, Aging, and Self-Regulation in the Elderly. Edited by Schaie KW, Carstensen L. New York, Springer, 2006, pp 189–208

Jackson JS, Torres M, Caldwell CH, et al: The National Survey of American Life: a study of racial, ethnic and cultural influences on mental disorders and mental health. Int J Methods Psychiatr Res 13:196–207, 2004

Jackson JS, Knight KM, Rafferty JA: Race and unhealthy behaviors: chronic stress, the HPA axis, and physical and mental health disparities over the life course. Am J Public Health 100:933–939, 2010

Karlsen S, Nazroo JY: Agency and structure: the impact of ethnic identity and racism on the health of ethnic minority people. Sociol Health Illn 24:1–20, 2002

Kent MM: Immigration and America's black population. Popul Bull 62:1–16, 2007

Kessler RC, Üstün TB: The World Mental Health (WMH) Survey Initiative Version of the World Health Organization (WHO) Composite International Diagnostic Interview (CIDI). Int J Methods Psychiatr Res 13:93–121, 2004

Kessler RC, Üstün TB (eds): The WHO Mental Health Surveys: Global Perspectives on the Epidemiology of Mental Disorders. New York, Cambridge University Press, 2008

Kessler RC, McGonagle KA, Zhao S, et al: Lifetime and 12-month prevalence of DSM-III-R psychiatric disorders in the United States: results from the National Comorbidity Survey. Arch Gen Psychiatry 51:8–19, 1994

Magee WJ, Eaton WW, Wittchen HU, et al: Agoraphobia, simple phobia, and social phobia in the National Comorbidity Survey. Arch Gen Psychiatry 53:159–168, 1996

Nazroo J: The structuring of ethnic inequalities in health economic position, racial discrimination, and racism. Am J Publ Health 93:277–284, 2003

Neighbors HW, Jackson JS, Campbell L, et al: The influence of racial factors on psychiatric diagnosis: a review and suggestions for research. Community Ment Health J 25:301–311, 1989

Noh S, Kaspar V: Perceived discrimination and depression: moderating effects of coping, acculturation, and ethnic support. Am J Public Health 93:232–238, 2003

Robins L, Regier DA (eds): Psychiatric Disorders in America: The Epidemiologic Catchment Area Study. New York, Free Press, 1991

Somervell PD, Leaf PJ, Weissman MM, et al: The prevalence of major depression in black and white adults in five United States communities. Am J Epidemiol 130:725–735, 1989

U.S. Department of Health and Human Services: Mental Health: Culture, Race, and Ethnicity—A Supplement to Mental Health: A Report of the Surgeon General. Rockville, MD, U.S. Department of Health and Human Services, Office of the Surgeon General, Substance Abuse and Mental Health Services Administration, 2001

Vega WA, Rumbaut RG: Ethnic minorities and mental health. Annu Rev Sociol 17:351–383, 1991

Williams DR, Harris-Reid M: Race and mental health: emerging patterns and promising approaches, in A Handbook for the Study of Mental Health: Social Contexts, Theories, and Systems. Edited by Horwitz AV, Scheid TL. Cambridge, UK, Cambridge University Press, 1999, pp 295–314

World Health Organization: International Statistical Classification of Diseases and Related Health Problems, 10th Revision. Geneva, World Health Organization, 1992

CHAPTER 13

Gender and Gender-Related Issues in DSM-5

Kimberly A. Yonkers, M.D.
Diana E. Clarke, Ph.D.

As the American Psychiatric Association constructs a new edition of the *Diagnostic and Statistical Manual of Mental Disorders* (DSM), DSM-5, it has an opportunity to address a number of issues that past iterations of the DSM did not include, or handled unevenly. The notion that there may be gender, race, or ethnic differences in the incidence, prevalence, or expression of psychiatric illness is not new. Similarly, there have been suggestions of the possibility of gender bias among some of the DSM categories (Kaplan 1983). Ongoing issues include how the criteria sets and the text of the manual can best impart the most accurate information and accommodate possible differences among the many subgroups. The focus of this chapter is on the inclusion of both gender differences and gender-related features in DSM-5. We use the term *gender,* rather than *sex,* because we discuss the psychological construct of gender rather than simply the biological determinism associated with birth as a male or female. However, we acknowledge that much of the "psychology" of gender derives from one's biological sex, as well as others' response to it. Moreover, some of the issues in DSM relate to biological (sexual) functioning, and not gender.

Historical Context for Gender Issues in DSM

Widiger and colleagues (Hartung and Widiger 1998; Widiger 2007) have reviewed the inclusion of gender issues in DSM in several reports that illustrate both an evolution in the way of handling gender issues and a deficit in available information among the various DSM editions. DSM-I included gender as one of the demographic variables that would be important to measure among populations with mental illnesses, but this edition did not include sex ratios or prevalence statistics (American Psychiatric Association 1952). DSM-II included a gender-specific category of psychosis with childbirth but did not retain the category in future iterations of DSM (American Psychiatric Association 1968). DSM-III improved on the information available about gender effects by including sections on "associated features," "age at onset," "complications and predisposing factors" and, in many sections, "sex ratio" (American Psychiatric Association 1980; Widiger 2007). However, much of the information was inaccurate and imprecise. To illustrate, the text included such statements as "The disorder is apparently equally common in males and females," or "The disorder is diagnosed more commonly in females than males" (American Psychiatric Association 1980). Such statements derive from clinical impression, rather than from research from representative community cohorts. DSM-III also included a number of categories that were either gender specific, such as "gender identity disorder of childhood," or relevant to individuals of one sex or the other, such as selected "psychosexual disorders" (American Psychiatric Association 1980). The authors removed the category for psychosis with childbirth in this iteration, and, as such, criteria sets that were gender specific were limited to those that involved sexual identity or sexual function.

The revision of DSM-III (DSM-III-R; American Psychiatric Association 1987) benefited from epidemiological study that occurred around that time and provided more information on sex ratios, although the data on sex ratios remained largely inadequate. For example, DSM-III-R indicated that "dissociative disorders" occurred three to nine times as often in females as males, a range so large that one cannot identify the estimate with certainty. Separate criteria for "gender identity disorders of childhood" in males and females and select "sexual disorders" (e.g., female sexual arousal disorder or male erectile disorder) were retained. However, there was consideration of another gender-specific category that was not simply a disorder of sexual functioning. This condition, late luteal phase dysphoric disorder, was eventually included in the appendix of DSM-III-R under "Proposed Diagnostic Categories Needing Further Study" (American Psychiatric

Association 1987). The proposed condition was included only in the appendix because some believed that more data needed to be collected before it qualified as a stand-alone disorder. There were also concerns among many on the task force that a gender-specific diagnosis such as this might stigmatize women.

DSM-IV (American Psychiatric Association 1994) provided more information on gender issues; this included prevalence data as well as descriptive information in the text of various disorders, under the section "Specific Culture, Age, and Gender Features." However, not all the information provided was well documented and accurate (Hartung and Widiger 1998). Despite substantially more available research on late luteal phase dysphoric disorder, it was not included as a regular category. Instead, it was renamed premenstrual dysphoric disorder and retained in the appendix. The text update for DSM-IV, DSM-IV-TR (American Psychiatric Association 2000), was designed to bring greater accuracy to statistical and other information. Literature reviews and evidence tables supported changes in the text. This volume also preserved different criteria sets for select "sexual disorders" that occur in either men or women. Interestingly, in this update, a specifier to indicate postpartum onset of major depressive disorder was added.

In summary, the various iterations of DSM have incorporated more plentiful and more accurate information about sex ratios for the various psychiatric conditions, although there are still deficiencies. For example, the current edition provides no ratio for posttraumatic stress disorder (PTSD), and some of the conditions simply state a majority in males or females, without specific ratios. DSM continues to include the gender-specific categories for select "sexual disorders." In one instance, a postpartum modifier for major depressive disorder was included as recognition of the role of reproductive events. Premenstrual dysphoric disorder, another gender-specific disorder, remains in the appendix, largely because of concerns about the stigma such a diagnosis might confer rather than the science associated with the category (Widiger 2007).

DSM-5 and Gender-Related Issues

The form of DSM-5 is a work in progress. Nonetheless, gender-related issues might be better integrated into DSM-5 in a number of ways, and this could be done with a greater level of sophistication than outlined in the previous section.

Epidemiological Data

We now have substantially more data on the incidence and prevalence of psychiatric disorders in men and women. Included in this database are cross-sectional studies, such as the Epidemiologic Catchment Area Study (Robins and Regier 1991), the National Comorbidity Study Replication (Kessler et al. 1994), and the National Epidemiologic Survey on Alcohol and Related Conditions (Grant et al. 2004). Some of these surveys have multiple waves of data collection, which, in conjunction with cohort studies, such as the Zurich Study (Angst and Dobler-Mikola 1985) and Dunedin Longitudinal Study (Hankin et al. 1998), can provide prospective estimates of incidence rates. Examples of relevant information include the finding that the community 12-month and lifetime prevalence of major depressive disorder in adult premenopausal women is approximately twofold higher than in men (Angst and Dobler-Mikola 1984; Hasin et al. 2005; Kessler et al. 1994, 2005; Klose and Jacobi 2004; Weissman et al. 1993). Similarly, attention-deficit/hyperactivity disorder occurs more often in boys than in girls, with a gender ratio of between 3:1 and 5:1 (Costello et al. 2003; Moffitt 1990).

As the strength of epidemiological information grows, it is important to consider additional issues (Rutter et al. 2003). First, it would be preferable if DSM-5 were to use data obtained from community cohorts rather than clinical settings, because factors that influence treatment attendance might bias information gathered from treatment settings. For example, DSM-III-R stated that social phobia was more common among males in clinical settings. DSM-IV clarified the bias found through use of clinical cohorts and stated that, in the community, the disorder is more common in women. In fact, several surveys found a gender ratio of approximately 1.5:1 for women compared with men, and convergence of findings strengthened the estimate (De Wit et al. 1999; Kessler et al. 1994). Second, epidemiological studies from several countries, cultures, or settings can identify stable gender differences and replicate findings. The two studies on social phobia mentioned previously are from the United States (Kessler et al. 1994) and Canada (De Wit et al. 1999), and although point estimates for prevalence of social phobia differ in these two countries, the gender ratio was about the same. Similarly, 12-month prevalence rates for major depressive disorder in premenopausal women vary across countries, but the gender ratio is strikingly similar (Weissman et al. 1993) and may indicate gender-related vulnerability factors that are relatively stable (Rutter et al. 2003). DSM-5 can continue to report gender ratios in conjunction with prevalence estimates.

A caveat to this is that the measurements and methods used to identify incidence and prevalence statistics—and, hence, estimates of gender differences—require consideration. Although randomly selected community participants will minimize selection bias, it is possible that there will be reporting bias and that individuals who are queried will supply more socially acceptable answers rather than historically accurate answers. For instance, men may be less likely to report symptoms of tearfulness (Salokangas et al. 2002) and, perhaps, other manifestations of depression, whereas women may be less apt to report substance misuse (Greenfield et al. 2007). DSM-5 authors can examine the methods that are used in epidemiological studies to identify possible sources of information bias.

Beyond Epidemiology and Gender Ratios: Gender and Construction of Criteria Sets

Several DSM disorders do not assume gender neutrality but rather are gender specific because biology indicates that individuals from only one sex can have the disorder. Examples include dyspareunia in women or male erectile disorder in men. On the other hand, whether conduct disorder is gender neutral, or *should* be gender neutral, has been controversial. The condition is more prevalent in males than in females, and the distribution of some features differ by sex in adolescents. Studies of conduct disorder find greater difficulties with physical aggression in males, and higher rates of sexual indiscretion as well as other relational forms of aggression in females (Rutter et al. 2003). Accordingly, some researchers advocate a lower "threshold" for diagnosis in females, compared with males, in order to render the diagnostic category gender neutral (Zoccolillo et al. 1996). Others find that that the criteria outlined in DSM-IV appropriately reflect the gender differences found for the essential components of the illness (Doyle et al. 2003; Lahey et al. 2006).

Questions have arisen about the gender neutrality of another condition, somatization disorder (Hartung and Widiger 1998). This category evolved from "hysteria," and its very basis was gender biased. Workers associated with DSM winnowed these gender-specific criteria over the various iterations the manual. DSM-IV added one criterion specific to men (ejaculatory dysfunction) and retained some female-specific criteria (irregular menses, excessive menstrual bleeding, vomiting throughout pregnancy) but eliminated others in an attempt to achieve gender neutrality (American Psychiatric Association 2000).

Gender neutrality has been questioned less for other DSM criteria sets, but this is a consideration for DSM-5. Empirical explorations to identify gender bias within individual categories will encounter a number of complexities. As mentioned, some symptoms *reported* by those with the true disease may be influenced by perceptions of social acceptability. Not only can these reported symptoms yield inaccurate estimates of the true disease—in either men or women (or both)—but they also may lead to inaccurate descriptions of the disease. To illustrate, some work shows that, compared with women with major depressive disorder, men with this illness are less likely to endorse problems with libido or somatic symptoms, such as appetite and sleep disturbance (Silverstein 1999). Does this mean that men with a depressive disorder are less likely to have impaired libido or be afflicted with sleep and appetite problems, or are they less likely to report such difficulties? If critical symptoms are underreported in some groups, researchers might miss less severe variants.

Figure 13–1 is a hypothetical illustration of how differences between genders in the endorsement of candidate symptoms could yield different illness rates. In the graph, a greater number of women reach criteria for the illness when they are less ill. This could occur if the critical symptoms men experience are not included in the threshold necessary to diagnose the disease or if men fail to report the symptoms. A similar result could occur if symptoms of nonspecific distress, which are more common in women than men, were included in a diagnostic criterion set, as illustrated in Figure 13–2. To use tearfulness as an example, if tearfulness is a common expression of emotionality in women (Williams and Morris 1996), and tearfulness were incorporated into the symptom checklist and criterion set for major depressive disorder, this would serve to perpetuate a gender-biased estimate of the prevalence of the disorder. Such an item would be described as being measurement non-invariant (i.e., having different probability of being endorsed by one group compared with another, despite similar underlying levels of the disorder). Tearfulness is not a DSM symptom of depression, but somatization disorder is a particularly relevant example of Figure 13–2. Not only was the disorder derived from a gender-biased perspective (e.g., from "hysteria"), but the inclusion of items that can be experienced only by women may have perpetuated the disproportionate rate of illness in women as compared with men. The fact that most of the research on this condition has included women only (Hartung and Widiger 1998) further ensures a higher representation of women among those with this disorder.

It is reasonable to wonder how colleagues involved with DSM-5 might determine which, if any, diagnostic criteria have been influenced by gender bias. We discussed examples of conduct disorder and somatization disorder in the previous paragraphs. Certainly, the inclusion of criteria that can be only, or are typically, experienced by individuals of one sex or another suggests the possibility of gender bias. Another indicator of possible gender bias lies within the epidemiology of the disorder and disproportionate prevalence rates between men and women, although such differences in illness rates might reflect actual illness in men and women. Given the availability of appropriate data sets, members of the DSM-5 work groups and study groups can statistically test the relevance of symptoms expressed in both men and women in relation to the diagnosis of an illness.

One approach is *latent-class analysis*. This analytic approach assumes that latent and unobservable variables (classes) represent the

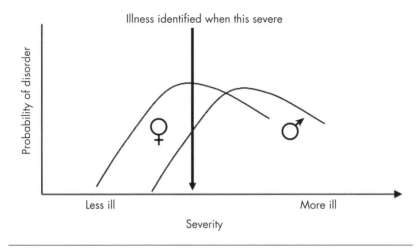

FIGURE 13–1. Gender-related measures of severity, leading to different illness detection rates.

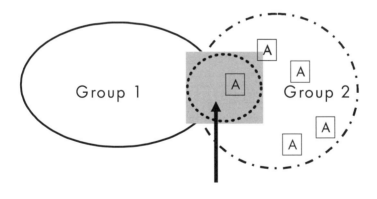

FIGURE 13–2. Criteria biased by prevalence of noncontributing symptoms in the group most likely to have the illness.

illness and that it is possible to model these variables through the structure of correlations between variables that are observable. If the composition of latent classes does not vary between men and women (measurement invariance), then it is likely that criterion items are relevant for both men and women. Chung and Breslau (2008) employed this approach to evaluate gender bias in the criterion set for PTSD. As context, numerous studies find that, after a traumatic event, women are more likely to develop PTSD than are men (Breslau et al. 1991; Fullerton et al. 2001; Holbrook et al. 2002; Norris 1992). Furthermore, the type of traumatic events to which women are typically exposed differs somewhat from that for men, because women have a greater likelihood of exposure to interpersonal violence, whereas men are more often exposed to other types of trauma (Breslau et al. 1991; Kimerling et al. 2000). Chung and Breslau (2008) used a community cohort of individuals who were queried about PTSD and explored measurement invariance according to groups that differed by trauma type and gender. They found that measurement of PTSD varied according to trauma type (assaultive violence vs. other traumatic events) but not according to gender. The implications suggest that, after taking type of trauma into consideration, the criteria set fits men and women equally well. Although reassuring, results such as this merit replication.

Another analytic approach useful in examining the presence of possible gender bias in the diagnostic criteria sets for different disorders is *item response theory* (IRT), in which the term *differential item functioning* (DIF) is synonymous with measurement non-invariance. IRT analysis also assumes that the disorder/illness is unobservable and represented by an underlying latent structure (i.e., θ), which is estimated by the observed variables (i.e., symptoms). Information about an individual's illness severity (or ability) and the test-item characteristics (i.e., item difficulty, or β parameters, and item discrimination, or α parameters) is used to predict the probability of a positive endorsement for a particular symptom and is displayed graphically by the item-characteristic curves. In the item-characteristic curve for each item or symptom, the severity of the condition, as represented by the underlying latent structure, θ, is constant, and group differences in the item difficulty, β parameters, and item discrimination, α parameters, are compared.

The use of IRT to assess gender-based DIF involves examining differences in the probability of endorsing an item between the reference group (i.e., females) and focal group (i.e., males), who both have the same underlying severity of the disorder. Symptoms that are more likely to be endorsed by one group (i.e., females) across all levels of the disorder, compared with another group (e.g., males) with the same underlying severity of the disorder (Figure 13–3), are said to have uniform DIF. *Uniform DIF* in IRT analysis is analogous to a significant main (group) effect in regression analysis predicting

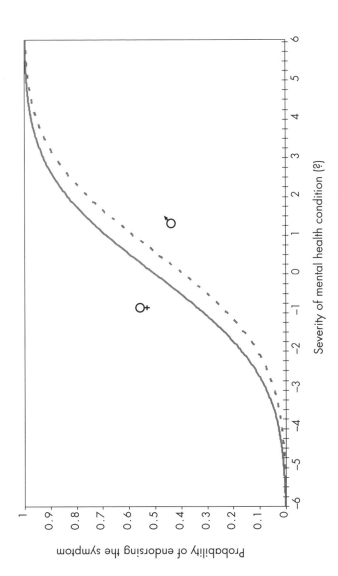

FIGURE 13–3.   Gender-based uniform differential item functioning in endorsing a symptom for hypothetical mental health condition.

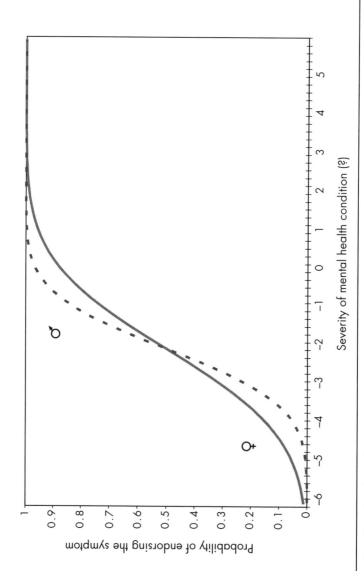

FIGURE 13–4. Gender-based non-uniform differential item functioning in endorsing a symptom for hypothetical mental health condition.

endorsement of specific symptoms. On the other hand, symptoms that are more likely to be endorsed by one group, compared with another, at high levels of the outcome but exhibit the reverse property at low levels of the outcome (or vice versa) are said to have *non-uniform DIF,* which is analogous to an interaction term in regression analysis (Figure 13–4). In assessment of gender-based measurement non-invariance, non-uniform DIF is investigated first, and if it is absent, uniform DIF is examined.

Preliminary examinations, by the DSM-5 Cross-Culture and Gender Study Group, of gender-based measurement non-invariance for the major depressive disorder symptoms specified in DSM-IV have shown a lack of non-uniform DIF. However, minimal—that is, not meaningful, based on less than 10% change in the β-parameter estimates (Moldonado and Greenland 1993)—gender-based uniform DIF occurred for some depressive symptoms. Such findings imply that the items specified for major depressive disorder do not favor one gender over the other and therefore have minimal effect on the observed differences between males and females in prevalence of the disorder. These observations warrant additional studies to replicate the findings.

Alternative Criterion Sets for Men and Women

As noted, some disorders have separate criterion sets for men and women, but these are mainly disorders for which sexual function differs by gender. Alternative diagnostic criteria sets for males and females with conduct disorder have been advocated by some (Zoccolillo et al. 1996), but this idea is not universally supported (Rutter et al. 2003). A high level of evidence to support a need for different criteria sets among males and females must exist. Such information may include evidence that 1) the same disorder is represented by a number of different symptoms in males and females; 2) there is underdiagnosis of one group, if these different symptoms are not considered; and 3) the clinical course of the disorder, operationalized under different criteria sets, has an analogous course, biology, and so on.

Gender Considerations and Diagnostic Specifiers

Past iterations of DSM have used diagnostic specifiers such as age at onset, severity, course specifiers, and characteristics ("type," such as "generalized" or "paranoid"). Specifiers can provide additional diagnostic information to the clinician and hence guide treatment. An example of a gender-related specifier is the "postpartum onset" specifier for major depressive disorder found in DSM-IV. It is possible that this and other reproductive events in women could add necessary diagnostic information; therefore, review of this information or additional data collection would be important for DSM-5. As an example, premenstrual worsening of a unipolar depressive disorder would be important to identify because it could identify a period of vulnerability for relapse (the premenstrual phase) and because it might have treatment implications. Women who are otherwise stable but experience premenstrual worsening of mood might require an increased dosage of medication, the addition of another medication, or a change to an agent that is effective for premenstrual symptoms as well as major depressive disorder. Gender-related specifiers may best be limited to those specifiers that indicate important diagnostic and management issues in women.

Integration of Gender-Related Issues Into the Text of DSM-5

A great deal of valuable information is included in the text of DSM and, in past iterations, this has included "gender features." The scientific literature on gender differences in the causes and expression of psychiatric disorders has increased substantially over the past decade, and the text would be an ideal place for new information. However, such information should hold to the principles outlined earlier: it should include data from community cohorts as well as clinical samples; it should be validated by replication; and it should be scientifically rigorous. Ideally, such information would help clinicians and researchers in their diagnostic endeavors and would indicate areas with treatment implications. We discussed gender differences in the presentation of conduct disorder and the differential exposure to various traumatic events for men and women. Information such as this would be helpful to include in the text of DSM-5.

Conclusion

The evolution of the DSM has included increased attention to gender issues. Comprehensive information about epidemiology is necessary and should be as accurate as possible. However, DSM-5 has an opportunity to go beyond rudimentary statistics and address whether categories are, or should be, gender neutral. Alignments in criteria sets also may reciprocally influence gender differences in the epidemiology of various diagnoses. DSM-5 could incorporate gender-related issues as "specifiers" or in text information. Attention to these details will render DSM-5 relevant to individuals of both genders.

References

American Psychiatric Association: Diagnostic and Statistical Manual: Mental Disorders. Washington, DC, American Psychiatric Association, 1952

American Psychiatric Association: Diagnostic and Statistical Manual of Mental Disorders, 2nd Edition. Washington, DC, American Psychiatric Association, 1968

American Psychiatric Association: Diagnostic and Statistical Manual of Mental Disorders, 3rd Edition. Washington, DC, American Psychiatric Association, 1980

American Psychiatric Association: Diagnostic and Statistical Manual of Mental Disorders, 3rd Edition, Revised. Washington, DC, American Psychiatric Association, 1987

American Psychiatric Association: Diagnostic and Statistical Manual of Mental Disorders, 4th Edition. Washington, DC, American Psychiatric Association, 1994

American Psychiatric Association: Diagnostic and Statistical Manual of Mental Disorders, 4th Edition, Text Revision. Washington, DC, American Psychiatric Association, 2000

Angst J, Dobler-Mikola A: Do the diagnostic criteria determine the sex ratio in depression? J Affect Disord 7:189–198, 1984

Angst J, Dobler-Mikola A: The Zurich Study—a prospective epidemiological study of depressive, neurotic and psychosomatic syndromes, IV: recurrent and nonrecurrent brief depression. Eur Arch Psychiatry Neurol Sci 234:408–416, 1985

Breslau N, Davis GC, Andreski P, et al: Traumatic events and posttraumatic stress disorder in an urban population of young adults. Arch Gen Psychiatry 48:216–222, 1991

Chung H, Breslau N: The latent structure of post-traumatic stress disorder: tests of invariance by gender and trauma type. Psychol Med 38:563–573, 2008

Costello EJ, Mustillo S, Erkanli A, et al: Prevalence and development of psychiatric disorders in childhood and adolescence. Arch Gen Psychiatry 60:837–844, 2003

De Wit DJ, Ogborne A, Offord DR, et al: Antecedents of the risk of recovery from DSM-III-R social phobia. Psychol Med 29:569–582, 1999

Doyle AE, Biederman J, Monuteaux M, et al: Diagnostic threshold for conduct disorder in girls and boys. J Nerv Ment Dis 191:379–386, 2003

Fullerton CS, Ursano RJ, Epstein RS, et al: Gender differences in posttraumatic stress disorder after motor vehicle accidents. Am J Psychiatry 158:1486–1491, 2001

Grant B, Stinson FS, Dawson DA, et al: Co-ocurrence of 12-month alcohol and drug use disorders and personality disorders in the United States: results from the National Epidemiologic Survey on Alcohol and Related Conditions (NESARC). Arch Gen Psychiatry 61:361–368, 2004

Greenfield SF, Brooks AJ, Gordon SM, et al: Substance abuse treatment entry, retention, and outcome in women: a review of the literature. Drug Alcohol Depend 86:1–21, 2007

Hankin BL, Abramson LY, Moffitt TE, et al: Development of depression from preadolescence to young adulthood: emerging gender differences in a 10-year longitudinal study. J Abnorm Psychol 107:128–140, 1998

Hartung CM, Widiger TA: Gender differences in the diagnosis of mental disorders: conclusions and controversies of the DSM-IV. Psychol Bull 123:260–278, 1998

Hasin DS, Goodwin RD, Stinson FS, et al: Epidemiology of major depressive disorder: results from the National Epidemiologic Survey on Alcoholism and Related Conditions. Arch Gen Psychiatry 62:1097–1106, 2005

Holbrook TL, Hoyt DB, Stein MB, et al: Gender difference in long-term posttraumatic stress disorder outcomes after major trauma: women are at higher risk of adverse outcomes than men. J Trauma 53:882–888, 2002

Kaplan M: A woman's view of DSM-III. Am Psychol 38:786–792, 1983

Kessler RC, McGonagle KA, Zhao S, et al: Lifetime and 12-month prevalence of DSM-III-R psychiatric disorders in the United States: results from the National Comorbidity Survey. Arch Gen Psychiatry 51:8–19, 1994

Kessler RC, Berglund P, Demler O, et al: Lifetime prevalence and age-of-onset distributions of DSM-IV disorders in the National Comorbidity Survey Replication (see comment). Arch Gen Psychiatry 62:593–602, 2005 (erratum in Arch Gen Psychiatry 62:768, 2005)

Kimerling R, Clum GA, Wolfe J: Relationships among trauma exposure, chronic posttraumatic stress disorder symptoms, and self-reported health in women: replication and extension. J Trauma Stress 13:115–128, 2000

Klose M, Jacobi F: Can gender differences in the prevalence of mental disorders be explained by sociodemographic factors? Arch Womens Ment Health 7:133–148, 2004

Lahey BB, Van Hulle CA, Waldman ID, et al: Testing descriptive hypotheses regarding sex differences in the development of conduct problems and delinquency. J Abnorm Child Psychol 34:737–755, 2006

Moffitt TE: Juvenile delinquency and attention deficit disorder: boys' developmental trajectories from age 3 to age 15. Child Dev 61:893–910, 1990

Moldonado G, Greenland S: Simulation study of confounder-selection strategies. Am J Epidemiol 138:923–936, 1993

Norris FH: Epidemiology of trauma: frequency and impact of different potentially traumatic events on different demographic groups. J Consult Clin Psychol 60:409–418, 1992

Robins L, Regier DA (eds): Psychiatric Disorders in America: The Epidemiologic Catchment Area Study. New York, Free Press, 1991

Rutter M, Caspi A, Moffitt TE: Using sex differences in psychopathology to study causal mechanisms: unifying issues and research strategies. J Child Psychol Psychiatry 44:1092–1115, 2003

Salokangas RK, Vaahtera K, Pacriev S, et al: Gender differences in depressive symptoms: an artifact caused by measurement instruments? J Affect Disord 68:215–220, 2002

Silverstein B: Gender difference in the prevalence of clinical depression: the role played by depression associated with somatic symptoms. Am J Psychiatry 156:480–482, 1999

Weissman MM, Bland R, Joyce PR, et al: Sex differences in rates of depression: cross-national perspectives. J Affect Disord 29:77–84, 1993

Widiger TA: DSM's approach to gender: history and controversies, in Age and Gender Consideration in Psychiatric Diagnosis: A Research Agenda for DSM-V. Edited by Narrow WE, First MB, Sirovatka PJ, et al. Arlington, VA, American Psychiatric Association, 2007, pp 19–31

Williams DG, Morris GH: Crying, weeping or tearfulness in British and Israeli adults. Br J Psychol 87:479–505, 1996

Zoccolillo M, Tremblay R, Vitaro F: DSM-III-R and DSM-III criteria for conduct disorder in preadolescent girls: specific but insensitive. J Am Acad Child Adolesc Psychiatry 35:461–470, 1996

PART V

INCORPORATING DEVELOPMENTAL
VARIATIONS OF DISORDER EXPRESSION
ACROSS THE LIFESPAN

CHAPTER 14

Increasing the Developmental Focus in DSM-5

Broad Issues and Specific Potential Applications in Anxiety

Daniel S. Pine, M.D.
E. Jane Costello, Ph.D.
Ron Dahl, M.D.
Regina James, M.D.
James F. Leckman, M.D.
Ellen Leibenluft, M.D.
Rachel G. Klein, Ph.D.
Judith L. Rapoport, M.D.
David Shaffer, M.D.
Eric Taylor, M.A, M.B.
Charles H. Zeanah, M.D.

As work on the fifth edition of the *Diagnostic and Statistical Manual of Mental Disorders* (DSM-5) progresses, discussions are intensifying concerning the need to implement major changes to nosology (Hyman 2007; Shear et al. 2007). In this chapter we consider procedures for implementing one set of potentially major changes that would increase focus on developmental themes.

We begin by delineating findings that have emerged since publication of DSM-IV (American Psychiatric Association 1994), which suggest a need to increase our focus on development in standard nomenclatures. This research consolidates a view of many mental syndromes, prevalent at various stages of life as disorders, with pathophysiological processes identifiable in childhood.

Following this brief review, we then describe three specific proposals for increasing a focus on developmental themes in DSM-5 relative to DSM-IV:

1. Revise the text sections of DSM-IV to increase focus on development.
2. Integrate explicit descriptions of *developmental manifestations* into DSM-5 as part of criteria for each mental disorder.
3. Implement procedures for considering and evaluating *developmental subtypes* of disorders.

Each of these proposed revisions is relatively complex, and the support for each varies as a function of individual disorder features. As a result, the revisions are not mutually exclusive; DSM-5 could incorporate any combination of the three, and different proposals may work better for one or another specific disorder. In this chapter, we maintain a primary focus on anxiety disorders—to exemplify procedures applicable to all mental disorders—with other disorders considered to illustrate specific points. Thus, we specifically review research emphasizing the importance of developmental perspectives on anxiety disorders in order to illustrate the broader importance of development in mental disorders. Moreover, we also describe potential changes in text, possible age-related manifestations, and proposals for age-related subtypes, specifically for anxiety disorders. Finally, these descriptions focus on specific anxiety disorders as narrowly as possible.

Obsessive-compulsive disorder (OCD) and posttraumatic stress disorder (PTSD) can be differentiated from other anxiety disorders (Pine 2007). For example, children presenting for treatment of anxiety can be divided, based on patterns of comorbidity, into three groups: those with OCD, those with PTSD, and those with other anxiety disorders (March et al. 1998; Pine and Cohen 2002; Research Units on Pediatric Psychopharmacology 2001). Studies of neurobiology and familial aggregation support a similar three-group division, where the correlates of OCD, PTSD, and other pediatric anxiety disorders appear to differ (De Bellis 2001; Pine 2007; Rosenberg and Hanna 2000). Given a narrow focus on particular conditions in this chapter, our specific examples primarily draw on data for particular anxiety disorders. In children and adolescents presenting for treatment, these anxiety disorders primarily comprise social anxiety disorder/ social phobia, separation anxiety disorder, and generalized anxiety disorder (GAD).

Emergence of Developmental Perspectives

Many changes in conceptualizations of mental disorders have emerged since revisions to the psychiatric nosology in the early 1980s with publication of DSM-III in 1980 (American Psychiatric Association 1980), followed by two subsequent revisions, DSM-III-R in 1987 (American Psychiatric Association 1987), and DSM-IV in 1994. However, few changes have been as dramatic as those associated with an increasing emphasis on development. DSM-III contained a relatively brief consideration of developmental themes, and the extent of this focus did not change appreciably in DSM-III-R or DSM-IV (Pine et al. 2002b). In the meantime, advances in research led to radical resculpting of developmental perspectives, leaving DSM-IV somewhat out of step with the current research base. This creates a need to markedly increase the focus on development in DSM-5.

In considering a broad perspective on mental illnesses, four areas of research emphasize the importance of development: 1) clinical presentation, 2) natural history, 3) developmental psychopathology, and 4) age at onset. As noted, to provide concrete examples, we focus in this chapter on anxiety, viewed developmentally. However, where particularly important data or major questions arise, we also discuss data in other areas.

Clinical Presentation

With the creation of disorder-specific criteria in DSM-III, attention began to focus on application to children, including children with anxiety disorders and related conditions, such as mood disorders (Costello et al. 2002). This attention alerted clinicians to the fact that differences in symptoms, or core features, of disorders often vary as a function of development. For example, in the anxiety disorders, most research on therapeutics in adults targets patients who present with relatively specific forms of anxiety disorders, such as panic disorder, GAD, or social anxiety/social phobia. Early attempts to conduct comparable studies in youths confronted the fact that children and adolescents typically present with more varied collections of anxiety symptoms encompassing several so-called specific disorders, such as social phobia, separation anxiety disorder, and

GAD. As a result, considerable research on therapeutics in pediatric anxiety disorders, unlike in adults, targeted patients presenting with various combinations of anxiety as opposed to one or another narrowly defined anxiety disorder (Pine et al. 2002a; Research Units on Pediatric Psychopharmacology 2001).

Clinicians need to be familiar with the varied ways in which development can affect the presentation of many disorders, beyond the anxiety disorders. DSM-IV also emphasized the role of impairment in psychopathology, but this edition does not discuss, in sufficient depth, the fact that patterns of impairment, much like symptoms, also can manifest in different ways at different ages. Changes in their environments can moderate levels of impairment in children, particularly when they are young. For example, for two children with identical biologically based predispositions to fear of dogs, impairment can be quite different if family circumstances force only one of these children consistently to be in the presence of dogs. Children's dependence on adults often forces them to confront situations such as these that older, more independent anxious individuals can choose to avoid. This leads to age-related differences in manifestations of impairment. As with developmental variations in symptomatic presentation, DSM-5 needs to consider developmental changes in manifestations of impairment.

Natural History

The creation of standard disorder-specific criteria in DSM-III set the stage for longitudinal research documenting the natural history of mental conditions. Perhaps more than any other advance, research following children as they matured called attention to the importance of developmental conceptualizations. Thus, research has linked virtually all forms of adult psychopathology to earlier manifestations of mental illness observable during childhood. This applies to research on the pediatric anxiety disorders (Beesdo et al. 2007; Costello et al. 2002; Pine et al. 1998). Family studies also extend these findings by demonstrating an association between mental disorders manifest across generations.

As with chronic medical illness, such as cardiovascular disease, data on anxiety disorders and other mental syndromes emphasize the importance of probabilistic perspectives and a focus on prevention. Thus, early problems with anxiety constrain patterns of function during adulthood and predict a statistically increased risk for later problems, but they do not *invariably* predict a chronic, unrelenting pattern of illness from childhood into adulthood (Pine et al. 1998). The increased risk of anxious children is statistical and probabilistic, not deterministic: although pediatric anxiety disorders precede most adult mood and anxiety disorders, pediatric anxiety disorders are highly prevalent and usually remit. However, a minority of children with persistent anxiety mature to account for most adults with mood and anxiety disorders.

Developmental Psychopathology

Formulations of mental illness have long recognized the salience of critical or sensitive periods, stages of development in which influences of the environment can appear particularly robust. These formulations resonate with views of normal development that also demonstrate a role for sensitive periods in core psychological functions, such as language acquisition. Particular experiences—such as brain injury or changes in the social environment—that cause early life disruptions in language acquisition have more marked effects on adult functioning than if these same experiences occur later in life. Moreover, charting children's ongoing development, as opposed to examining their functioning at any one specific point in time, is the best way to characterize such adverse effects. This reflects the fact that risk for poor outcome is higher among children who show consistent patterns of dysfunction over time than among children who show dysfunction at only one point in time (Costello et al. 2002; Pine et al. 1998). This suggests a view of psychopathology that highlights as abnormal a child's failure to undergo typical, expected changes in behavior and cognition with maturation or a child's failure to overcome transient perturbations in function. To understand mental illness, one needs to understand normal changes in development.

The developmental psychopathology perspective emphasizes the need to understand typical development when considering one, or another, behavioral profile as atypical. This theoretical school recognizes the importance of understanding mental illnesses as failures in maturation whereby pathology can either reflect a failure of mature behaviors to unfold or of immature behaviors to vanish. Thus, applied to the anxiety disorders, periods of intensified fear represent a normal stage of development across virtually all cultures, in which children manifest stereotypical fears at specific ages, such as an early emerging fear of separation in toddlers and an adolescent emergence of social fear, particularly when meeting unfamiliar peers (Ollendick et al. 1996). We can view anxiety disorders as exaggerated forms of these typical fears or as failed extinctions of the fears during development.

A focus on critical periods has intensified in light of recent breakthroughs. These advances have stimulated new ways of understanding evolving individual differences in thought and behavior through a focus on genomic features and their interactions with the environment (Meaney 2001; Rutter et al. 2006). Research on anxiety specifically demonstrates how genetic and environmental influences sculpt the development of the brain circuitry devoted to processing danger; these developmental effects have been linked to developmental manifestations of clinically significant anxiety (Pine 2007). Although such advances are likely to impact current conceptualizations contained in DSM-5, their reverberating influences are likely to exert increasingly profound effects in future years.

Age at Onset

One set of questions, emerging in light of recent developmental research, concerns the degree to which age at onset moderates the presentation of mental illnesses. Perhaps the most compelling theme in research on this issue focuses on conduct problems in children. Here, a growing consensus suggests that problems that emerge early identify a unique subgroup with particularly malignant conditions distinct from those whose problems first manifest later in development (Moffitt et al. 2002). These findings raise broader questions on the degree to which other conditions in DSM-5, contained under a single mental disorder heading, identify heterogeneous collection and could be parsed based on age at onset.

Integrating Developmental Data Into Text Revisions

A careful revision of disorder-associated text probably represents the easiest way to increase the focus on development in DSM. DSM-IV contains text discussions of developmental themes. However, this text often includes discussions of development under the same headings as features related to culture and gender. Clearly, separate text sections specifically focused on development would call increasing attention to developmental themes.

What type of material could be included in text sections focused on development? In terms of the three anxiety disorders described illustratively in this chapter, a few potential organizational principles emerge. First, text sections on developmental conceptualizations should alert clinicians to the changing clinical manifestations of specific syndromes. For example, the section on separation anxiety disorder could describe clues for differentiating normal separation anxiety from the disorder. This could include descriptions of the age at which typical separation anxiety disappears and summaries of situations in which impairing separation anxiety disrupts normal function. Similarly, the text on social phobia could describe normal adolescent increases in social anxiety and provide clues for differentiating such normal adolescent fluctuations in social fears from impairing social anxiety. The text on GAD could differentiate normal from abnormal age-related worries.

Second, text sections should review data on natural course. Thus, as noted, considerable data document the long-term outcome of anxiety disorders in children and adolescents (Beesdo et al. 2007; Gregory et al. 2007; Moffitt et al. 2007; Pine et al. 1998). These data provide important clues about points during the course of a child's or an adolescent's disorder when the clinician might expect a level of stability, improvement, or deterioration. For example, text should note that risk for major depression increases in adolescence, particularly among girls, and that clinicians should be aware of particularly high risks in girls with a history of an anxiety disorder. Data on associations between anxiety in children or adolescents and psychopathology in their parents might also be contained within text revisions. Much like data on natural history, data on parent–child associations serve to alert clinicians to the fact that pediatric anxiety disorders are associated with adult mood and anxiety disorders. These associations manifest both in the same child followed longitudinally into adulthood and in the child's parents, who face high risks for mood and anxiety disorders.

Finally, text revisions might call attention to associated features that manifest at specific points in development. For example, an increasing focus on developmental themes has called attention to increasingly early manifestations of psychopathology. In terms of the anxiety disorders, this includes a focus on the temperamental antecedents of frank anxiety disorders. The term *behavioral inhibition* has been used to describe a group of toddlers and preschoolers who manifest extreme shyness and wariness when confronted with novelty, particularly social novelty (Fox et al. 2005; Kagan 1994). Because it is not associated with clinically significant distress or impairment, we do not consider behavioral inhibition an anxiety disorder, per se, but rather a risk factor for later anxiety disorders, particularly social phobia, based on longitudinal and family-based data (Rosenbaum et al. 2000; Schwartz et al. 1999). Calling attention to this research in the text for social phobia could alert clinicians to early subclinical manifestations of overt anxiety disorders, increasing the focus more broadly on development as well as on associated themes, such as prevention. Other research focused on risk factors or disorder-related correlates beyond early childhood behavior could be similarly important. For example, considerable prospective work implicates adverse life events—particularly when they occur at key developmental stages—in a range of pediatric mental syndromes, including anxiety disorders, particularly GAD (Moffitt et al. 2007; Pine et al. 2002b). Again, describing this work in DSM-5 text for specific disorders could increase clinicians' attention to important, potentially modifiable risk factors or to groups of children facing high risk for future disorders.

Age-Related Manifestations

Beyond Text Revisions: Is There a Need for Major Changes?

Text revisions surely will increase focus on development to a degree, but the impact of text revisions alone is likely to be no more than moderate on clinicians' thoughts and practices. This reflects the limited evidence of any marked impact on clinical thinking following a text revision to DSM-IV in 2000 (DSM-IV-TR; American Psychiatric Association 2000). Thus, text revisions might have less impact than is warranted by recent research findings regarding developmental conceptualizations of mental illness. We should consider more extensive, major changes for DSM-5.

One major issue, in the context of considering a potentially broad reorganization of DSM-5, concerns the placement of individual disorders that are highly prevalent during childhood. In DSM-IV, disorders we have long recognized as manifesting during childhood are placed in a separate category, "Disorders Usually First Diagnosed in Infancy, Childhood, or Adolescence." For the anxiety disorders, this includes only separation anxiety disorder in DSM-IV, although avoidant disorder and overanxious disorder also appeared in DSM-III and DSM-III-R. In one sense, retention of this broad category in DSM-5 would maintain a focus on at least some disorders viewed from developmental perspectives. However, research during the past two decades suggests that developmental conceptualizations extend far beyond the disorders encompassed in this explicitly developmental category. Thus, we also should consider eliminating this DSM-IV category and instead replacing it with an increased focus on developmental themes in many, if not all, of the conditions listed in DSM-5.

Three DSM-5 work groups focus on development, comprising one group focused on overarching issues, a second on disruptive behavior disorders, and a third on autism spectrum and learning disorders. These three groups have begun to discuss the advantages and disadvantages of eliminating or retaining a separate category of developmental disorders in DSM-5. The main advantage stems from the opportunity to increase attention to the developmental features of many conditions, beyond those currently viewed as developmental. This might occur if many other disorders in DSM-5—beyond those classified in DSM-IV as usually diagnosed in infancy, childhood, or adolescence—included a prominent developmental focus. For example, major depression does not appear in the section on conditions manifest in infancy, childhood, or adolescence. Yet recent and current research is increasingly demonstrating that major depression typically arises in adolescence. DSM-5 could better acknowledge this fact. Such a broadening of a focus on development would be consistent with research emphasizing the broad applicability of developmental perspectives in many disorders, such as major depression.

The main disadvantage with such broadening relates to the possibility of unintentionally reducing a focus on development. A separate category in DSM-IV focused on development represents the place where developmental perspectives appear most prominently. At this stage, work group members appear willing only to consider eliminating the category "Disorders Usually First Diagnosed in Infancy, Childhood, or Adolescence" if other major changes in DSM-5 increase the focus on development in a range of disorders. Moreover, even in this instance, it still may be advantageous to retain the category to ensure at least as strong a focus on development in DSM-5 as exists in DSM-IV.

Defining Age-Related Manifestations

Another way to increase the focus on development in DSM-5 would involve including sections that illustrate how a particular criterion might manifest at different ages. These novel sections, termed "age-related manifestations," could appear not only in text but also alongside criteria, thus emphasizing their importance. DSM-5 could provide this feature for all disorders, basing inclusions on general clinical support as opposed to a systematic review of data. Even for disorders for which no such support emerges, a statement to this effect could still be included in the relevant DSM-5 disorder criteria set to facilitate a focus on developmental aspects for all mental disorders.

DSM-IV subtly implies the existence of developmental manifestations, mostly in text sections, but also in a few isolated instances where disorder-specific criteria refer to developmental features. For example, the DSM-IV text on attention-deficit/hyperactivity disorder (ADHD) notes that symptoms become less conspicuous as children mature, even noting that adult manifestations may involve feelings of restlessness as opposed to overt hyperactivity observable to others. Similarly, some ADHD criteria include age-sensitive examples, by referring to schoolwork. A major change for DSM-5 could involve more explicit, detailed, and in-depth discussion of age-related manifestations across virtually all families of mental disorders.

It is important to distinguish so-called age-related *manifestations* of mental disorders from age-related *subtypes,* as is discussed in the next section of this chapter. For age-related manifestations, identical criteria indicate distinct age-related manifestations of each particular symptom. Age-related manifestations identify developmentally unique presentations of one or another clinical feature that characterizes the same underlying construct at distinct points in development; these manifestations represent examples of symptomatic expressions at different ages, placed alongside criteria. Age-related subtypes, in contrast, identify unique forms of disorders. As such, they refer to clinical presentations at specific ages that differ fundamentally across age groups in terms of the associated validating features. Moreover, whereas age-related manifestations could occur for most, if not all, disorders based on clinical supporting evidence, age-related subtypes should occur only for disorders for which strong support emerges, based on systematic evidence of their occurrence and validity. Thus, although both age-related constructs increase a focus on development in DSM-5, the change in developmental focus from DSM-IV to DSM-5 will be broader across disorders because of additions of age-related manifestations as opposed to age-related features.

Applications in Anxiety

In terms of potential age-related manifestations of anxiety disorders, available data on social anxiety/social phobia provide clues for potential revisions whereby DSM-5 might express age-related manifestations in three specific ways:

1. *Give age-sensitive examples for particular criteria.* Thus, Criterion A for social anxiety/social phobia calls for a "marked and persistent fear of one or more social or performance situations." Major changes occur with development, in terms of the types of exposures of individuals in whom social anxiety might manifest. Age-related manifestations might describe specific instances in which aspects of age-specific situations commonly precipitate anxiety, in order to assist clinicians in correctly identifying social anxiety at particular development periods. For example, text might suggest that it manifests in young children, when they attend birthday parties or make presentations at school, but that it manifests in adults when they are required to make oral presentations at work.

2. *More explicitly link some disorder-specific criteria to designations of developmentally appropriate behaviors so that clinicians can better appreciate the differences between typical and atypical development.* The manual could note some explicit reference to increases in anxiety during adolescence in social anxiety/social phobia Criterion A, which describes marked, persistent fear of social situations, alongside descriptions of features that differentiate appropriate from inappropriate increases in social anxiety during adolescence. Criterion A goes on to note that children must manifest the capacity for age-appropriate social relationships and manifest anxiety in peer settings; it could provide richer descriptions of these developmental features. DSM-5 also could revise Criterion B, which notes that exposure to social situations almost invariably

provokes anxiety, to note the varied ways in which exposure to feared situations might lead to anxiety provocation, manifest in unique ways across development. For example, although adolescents may talk about the specific aspects of social situations they most fear, younger children may present only with a pattern of avoidance when confronted with specific scenarios, such as oral presentations in school or other group settings.

3. *Delineate features of conditions for which there is evidence of age-related changes in a high proportion of cases.* For example, again considering social anxiety/social phobia, symptoms of selective mutism can be a manifestation of extreme social anxiety in young children; however, this symptom is relatively rare in older children. Thus, explicit reference to this developmental feature could be included when describing age-related manifestations of pathological social anxiety in specific situations.

Similar opportunities abound for the other anxiety disorders, including separation anxiety disorder and GAD. As with social anxiety, DSM-5 could incorporate age-related manifestations by focusing on how specific criteria manifest in distinct age groups. In separation anxiety disorder, for example, age-related manifestations could reflect the increasing emphasis placed on independent activities as children transition toward adolescence. Young children spend more time with parents than do older children and adolescents. Hence opportunities for separation may manifest in different scenarios. A young child may manifest severe separation anxiety when initiating first grade, an older child when leaving for sleep-away camp, and a late adolescent when leaving for college. Similarly, considerable data document robust decreases in separation anxiety disorder prevalence, as reflected in the DSM-IV text. DSM-5 might specifically mention this feature as an age-related manifestation, perhaps to call clinicians' attention to the fact that relatively few separation anxiety cases persist into adolescence.

Age-Related Disorder Subtypes

The inclusion of age-related subtypes in DSM-5 might augment both text revisions and the specifications of age-related manifestations. Age-related disorder subtypes differ from age-related manifestations in crucial respects. Namely, age-related disorder subtypes will only appear for isolated conditions for which strong support emerges for inclusion based on systematic evidence for their occurrence and validity. The example of DSM-IV conduct disorder provides a framework for evaluating such systematic evidence.

Conduct Disorder: The Prototypical Example

Conduct disorder represents the prototypical condition in DSM-IV for which data exist to support the validity of an age-related subtype. Thus, considerable research demonstrates meaningful distinctions between individuals who first manifest significant conduct problems before age 10 years and individuals who manifest such problems only at later developmental stages. This includes data on longitudinal outcome, familial aggregation, associated risk factors, and neuropsychological profiles (Moffitt et al. 2002). Although few randomized controlled trials directly compare treatment responses in individuals with early- and late-onset varieties of conduct disorder, the two forms also may differ in terms of treatment response, based on differences in long-term prognosis from naturalistic studies. As such, early- and late-onset varieties of conduct disorder are likely to be distinct pathophysiological conditions, despite the fact that DSM-IV identifies them with identical criteria. The case of conduct disorder provides a prototypical example against which other age-related subtypes to be added to DSM-5 should be considered. Thus, DSM-5 should consider age-related subtypes in instances, such as conduct disorder, in which a fundamental aspect of a clinical syndrome is likely to differ as a function of age at onset. Moreover, support for inclusion of a new subtype requires data on a range of external validators, such as those examined for early- and late-onset conduct disorder.

Anxiety: Examples

DSM-5 might consider two types of age-related subtypes. One type is analogous to the example of conduct disorder. This concerns instances in which criteria are identical across age groups but appear to identify conditions that have meaningful differences in pathophysiology. Again, conduct disorder represents the best example of disorders considered distinct, based on a broad pattern of results from a series of external validators. In terms of anxiety disorders, probably the strongest data on this form of age-related subtype emerges for OCD, which, like PTSD, we do not consider otherwise in this chapter. Here, data document age-related differences in comorbidity with tic disorders as well as gender ratios or other risk factors that suggest distinctions in pathophysiology between early- and late-onset forms of the condition. In terms of the three anxiety disorders that form the focus of this chapter, less research suggests the utility of this form of age-related subtype than for PTSD or OCD. Nevertheless, some evidence suggests considering the utility of developmental subtypes of separation anxiety disorder as they relate to panic disorder. As noted, DSM-IV implicitly recognizes the heterogeneity in separation anxiety disorder by calling attention to the strong associations with age. Separation anxiety disorder relates to panic disorder in family-based, longitudinal, and physiology studies (Pine and Klein 2008). Longitudinal and family-based data suggest that separation anxiety disorder, specifically manifest relatively late in development, may show a particularly strong relationship to panic disorder (Bruckl et al. 2007; Nocon et al. 2008; Wittchen et al. 2008).

The second variant of age-related subtypes applies to conditions for which criteria differ in distinct age groups for conditions considered "the same," from the perspective of pathophysiology. Probably the closest example in DSM-IV pertains to GAD, where three "associated features," such as irritability, sleep disturbance, or muscle tension, are required to fulfill Criterion C in adults, but only one such associated feature is required in children. Without question, such a subtle distinction in only one criterion represents a less dramatic instance of an age-related subtype, relative to potential changes for other disorders, where a large proportion of criteria might differ as a function of age. For example, for PTSD, data suggest that manifestations of the same underlying syndrome can be quite different in young children, relative to adults, calling for the use of quite different criteria at different ages. Thus, if data support the validity of these differences, PTSD would represent an instance of an age-related subtype for which different criteria identify conditions viewed as alternative manifestations of the same underlying syndrome, with distinct symptomatic expressions at specific ages. Nevertheless, the example of GAD, although less dramatic, also is illustrative as it does represent an instance in which criteria in DSM-IV already diverge, as a function of age group.

As delineated earlier, two forms of age-related subtypes exist: one characterized by similar symptoms, with distinct validators, and the other by different symptoms but similar validators. Beyond such age-related subtypes of disorders, other aspects of discussion on subtypes among members of the DSM-5 Task Force emphasize the importance of incorporating perspectives from prevention into nosology. Hence some members suggest the potential usefulness, as part of an increasing focus on dimensional perspectives, of calling attention to early, subclinical, symptomatic presentations of disorders. Some people have conceptualized these presentations, on occasion, as prodromal forms of specific DSM-IV disorders.

Probably the most extensive research considers the utility of the so-called schizophrenia prodrome. Any consideration of including criteria for subclinical entities as part of a broader focus on development in DSM-5 should begin by considering the utility of creating a "schizophrenia prodrome" before considering other prodromes. In-depth discussion of the advantages and disadvantages of this issue is beyond the scope of this chapter, with its focus on anxiety. However, as with other age-related subtypes, the threshold for adding any prodrome, including one for schizophrenia, should be very high in terms of data demonstrating validity and clinical utility. Moreover, these discussions should consider the possible disadvantages associated with calling attention to prodromal forms of disorders. For example, one can imagine many situations in which families could become quite distressed when being told that one or another set of behaviors predicts high risk for serious life-altering conditions, such as schizophrenia. This could be particularly distressing because the meaning of "high-risk" in this context refers to a relative increase over the risk in the population at large but not a high absolute risk (e.g., less than 50% chance of developing the full-blown syndrome).

In terms of prodromal forms of anxiety, behavioral inhibition emerges as the one phenotype for which some discussion seems worthwhile. As noted, both family based and longitudinal studies show an association between early childhood behavioral inhibition and adolescent or adult anxiety disorders manifest either in children followed prospectively or in their parents. Similarly, brain imaging studies document strong parallels in the underlying physiological correlates of behavioral inhibition and anxiety disorders (Pérez-Edgar et al. 2007).

In considering a specific "behavioral inhibition" prodrome as a phenomenon to be included in DSM-5, two key features arise. First, as with the schizophrenia prodrome, questions arise on weighing advantages associated with improved prevention and identification against potential adverse unintended consequences. The latter might emerge when the field calls attention to normal variations in temperament as associated features of psychopathology. Very high rates of anxiety disorder diagnosis in children and adolescents already raise questions on the degree to which current diagnostic criteria blur the boundaries between normal behavioral variation and frank pathology, thus trivializing severe clinical problems (Kessler et al. 2005; Shaffer et al. 1996). Expanding the range of conditions categorized in DSM-5 to encompass normal variations in temperament, even if they are associated with mental illnesses, would be likely to increase the force of such questions.

Second, we should consider the incremental utility for the clinician of adding such categories, given both methodological and theoretical differences between the construct of temperament and that of anxiety disorders. From a methodological standpoint, behavior inhibition typically is identified using direct observation measures, and clinical settings do not frequently employ such measures; complications are likely to arise when trying to integrate these measures into the clinic. From a theoretical perspective, research studies on anxiety disorders and on temperament both attempt to identify behavioral extremes associated with children's responses to threats. The degree to which researchers in both areas identify truly distinct, or overlapping, constructs remains unclear because there has been insufficient research examining incremental validity and assessing both constructs in the same group of children, in samples with clinically significant anxiety.

Conclusion

In this chapter, we have undertaken to delineate particularly pressing issues related to increasing developmental themes, through revisions from DSM-IV to DSM-5. Although we call most attention to specific changes in the anxiety disorders, these specific changes relate, more comprehensively, to a systematic series of broader changes throughout the nosology. It will be necessary to evaluate the advantages and disadvantages of each specific change, for each condition in DSM-5.

References

American Psychiatric Association: Diagnostic and Statistical Manual of Mental Disorders, 3rd Edition. Washington, DC, American Psychiatric Association, 1980

American Psychiatric Association: Diagnostic and Statistical Manual of Mental Disorders, 3rd Edition, Revised. Washington, DC, American Psychiatric Association, 1987

American Psychiatric Association: Diagnostic and Statistical Manual of Mental Disorders, 4th Edition. Washington, DC, American Psychiatric Association, 1994

American Psychiatric Association: Diagnostic and Statistical Manual of Mental Disorders, 4th Edition, Text Revision. Washington, DC, American Psychiatric Association, 2000

Beesdo K, Bittner A, Pine DS, et al: Incidence of social anxiety disorder and the consistent risk for secondary depression in the first three decades of life. Arch Gen Psychiatry 64:903–912, 2007

Bruckl TM, Wittchen HU, Hoffler M, et al: Childhood separation anxiety and the risk of subsequent psychopathology: results from a community study. Psychother Psychosom 76:47–56, 2007

Costello EJ, Pine DS, Hammen C, et al: Development and natural history of mood disorders. Biol Psychiatry 52:529–542, 2002

De Bellis MD: Developmental traumatology: the psychobiological development of maltreated children and its implications for research, treatment, and policy. Dev Psychopathol 13:539–564, 2001

Fox NA, Henderson HA, Marshall PJ, et al: Behavioral inhibition: linking biology and behavior within a developmental framework. Annu Rev Psychol 56:235–262, 2005

Gregory AM, Caspi A, Moffitt TE, et al: Juvenile mental health histories of adults with anxiety disorders. Am J Psychiatry 164:301–308, 2007

Hyman SE: Can neuroscience be integrated into the DSM-V? Nat Rev Neurosci 8:725–732, 2007

Kagan J: Galen's Prophecy. New York, Basic Books, 1994

Kessler RC, Chiu WT, Demler O, et al: Prevalence, severity, and comorbidity of 12-month DSM-IV disorders in the National Comorbidity Survey Replication. Arch Gen Psychiatry 62:617–627, 2005

March JS, Biederman J, Wolkow R, et al: Sertraline in children and adolescents with obsessive-compulsive disorder: a multicenter randomized controlled trial. JAMA 280:1752–1756, 1998

Meaney MJ: Maternal care, gene expression, and the transmission of individual differences in stress reactivity across generations. Annu Rev Neurosci 24:1161–1192, 2001

Moffitt TE, Caspi A, Harrington H, et al: Males on the life-course-persistent and adolescence-limited antisocial pathways: follow-up at age 26 years. Dev Psychopathol 14:179–207, 2002

Moffitt TE, Caspi A, Harrington H, et al: Generalized anxiety disorder and depression: childhood risk factors in a birth cohort followed to age 32. Psychol Med 37:441–452, 2007

Nocon A, Wittchen HU, Beesdo K, et al: Differential familial liability of panic disorder and agoraphobia. Depress Anxiety 25:422–434, 2008

Ollendick TH, Yang B, King NJ, et al: Fears in American, Australian, Chinese, and Nigerian children and adolescents: a cross-cultural study. J Child Psychol Psychiatry 37:213–220, 1996

Pérez-Edgar K, Roberson-Nay R, Hardin MG, et al: Attention alters neural responses to evocative faces in behaviorally inhibited adolescents. Neuroimage 35:1538–1546, 2007

Pine DS: Research review: a neuroscience framework for pediatric anxiety disorders. J Child Psychol Psychiatry 48:631–648, 2007

Pine DS, Cohen JA: Trauma in children and adolescents: risk and treatment of psychiatric sequelae. Biol Psychiatry 51:519–531, 2002

Pine DS, Klein RG: Anxiety disorders, in Rutter's Child and Adolescent Psychiatry, 5th Edition. Edited by Rutter M, Bishop D, Pine D, et al. Oxford, UK, Blackwell, 2008, pp 628–647

Pine DS, Cohen P, Gurley D, et al: The risk for early adulthood anxiety and depressive disorders in adolescents with anxiety and depressive disorders. Arch Gen Psychiatry 55:56–64, 1998

Pine DS, Alegria M, Cook EH Jr: Advances in developmental science and DSM-V, in A Research Agenda for DSM-V. Edited by Kupfer DJ, First MB, Regier DA. Washington, DC, American Psychiatric Association, 2002a, pp 85–122

Pine DS, Cohen P, Johnson JG, et al: Adolescent life events as predictors of adult depression. J Affect Disord 68:49–57, 2002b

Research Units on Pediatric Psychopharmacology: Fluvoxamine for the treatment of anxiety disorders in children and adolescents. The Research Unit on Pediatric Psychopharmacology Anxiety Study Group. N Engl J Med 344:1279–1285, 2001

Rosenbaum JF, Biederman J, Hirshfeld-Becker DR, et al: A controlled study of behavioral inhibition in children of parents with panic disorder and depression. Am J Psychiatry 157:2002–2010, 2000

Rosenberg DR, Hanna GL: Genetic and imaging strategies in obsessive-compulsive disorder: potential implications for treatment development. Biol Psychiatry 48:1210–1222, 2000

Rutter M, Moffitt TE, Caspi A, et al: Gene-environment interplay and psychopathology: multiple varieties but real effects. J Child Psychol Psychiatry 47:226–261, 2006

Schwartz CE, Snidman N, Kagan J, et al: Adolescent social anxiety as an outcome of inhibited temperament in childhood. J Am Acad Child Adolesc Psychiatry 38:1008–1015, 1999

Shaffer D, Fisher P, Dulcan MK, et al: The NIMH Diagnostic Interview Schedule for Children Version 2.3 (DISC-2.3): description, acceptability, prevalence rates, and performance in the MECA Study. Methods for the Epidemiology of Child and Adolescent Mental Disorders Study. J Am Acad Child Adolesc Psychiatry 35:865–877, 1996

Shear MK, Bjelland I, Beesdo K, et al: Supplementary dimensional assessment in anxiety disorders. Int J Methods Psychiatr Res 16(suppl):S52–S64, 2007

Wittchen HU, Nocon A, Beesdo K, et al: Agoraphobia and panic: prospective-longitudinal relations suggest a rethinking of diagnostic concepts. Psychother Psychosom 77:147–157, 2008

CHAPTER 15

Diagnostic Issues Relating to Lifespan From Adulthood Into Later Life

Warachal Eileen Faison, M.D.
Susan K. Schultz, M.D.

As the graying of our population continues, it is of utmost importance to turn our attention to lifespan issues that encompass not only mid-adulthood but also the later years of life. We have much to learn from our colleagues in the area of child and adolescent development, who are adept at adjusting their clinical lens to focus on the most appropriate assessments for varying stages of early life development. Thus, the proposals of the DSM-5 Work Group on Child and Adolescent Disorders provide an important model that we look to in defining our approach to diagnosis of later-life syndromes. In this chapter, we review the four aspects of development that this work group has focused on (i.e., clinical presentation, natural history, developmental psychopathology, and age at onset) and discuss how consideration of these four aspects may be relevant to assessment and diagnosis of the older adult.

Following our discussion of the four phases of development, we survey three methods by which DSM-5 might incorporate aging in-

The authors would like to acknowledge Daniel Pine, Dilip Jeste, and Dan Blazer, who provided the original conceptual framework behind the ideas discussed here.

formation into diagnostic decision making across all diagnoses, based on information we can discern by examining the lifespan aspects of each disorder. These three implementation methods involve a graded approach, ranging from simple modification of the DSM text accompanying a disorder, through identification of age-related manifestations that modify specific diagnostic criteria, to adoption of age-related subtypes considered distinct clinical entities, based on the highest level of evidence.

In this chapter, we also discuss these three potential methods of integrating lifespan information into DSM-5, in view of a few selected disorders. We survey information on depression and schizophrenia and illustrate how we might use current knowledge of lifespan expression in those two disorders to introduce text revisions and potentially age-related manifestations, respectively. We also briefly discuss diagnostic issues in substance abuse that could lead to fairly modest text revisions, which represent relatively subtle clinical differences in diagnostic decision making across the lifespan. Our intention in this chapter is not to conduct a comprehensive literature review but rather to illustrate how each work group may use information best to inform the development of DSM-5 text. In this chapter, we also raise questions about what information may yet be needed before diagnostic methods can fully accommodate age-associated variation in the clinical expression of mental disorders.

Four Phases of Development: Specific Issues Related to Characterization of Clinical Expression of Illness From Adulthood Into Later Life

Clinical Presentation

As in the disorders with onset in childhood, there are differences in clinical expression and severity of symptoms with increasing age. However, in late life, symptom expression must be disaggregated from aging factors that are often medical in nature as compared with child and adolescent disorders. With aging, symptom expression may undergo substantial variance due to interactions with medical comorbidity and functional changes related to "normal" age-related physiological variation, such as changes in sleep regulation, cognitive function, and comorbid medical conditions. Historically, an integral feature used to define the presence of a disorder has been its ability to incur functional impairment, yet patterns of impairment vary significantly with advancing age. Hence we must interpret functional impairments against the backdrop of changes that may be related to chronic disease, mobility limitation, and changes in social role functioning, such as retirement and bereavement. Additionally, in the older adult there may be disproportionate functional impairment in the face of subsyndromal symptoms; for example, among patients with subsyndromal mood disorders, the degree of functional impairment may be in excess of what would be expected for the depression severity and may be comparable to impairment seen in a full depressive syndrome (e.g., Chuan et al. 2008).

In this chapter, we discuss age differences in clinical presentation in the context of depression and schizophrenia; however, the extent to which these and other disorders warrant more extensive DSM-5 modification (including age-specific diagnostic criteria or age-related subtypes) remains to be clarified by each of the individual DSM-5 work groups, in collaboration with their advisers and feedback from the field.

Natural History

Increasingly, longitudinal studies are providing information on the mid- to late-life course of psychiatric illnesses, particularly in depressive and psychotic disorders. The natural history of mental disorders across the lifespan may include a spectrum of life histories, such as 1) childhood disorders as they evolve into adulthood and late life (e.g., autism into adulthood), and 2) childhood onset of typically adult disorders (e.g., childhood-onset schizophrenia across the lifespan). These two scenarios are presently undergoing extensive discussion by the Child and Adolescent Work Group, and their narratives will provide more detail in this area.

As one considers the aged end of the lifespan, there remain challenges to better characterize "adult" disorders—such as chronic schizophrenia, somatization disorder, substance abuse, and anxiety and mood disorders— into late life, that is, from adulthood into senescence. The episodic and cross-sectional nature of much of medical practice is such that the same clinician often does not have the luxury of observing each patient's course from first episode of illness through the later-life course of the disorder. Hence there is an important opportunity for DSM-5 to describe how illnesses may appear decades into the life course by detailing characteristic features of each illness across the lifespan; for example, features that tend to be treatment responsive versus features that may tend to be persistent, residual, or exacerbate into later years of a given illness. Lifespan variations are relevant across nearly all DSM disorders and, in most cases, may warrant text revisions that serve to facilitate awareness on the part of the clinician.

When one is considering the natural history of psychiatric illnesses, it is particularly important to consider cohort effects. For example, in the case of schizophrenia, Harvey (2001) described eloquently how a number of patients residing at Pilgrim State Psychiatric Center resisted vigorous attempts at deinstitutionalization and subsequently became participants in late-life studies. Similarly, Arnold (2001) noted that effects of institutionalization may account for the severely impaired cognitive state documented in many antemortem assessments, thus affecting the conclusions of postmortem studies of schizophrenia. It is apparent that the atypical deterioration occurring in some patient populations may have created a more pessimistic picture of the outcome of young-onset schizophrenia in late life. The pessimistic view is at odds with the works of Harding et al. (1987), McGlashan (1988), Huber et al. (1980), Ciompi (1980), and others who have suggested that the outcome of young-onset schizophrenia may, in fact, be associated with an amelioration of symptoms and improvement or stabilization in social function in later life. Ideally, this important area will benefit from larger-scale epidemiological studies able to identify and characterize subjects with schizophrenia who have remained in the community, with sufficient support to maintain treatment compliance and optimal socialization, over a lifetime. Presently, we are at a very interesting juncture in history, where we are able to encounter individuals with schizophrenia entering late life who have had successful treatment with antipsychotic medication and have maintained community living throughout the entire course of their illness. Although the fundamental diagnostic criteria for schizophrenia may be sufficient for diagnostic reliability regardless of the age at which one encounters an individual patient, nonetheless it may be very helpful for DSM-5 to include text that addresses how age may affect clinical expression of illness. Field trial studies designed to test diagnostic criteria are likely to have similar reliability in both younger and older adults—provided the studies examine all ages; therefore, we may not be able to test the nuances of age-related variation, necessarily, via that particular process. However, there is an opportunity to infuse DSM-5 text with a variety of important observations regarding lifespan variation from findings of recent decades of clinical and epidemiological research.

Developmental Psychopathology

The DSM-5 Child and Adolescent Work Group has emphasized the opportunity to go beyond developmental aspects of social environment and psychological exposures to implement more refined ways of assessing individual differences (e.g., genetic features) in DSM-5. In a similar manner, research on late-life expression of illness also will benefit from characterizing critical exposures, and their interactions with genetic features of an individual, across the lifespan.

We are most likely to find evidence for significant interactions of environment and genotype in later life in the neurodegenerative/ neurocognitive disorders. Furthermore, an interaction between a critical period of environmental exposures and subsequent life course, potentially, may occur in substance use behaviors in late life; for example, when alcohol use may begin, or reactivate, in the context of bereavement or new social isolation in late life.

Along these lines, analysis of the National Epidemiologic Survey on Alcohol and Related Conditions data set, from the National Institute on Alcohol Abuse and Alcoholism (Grant and Dawson 2006), has shown that the large majority of all lifetime substance abuse or substance dependence diagnoses were first contracted between the ages of approximately 15 and 21 years. Among adults older than 40 years, less than 15% of all individuals who met criteria for abuse of, or dependence on, any substance first met the criteria after age 21 years. Researchers have observed similar age-at-onset patterns for tobacco, alcohol, and other substance use disorders. These patterns appear consistent for both genders, although potentially more so for men than women. Furthermore, these findings also appear to remain consistent across most ethnic groups (http://www.niaaa.nih. gov/Resources/DatabaseResources). These and other findings have been widely interpreted as evidence for the "time limited" nature of substance use disorders, and there has been much discussion regarding efforts to delay use of substances among those younger than 21 years as a way of forestalling new cases of abuse and dependence. Interestingly, within the substance use disorders there have been reports of a cohort effect showing increased rates of alcohol abuse and dependence among men and women who were born between 1944 and 1953, as compared with rates seen in prior cohorts (Grucza et al. 2008). At the same time, these rates appear to reflect a reappearance of a preexisting vulnerability and are highest among those who originally met criteria earlier in their lives (usually in their teens). Recent findings support a potential cohort effect of the 1940– 1955 birth group. A report on the epidemiology of substance abuse among middle-age and elderly community-dwelling adults observed that alcohol use, as well as overall drug use, was more common among respondents ages 50–64 years when compared with those older than 65 years, although younger age groups were not compared (Blazer and Wu 2009). Additional evidence that there may be clinical variation imposed by cohort effects in younger populations may be inferred from findings of the U.S. National Alcohol Surveys, which have suggested that more recent birth cohorts (after 1975) have shown increased volume of alcohol intake compared with older birth cohorts when age, period, and demographic effects were controlled. A study by Kerr et al. (2009) also suggested that for women, the 1956–1960 birth cohort stands out from adjacent cohorts as being higher in volume of alcohol intake.

Taken together, these findings suggest that substance abuse may serve as an excellent example of a syndrome that appears to have a time-limited risk period in late adolescence but in the context of environmental factors has the capability to reactivate the fundamental vulnerability in later years or to display unique patterns among specific birth cohorts. Hence substance abuse disorders likely do not have sufficient evidence to warrant age-related manifestations or age-related subtypes, but there is important information regarding the risk window in early life as well as clinically relevant observations regarding potential variation later in life. Although these observations may not change the core criteria needed to diagnose substance use disorders, it may be fruitful to discuss these observations in the text of the manual.

Impact of Age at Onset

The age at first onset of a disorder may influence, significantly, variations across the natural history of the disorder. There has been evidence, particularly in the case of depressive illness, that the age at onset may incur variance in the expression of illness, in the nature of symptoms, symptom severity, and treatment responsiveness. For example, differences in clinical expression and natural course have been reported between early- (age <60 years) and late-onset depression (age >60 years). Using the criteria of greater or less than 60 years, one study demonstrated that patients with early-onset depression had more frequent depressive episodes as well as more prescribed medications. Interestingly, this study also noted that early onset of depression was associated with a greater prevalence of cardiac disease, diabetes mellitus, gastrointestinal disorders, and arthritis when individuals reached late life (Holroyd and Duryee 1997). A number of clinical features suggest a greater burden of depression severity in younger-onset cases, as well as more psychosocial dysfunction; for example, personality abnormalities and dysfunctional past marital relationships have been associated with younger-onset illness (Brodaty et al. 2001). Similarly, a large study recently reported by Kovacs et al. (2009) longitudinally examined adults who had childhood-onset depressive disorder and control subjects with no history of major mental disorder. These researchers observed that adults with previous depressive episodes, beginning in childhood, had greater maladaptive responses to their own sadness than did control subjects, suggesting more pervasive dysfunction and a poorer prognostic course (Kovacs et al. 2009).

Despite these interesting findings, one may argue that the fundamental phenomenology of depressive illness is essentially the same in terms of diagnostic criteria, involving relatively cohesive core symptoms regardless of age at onset or nature of relapses. Along these lines, Nelson et al. (2005) reported that the symptoms most frequent in patients with late-life depression were similar to those in mixed-aged samples in a study of 728 patients older than 60 years. Hence the impact of age at onset in depression may affect the life course and propensity to comorbidity, but it may not reach a level of evidence for an age-related diagnostic subtype. Yet there remains an important opportunity for DSM-5 to provide descriptive material to highlight the prognostic implications of early onset illness. For example, an intriguing recent latent cluster analysis supported the oft-observed phenomenon that overt sadness may be less prominent and less severe among adults experiencing depression in later life, providing evidence for the notion of "depression without sadness" (Hybels et al. 2009). This area remains a dynamic field that may lend itself to ongoing revisions as new longitudinal data unfold. In a recent review, Beard et al. (2008) suggested that "many important, and in some respects quite basic, questions remain about the trajectory of depression and anxiety disorders over the life course and the factors that influence their incidence, recurrence and prognosis" (p. 83).

In addition to ongoing active work describing the life course of depression, for more than a century a substantial body of work has examined how age at onset may influence the clinical expression of schizophrenia. Perhaps because of its more severe and recalcitrant nature, there are extensive observational data on the natural course of illness for schizophrenia, alluded to earlier in this chapter. We discuss here the impact of age at onset in schizophrenia as a potential example of a disorder in which age-specific manifestations may potentially warrant mention in DSM-5. As noted by the Child and Adolescent Work Group, the impact of age at onset should be carefully addressed, with operational principles applied so that the nature of supporting evidence can be fully delineated.

Proposed Approaches

The DSM-5 Child and Adolescent Work Group has suggested the following three approaches for estimating the level of evidence, for each aspect of the lifespan issues described earlier. DSM-5 could use one or more of these approaches simultaneously, depending on level of clinical evidence for lifespan implications, for the clinical condition at hand. We summarize below the three methods, with reference to their applications for adult patients, including those in later life.

Text Revisions

The text section of DSM-5 could extend the current DSM-IV-TR section "Specific Culture and Age and Gender Features" (American Psychiatric Association 2000). That is, all disorders could have a text section reviewing age-related features more completely than does the text section that deals with age-specific features in DSM-IV-TR. Text should draw on literature reviews currently being prepared for DSM-5 and, ideally, should address all DSM disorders. For example, in revising text sections to specifically address aging issues, the developers of DSM-5 could

- Describe variance in clinical expression due to the age of the patient; for example, the tendency of an older adult to express "depression without sadness" or the tendency of patients with later-onset schizophrenia to display less affective restriction and less disorganization.
- Characterize interactions of advancing age and comorbid illness. Examples include the effects of comorbid neurocognitive disorders, such as dementia, on the expression of mood symptoms or the interaction between the presence of mood symptoms in late life and the emergence of somatic complaints.
- Emphasize that interactions between age and gender may play an important role in the expression of disorders in late life.

The presence of text revisions will permit a dimensional description that will facilitate awareness by clinicians of multiple interacting factors (e.g., age, gender, brain changes, and comorbidity).

Age-Related Manifestations

Additionally, DSM-5 may contain sections that illustrate how a particular criterion may manifest at different ages. These sections may be titled "Age-Related Manifestations." The DSM-5 Child and Adolescent Work Group suggested that sections on age-related manifestations may appear next to where diagnostic criteria appear as well as in the text of the manual. Age-specific manifestations presented next to diagnostic criteria will occur only for those diagnoses for which there is strong supporting evidence that such manifestations may increase diagnostic reliability. DSM-5 age-related manifestations would serve to illustrate how a particular criterion may manifest at different ages. Examples of how later-life age-related manifestations of illness may influence criteria development include

- Criteria should be more inclusive and include age-sensitive examples, where appropriate; for example, if criteria are employed that reflect functional impairment in social or occupational function, these criteria might address role-functioning thresholds for persons who are retired.

- Some criteria may link to norms of what we consider appropriate for a given disorder; for example, the diagnosis of late-life dementia in the context of preexisting mental retardation, autism, or other developmental disorder may require adjustment for the underlying disorder.
- Diagnostic criteria may potentially be adjusted when there is evidence of age-related changes in a high proportion, but not all instances, of cases; for example, possible attenuation of symptom severity of some personality disorders in late life.

Age-related manifestations differ from age-related subtypes. Age-related *manifestations* will be appropriate when there is general clinical support for descriptive modifiers that may enhance interpretation and application of diagnostic criteria, based on current evidence for differences, as reflected in the views of the DSM-5 work groups. In contrast, age-specific *subtypes* should appear only for disorders for which there is strong, systematic evidence for the occurrence of a separate subtype based on age or there is strong evidence for distinct differences in criteria necessary to identify the syndrome.

Age-Related Subtypes

There are two types of age-related subtypes to consider. Age-related subtypes should be considered for conditions for which criteria differ, in distinct age groups, for "the same" condition (e.g., irritability is a depressive symptom equivalent in child mood syndromes). Thus, the same diagnostic conclusion may arise from different criteria, depending on the age group to which they are applied. Although the Childhood and Adolescent Disorders Work Group has been actively identifying instances in which distinct criteria may be necessary for diagnostic accuracy among children, when diagnostic criteria are applied in adult and later-life patients, for the most part, diagnostic variation is relatively attenuated such that age-related subtypes may be less essential, relative to diagnostic assessments among children. Despite discrete diagnostic criteria, conditions can be "the same" if clinical criteria vary slightly but validity data (e.g., course, neuropsychology and other indicators of pathophysiology, and family genetics) document similarities within the disorder across age groups.

Age-related subtypes should also be considered for conditions for which work groups have proposed that criteria should be identical in two or more age groups but the disorders still appear "distinct." Disorders with identical criteria in different age groups can be considered "distinct" when evidence from multiple sources has shown that key features, such as longitudinal outcomes, family genetics, or physiological correlates, differ in individuals whose condition presents at different ages (e.g., early- vs. late-onset Alzheimer's disease).

Depression Across the Lifespan

Along the lines of the previous discussion regarding age at onset in depression, symptom expression of depression appears to follow a similar phenomenology across the lifespan of an individual, with relatively subtle variation in core features of the illness. Medical comorbidity, however, may play a significant role in influencing vulnerability to depression as well as influencing treatment response and self-reported well-being (Pirkola et al. 2009).

In addition to subtle differences in symptom character, there may be differences in the episodic nature, or lack thereof, among older adults with depression. For example, a 6-year follow-up of community-dwelling older adults in the Netherlands illustrates the chronicity of late-life depression. Among those with clinically significant depressive symptoms, 23% had remission of symptoms, 44% displayed an unfavorable but fluctuating course, and 33% demonstrated a severe chronic course. In the group diagnosed with subthreshold depression, 25% experienced a chronic course (Beekman et al. 2002). This is consistent with findings of previous work in this area demonstrating that depression in older persons, over longer follow-up periods, has a chronic, remitting course (Alexopoulos et al. 1996; Baldwin and Jolley 1986; Blazer et al. 1992; Murphy 1983; Post 1962; Reynolds et al. 1992).

In the Berlin Aging Study, research psychiatrists made a diagnosis of subthreshold depression for case patients in which no DSM-III-R criteria (American Psychiatric Association 1987) were fulfilled but who nevertheless presented with depressed mood, loss of energy and/or interest, and at least two further depressive symptoms during the past 4 weeks or longer (Schaub et al. 2003). In addition, psychiatrists rated whether current signs and symptoms were severe enough to justify or require antidepressant intervention (Geiselmann et al. 2001; Helmchen et al. 1999). Subthreshold depression, as defined in the Berlin Aging Study, seems to represent a diagnostic concept that occurs preferentially in the elderly patient and may benefit from discussion in DSM-5 text (Geiselmann and Bauer 2000). Whether the entity of subthreshold depression warrants discrete representation in DSM-5 is an interesting area that may benefit from further discussion.

Similarly, the Automated Geriatric Examination for Computer Assisted Taxonomy (AGECAT; Copeland et al. 1986) offers advantages for greater detection of clinically important conditions that may escape detection of current DSM criteria. The advantage of categories generated by the AGECAT, for example, is that they are more likely to pick up on syndromes rather than highly discrete nosological categories. For example, AGECAT uses the necessity of intervention as a criterion for caseness and, hence, has a clinical-entity approach as opposed to a nosologic framework based entirely on psychopathology. In a study including the oldest old (Schaub et al. 2003), when the AGECAT was used, depression was diagnosed in 12.4% and 19.4% of males and females, respectively, between ages 70 and 84 years. By contrast, fewer cases were diagnosed with DSM-III-R: 5.4% and 8.5% of men and women, respectively, in the same age group. Among subjects between ages 83 and 103 years, a diagnosis of depression based on the AGECAT was made in 14.7% of men and 19.4% of women. With DSM-III-R, again, fewer cases were diagnosed: 6.2% of men and 17.1% of women in this age group. This issue of "clinical need" versus nosologic distinctness is a key issue relating to the older adult and an important challenge for DSM-5.

Older adults are particularly vulnerable to distress, functional impairment, and a need for care in the context of symptoms that may be both subsyndromal and highly comorbid with other psychiatric or physical symptoms. Löwe et al. (2008) addressed this scenario; although their study did not focus on elderly subjects, this group's observations are quite relevant to aging. Specifically, the authors reported findings—from 2,091 consecutive patients presenting to 15 different primary care clinics—that documented the co-occurrence of depression, anxiety, and somatization in more than half of patients. Furthermore, these authors observed that there was a contribution of the overlap of these disorders, such that functional impairment from their co-occurrence substantially exceeded the individual contribution of each disorder. Specifically, the authors used two measures of functional impairment: the Medical Outcomes Study Short-Form General Health Survey and self-reported disability days. The overlap of these syndromes resulted in a contribution of 24.5% to the explained variance, as compared with 2.3% for depression alone, 0% for anxiety alone, and 7.1% for somatization alone. Although there remains active discussion as to how to integrate functional impairment into DSM-5 formulations, it is clear that subthreshold symptoms, as well as comorbidity, are important clinical patterns that have an impact on the older adult, and a reflection of this observation would likely enhance DSM-5. The National Institutes of Health Patient-Reported Outcomes Measurement Information System may potentially be a useful tool in DSM field trials to help reflect comorbidity across psychiatric symptoms, as well as their overlap with measures of global health, physical, and social function.

Taken together, the evidence suggests that there may be substantive differences in clinical expression and life course (i.e., a tendency for subsyndromal symptoms that are a focus of clinical care and a tendency for chronicity in life course) that may characterize depression in the older adult. This likely rises to a level of text revision to help capture these important clinical differences. In addition, recent reports from the Collaborative Study of Depression (Coryell et al. 2009) suggest that younger age at onset may affect symptom persistence into later life. This 20-year follow-up study examined the long-term persistence of symptoms in major depressive disorder. Assessments were conducted among patients who were divided by their ages at intake, reflecting their age at onset: youngest (18–29 years), middle (30–44 years), and oldest (45 years or older). In this study, earlier ages at onset were associated with greater symptom persistence, particularly in the youngest group. The proportions of "weeks ill" showed intra-individual stability over time that was most evident in the oldest group. Hence an early age at onset, rather than youth per se, was associated with greater depression morbidity over two decades in largely midlife. Similarly, Driscoll et al. (2005) observed that late-life recurrent depression takes longer to respond to treatment than late-onset single-episode depression. The natural course of mood disorders, then, appears to be significantly influenced by interactions between age at onset, effects of aging, and diagnostic systems (AGECAT vs. DSM) used among older individuals.

Finally, Temple University researchers examined depression in a sample of 244 people who were age 100 or older (Davey et al. 2008). More than 25% of the people showed clinically relevant depressive symptoms, but only 8% reported a diagnosis of depression. The authors noted that depression in centenarians could be linked to a number of factors, including poor nutritional status, urinary incontinence, limited physical activity, and a past history of anxiety, highlighting the additional factors of comorbidity that may account for greater variance in symptoms, with increasing age.

To bring this discussion back to the three approaches suggested for integrating aging information into DSM-5, it appears that depressive disorders have specific features of increased chronicity and subthreshold features, which DSM text revisions most likely could specify. However, we may also consider the incorporation of age-specific manifestations that may help to specify diagnostic criteria, when applied to the older adult, such as consideration of a lower threshold of symptoms as diagnostic when impairment or distress suggests that treatment is warranted.

Schizophrenia Across the Lifespan

The International Late-Onset Schizophrenia Group summarized the clinical characteristics of late-onset schizophrenia (beginning after age 40 years) and concluded that there is evidence for its diagnostic validity as well as for very-late-onset schizophrenia-like psychosis (i.e., onset after age 60 years) (Howard et al. 2000). Defining the influence of age at onset on the course of schizophrenia has long been a source of study, beginning with Kraepelin in 1902, who suggested that only a small percentage of patients experienced the onset of dementia praecox symptoms after age 40 years.

Ensuing studies suggested that late-onset schizophrenia (i..e., onset after age 45 years) tends to have less affective flattening, less disorganization, fewer negative symptoms, a greater likelihood of paranoid delusions, and, overall, a less deteriorative course (Jeste et al. 1995; Riecher-Rossler et al. 1995). Consequently, DSM-III-R specified illness onset after age 45 years as a separate category. There also are demographic differences; for example, patients with late onset appear to include a preponderance of women with higher social and occupational functioning. DSM-III-R included "late onset" as a distinct category; however, by consensus, DSM-IV (American Psychiatric Association 1994) and ICD-10 (World Health Organization 1992) omitted this category. Similarly, DSM-IV-TR does not include a "late-onset" subtype but does include specific text in the section "Specific Culture, Age, and Gender Features" describing clinical characteristics that occur more commonly in patients with late illness onset.

In 2000, Howard et al. concluded that "in terms of the epidemiology, symptom profile, and identified pathophysiologies, the diagnoses of late-onset schizophrenia (>age 40 years) and very-late-onset schizophrenia-like psychosis (>age 60 years) have face validity and clinical utility" (p. 1334). Clinical features identified by the International Consensus group involved, primarily, a relative absence of formal thought disorder and fewer negative symptoms, with an overall better prognosis, relative to young-onset illness. From an epidemiological perspective, Harris and Jeste (1988) estimated the proportion of patients whose illness first emerged after age 40 years to be 23.5% of all persons with schizophrenia. Late-onset schizophrenia also afflicts women more frequently than men, to the extent that female gender may constitute a risk factor. Additionally, Pearlson et al. (1989) observed a lower morbid risk among relatives of patients with late onset. In terms of physiological parameters, brain imaging studies have found more frequent nonspecific structural changes among persons with late-onset illness (Krull et al. 1991), which provides some evidence that there may be differences in pathoetiology. Treatment responsiveness in patient with late-onset illness might follow a somewhat more favorable course, with 48%–61% of patients showing full remission of psychotic symptoms, which suggests a better response than young-onset illness and a better response when compared with delusional disorder (Jeste et al. 1993; Pearlson et al. 1989).

A recent study, however, examined 52 patients age 60 years and older and compared treatment outcomes in those patients with onset before age 40 with outcomes in patients with onset after age 40

(Huang and Zhang 2009). This study showed no difference in overall symptom severity between groups, and there were no significant differences with respect to cognitive impairment, daily functioning, and global outcome, with the exception that the mean antipsychotic dosage was nonsignificantly higher for the early onset patients. A helpful review by Tune and Salzman (2003) suggested that although late-onset illness may be more responsive to treatment, there may be a greater risk for treatment-emergent adverse effects such as tardive dyskinesia.

Schultz et al. (2000) compared symptom characteristics between early and intermediate-onset patients (N=259) to determine whether clinical features distinguished differences within younger populations. This study dichotomized subjects into "young" onset and "intermediate" onset groups, with ages at onset of 20–29 and 30–45 years, respectively. On global measures of psychotic, disorganized, and negative symptoms, early-onset patients had greater disorganized and negative symptoms but did not differ in hallucinations and delusions. These findings are consistent with a continuum of age at onset–associated variation that follows the same pattern observed with other thresholds for later onset.

To move still further along the continuum, the syndrome of "very-late-onset schizophrenia-like psychosis (>age 60 years)" proposed by Howard et al. (2000) represents an intriguing entity that has had relatively less scrutiny. In general, those who develop a chronic psychotic syndrome at age 60 years or older are at risk for a variety of comorbid factors that may substantially influence the clinical presentation. For example, a combination of additional neuropathological processes (i.e., vascular changes, Alzheimer's disease, or other age-related changes) may influence the presentation, course, and outcome of the illness sufficiently to warrant a separate nosologic entity, as Howard et al. (2000) suggests. However, it still may be beneficial to consider applying a dimensional view to the "late- to very-late" life transition, much like the young to midlife study noted earlier. That is, among those with onset at ages 45–60 years, a subgroup may have the same pathoetiological process operative among young-onset patients, but with illness onset delayed as a result of some protective factor or combination of protective factors. For example, the presence of estrogen might be a protective factor for development of psychosis, such that the perimenopausal phase introduces a new risk for older women. In contrast, another subgroup of patients with onset in the age range 45–60 years may be at risk for a degenerative psychosis related to cerebrovascular changes or other age-related comorbidity.

In terms of the "very late" psychoses, in the broader neurodegenerative sense, identified risk factors, such as a family history of schizophrenia, suggest that there may be a genetically mediated vulnerability to psychosis in late life, much like that seen in early-onset illness. Tsuang et al. (2000) have suggested that, in conjunction with appropriate factors activating a putative psychosis gene, a clinical picture of psychosis may emerge as a result of a number of underlying processes (e.g., Huntington's disease). This creates a "degenerative psychosis" model, such that in the context of an appropriate degenerative insult, certain genetically predisposed individuals manifest clinically distinguishable syndromes of late-life psychosis. These syndromes have unique features, such as a greater affective component, delusions of infidelity, and persecutory ideas. Diagnostic assessment of the neurocognitive disorders will likely encompass these conditions, and future discussion by the DSM-5 Neurocognitive Disorders Work Group will address these issues. Current estimates from the Alzheimer's Association indicate that Alzheimer's disease affects five million persons in the United States; this scenario, combined with the observation that psychosis may occur in 40% or more of those afflicted (Ropacki and Jeste 2005), makes it quite clear that this condition will become an increasingly important focus of diagnostic assessment and intervention.

To bring the discussion back to the diagnosis of schizophrenia, text revisions to DSM-5 may help characterize clinical differences in late-onset illness. Regarding diagnostic criteria, given that there is no symptom feature of late-onset schizophrenia outside the boundaries of clinical variation in the core illness, one might posit that text modifications or age-related manifestations may suffice. However, there may be sufficient syndromic coherence to late-onset schizophrenia (after age 40 years), or the very late schizophrenia-like psychosis (after age 60 years), that DSM-5 might discuss age-related subtypes. There also may be an opportunity in DSM-5 to shine more light on this subgroup by adding more information, in the form of "age-related manifestations," that tailors the clinical features of the diagnostic schema toward the age of a patient. Overall, a wealth of information exists on late-onset psychosis that provides a variety of opportunities to enhance DSM-5 text.

Conclusion

The three methods for implementing the addition of age-specific content to the DSM may involve a graded approach, including

1. Simple modification of text accompanying a disorder.
2. Inclusion of age-related manifestations that may be used to qualify/characterize specific diagnostic criteria.
3. Adoption of age-related subtypes, which have discrete diagnostic criteria of their own and may involve specific pathoetiologies, supported by the highest level of evidence.

This discussion illustrates some of the current issues surrounding the interpretation of evidence for any text modifications. One must bear in mind the complexity of cohort effects, the challenges of longitudinal studies, and the influences of medical comorbidity that create special issues in addressing later-life issues in psychiatric diagnoses. Our aging population is dramatically changing the face of mental health; hence, there is a great need for attention to later life. The National Institute on Aging (2007) recently noted that "people age 85 and over are now the fastest growing portion of many national populations" and for "the first time in history, and probably for the rest of human history, people age 65 and over will outnumber children under age 5" (p. 3). The implications of these facts are perhaps just beginning to rise to awareness in our field; where the burden of illness has historically drawn our gaze to look at early life, we must now turn our attention to the full lifespan.

References

Alexopoulos GS, Meyers BS, Young RC, et al: Recovery in geriatric depression. Arch Gen Psychiatry 53:305–312, 1996

American Psychiatric Association: Diagnostic and Statistical Manual of Mental Disorders, 3rd Edition, Revised. Washington, DC, American Psychiatric Association, 1987

American Psychiatric Association: Diagnostic and Statistical Manual of Mental Disorders, 4th Edition. Washington, DC, American Psychiatric Association, 1994

American Psychiatric Association: Diagnostic and Statistical Manual of Mental Disorders, 4th Edition, Text Revision. Washington, DC, American Psychiatric Association, 2000

Arnold SE: Contributions of neuropathology to understanding schizophrenia in late life. Harv Rev Psychiatry 9:69–76, 2001

Baldwin RC, Jolley DJ: The prognosis of depression in old age. Br J Psychiatry 149:574–583, 1986

Beard JR, Galea S, Vlahov D: Longitudinal population-based studies of affective disorders: where to from here? BMC Psychiatry 8:83, 2008

Beekman AT, Geerlings SW, Deeg DJ, et al: The natural history of late-life depression: a 6-year prospective study in the community. Arch Gen Psychiatry 59:605–611, 2002

Blazer D, Hughes DC, George LK: Age and impaired subjective support: predictors of depressive symptoms at one-year follow-up. J Nerv Ment Dis 180:172–178, 1992

Blazer DG, Wu LT: The epidemiology of substance use and disorders among middle-aged and elderly community adults: national survey on drug use and health. Am J Geriatr Psychiatry 17:237–245, 2009

Brodaty H, Luscombe G, Parker G, et al: Early and late onset depression in old age: different aetiologies, same phenomenology. J Affect Disord 66:225–236, 2001

Chuan SK, Kumar R, Matthew N, et al: Subsyndromal depression in old age: clinical significance and impact in a multi-ethnic community sample of elderly Singaporeans. Int Psychogeriatr 20:188–200, 2008

Ciompi L: Catamnestic long-term study on the course of life and aging of schizophrenics. Schizophr Bull 6:606–618, 1980

Copeland JR, Dewey ME, Griffiths-Jones HM: A computerized psychiatric diagnostic system and case nomenclature for elderly subjects: GMS and AGECAT. Psychol Med 16:89–99, 1986

Coryell W, Solomon D, Leon A, et al: Does major depressive disorder change with age? Psychol Med 19:1–7, 2009

Davey A, Siegler I, Martin P, et al: Centenarians 'grossly' underdiagnosed for depression. ScienceDaily, Nov 24, 2008. Available at: http://www.sciencedaily.com/releases/2008/11/081124080810.htm/releases/2008/11/081124080810.htm. Accessed August 31, 2009.

Driscoll HC, Basinski J, Mulsant BH, et al: Late-onset major depression: clinical and treatment-response variability. Int J Geriatr Psychiatry 20:661–667, 2005

Geiselmann B, Bauer M: Subthreshold depression in the elderly: qualitative or quantitative distinction? Compr Psychiatry 41:32–38, 2000

Geiselmann B, Linden M, Helmchen H: Psychiatrists' diagnoses of subthreshold depression in old age: frequency and correlates. Psychol Med 31:51–63, 2001

Grant BF, Dawson DA: Introduction to the National Epidemiologic Survey on Alcohol and Related Conditions. Alcohol Research & Health 29(2):74–78, 2006

Grucza RA, Bucholz KK, Rice JP, et al: Secular trends in the lifetime prevalence of alcohol dependence in the United States: a re-evaluation. Alcohol Clin Exp Res 32:763–770, 2008

Harding CM, Brooks GW, Ashikaga T, et al:. The Vermont longitudinal study of persons with severe mental illness, II: long-term outcome of subjects who retrospectively met DSM-III criteria for schizophrenia. Am J Psychiatry 144:727–735, 1987

Harris MJ, Jeste DV: Late-onset schizophrenia: an overview. Schizophr Bull 14:39–55, 1988

Harvey PD: Cognitive and functional impairments in elderly patients with schizophrenia: a review of the recent literature. Harv Rev Psychiatry 9:59–68, 2001

Helmchen H, Baltes MM, Geiselmann B, et al: Psychiatric illnesses in old age, in The Berlin Aging Study: Aging From 70 to 100. Edited by Baltes PB, Mayer KU. New York, Cambridge University Press, 1999, pp 167–196

Holroyd S, Duryee JJ: Differences in geriatric psychiatry outpatients with early vs late-onset depression. Int J Geriatr Psychiatry 12:1100–1106, 1997

Howard R, Rabins PV, Seeman MV, et al: Late-onset schizophrenia and very-late-onset schizophrenia-like psychosis: an international consensus. The International Late-Onset Schizophrenia Group. Am J Psychiatry 157:172–178, 2000

Huang C, Zhang YL: Clinical differences between late-onset and early onset chronically hospitalized elderly schizophrenic patients in Taiwan. Int J Geriatr Psychiatry 24:1166–1172, 2009

Huber G, Gross G, Schuttler R, et al: Longitudinal studies of schizophrenic patients. Schizophr Bull 6:592–605, 1980

Hybels CF, Blazer DG, Pieper CF, et al: Profiles of depressive symptoms in older adults diagnosed with major depression: latent cluster analysis: Am J Geriatr Psychiatry 17:387–396, 2009

Jeste DV, Lacro JP, Gilbert PL, et al: Treatment of late-life schizophrenia with neuroleptics. Schizophr Bull 19:817–830, 1993

Jeste DV, Harris MJ, Krull A, et al: Clinical and neuropsychological characteristics of patients with late-onset schizophrenia. Am J Psychiatry 152:722–730, 1995

Kerr WC, Greenfield TK, Bond J, et al: Age-period-cohort modeling of alcohol volume and heavy drinking days in the US National Alcohol Surveys: divergence in younger and older adult trends. Addiction 104:27–37, 2009

Kovacs M, Rottenberg J, George C: Maladaptive mood repair responses distinguish young adults with early onset depressive disorders and predict future depression outcomes. Psychol Med 20:1–14, 2009

Kraepelin E: Dementia praecox, in Clinical Psychiatry: A Textbook For Students And Physicians, 6th Edition. Translated by Diefendorf AR. New York, Macmillan, 1902

Krull AJ, Press G, Dupont R, et al: Brain imaging in late-onset schizophrenia and related psychoses. Int J Geriatr Psychiatry 6:651–658, 1991

Löwe B, Spitzer RL, Williams JB, et al: Depression, anxiety and somatization in primary care: syndrome overlap and functional impairment. Gen Hosp Psychiatry 30:191–199, 2008

McGlashan TH: A selective review of recent North American long-term followup studies of schizophrenia. Schizophr Bull 14:515–542, 1988

Murphy E: The prognosis of depression in old age. Br J Psychiatry 142:111–119, 1983

National Institute on Aging: Why Population Aging Matters: A Global Perspective. National Institute on Aging, National Institutes of Health, U.S. Department of Health and Human Services. Publication No. 07–6134, March 2007. Available at: http://www.nia.nih.gov/researchinformation/extramuralprograms/behavioralandsocialresearch/GlobalAging.htm. Accessed August 31, 2009.

Nelson JC, Clary CM, Leon AC, et al: Symptoms of late-life depression: frequency and change during treatment. Am J Geriatr Psychiatry 13:520–526, 2005

Pearlson GD, Kreger L, Rabins PV, et al: A chart review study of late-onset and early onset schizophrenia. Am J Psychiatry 146:1568–1574, 1989

Pirkola S, Saarni S, Suvisaari J, et al: General health and quality-of-life measures in active, recent, and comorbid mental disorders: a population-based health 2000 study. Compr Psychiatry 50:108–114, 2009

Post F: The Significance of Affective Symptoms at Old Age. Oxford, UK, Oxford University Press, 1962

Reynolds CF 3rd, Frank E, Pereil JM, et al: Combined pharmacotherapy and psychotherapy in the acute and continuation treatment of elderly patients with recurrent major depression: a preliminary report. Am J Psychiatry 149:1687–1692, 1992

Riecher-Rossler A, Rossler W, Forstl H, et al: Late-onset schizophrenia and late paraphrenia. Schizophr Bull 21:345–354, discussion 355–356, 1995

Ropacki SA, Jeste DV: Epidemiology of and risk factors for psychosis of Alzheimer's disease: a review of 55 studies published from 1990 to 2003. Am J Psychiatry 162:2022–2030, 2005

Schaub RT, Linden M, Copeland JR: A comparison of GMS-A/AGECAT, DSM-III-R for dementia and depression, including subthreshold depression (SD): results from the Berlin Aging Study (BASE). Int J Geriatr Psychiatry 18:109–117, 2003

Schultz SK, Ho BC, Andreasen NC: Clinical features characterizing young-onset and intermediate-onset schizophrenia J Neuropsychiatry Clin Neurosci 12:502–505, 2000

Tsuang MT, Stone WS, Faraone SV: Toward reformulating the diagnosis of schizophrenia. Am J Psychiatry 157:1041–1050, 2000

Tune LE, Salzman C: Schizophrenia in late life. Psychiatr Clin North Am 26:103–113, 2003

World Health Organization: International Statistical Classification of Diseases and Related Health Problems, 10th Revision. Geneva, World Health Organization, 1992

Index

*Page numbers printed in **boldface** type refer to tables or figures.*